KIDS
Having Kids

Also of interest from the Urban Institute Press:

Reconnecting Disadvantaged Young Men, by Peter Edelman, Harry Holzer, and Paul Offner

Black Males Left Behind, edited by Ronald B. Mincy

Digest of Social Experiments, third edition, by David H. Greenberg and Mark Shroder

SECOND EDITION

KIDS
Having Kids

Economic Costs &
Social Consequences
of Teen Pregnancy

Edited by
Saul D. Hoffman &
Rebecca A. Maynard

THE URBAN INSTITUTE PRESS
Washington, D.C.

THE URBAN INSTITUTE PRESS
2100 M Street, N.W.
Washington, D.C. 20037

Library of Congress Cataloging-in-Publication Data

Kids having kids : economic costs and social consequences of teen pregnancy / edited by Saul D. Hoffman and Rebecca A. Maynard. — 2nd ed.
        p. cm.
   Includes bibliographical references and index.
   ISBN 978-0-87766-745-2 (alk. paper)
   1. Teenage parents—United States. 2. Teenage pregnancy—Economic aspects—United States. 3. Teenage pregnancy—Social aspects—United States. I. Hoffman, Saul D., 1949- II. Maynard, Rebecca A.
   HQ759.64.K53 2008
   362.82'9—dc22

                                                           2008035051

Printed in the United States of America

12 11 10 09 08   1 2 3 4 5

THE URBAN INSTITUTE is a nonprofit, nonpartisan policy research and educational organization established in Washington, D.C., in 1968. Its staff investigates the social, economic, and governance problems confronting the nation and evaluates the public and private means to alleviate them. The Institute disseminates its research findings through publications, its web site, the media, seminars, and forums.

Through work that ranges from broad conceptual studies to administrative and technical assistance, Institute researchers contribute to the stock of knowledge available to guide decisionmaking in the public interest.

Conclusions or opinions expressed in Institute publications are those of the authors and do not necessarily reflect the views of officers or trustees of the Institute, advisory groups, or any organizations that provide financial support to the Institute.

Contents

      of Programs Aimed at Reducing Teen
      Sexual Risk-Taking?   403
      Lauren Sue Scher

      About the Editors   435

      About the Contributors   437

      Index   441

Acknowledgments

I n 1997, a group of researchers organized by the Robin Hood Foundation published *Kids Having Kids,* a volume that was the first comprehensive effort to identify the consequences of teenage births for the mothers, the fathers, and the children themselves. It examined a very wide range of outcomes: earnings of fathers; education, earnings, employment, welfare use, fertility, and marriage of mothers; health care, foster care, educational attainment, and even incarceration of the children as adolescents and adults. The researchers took great care to distinguish as well as possible the causal impact of a teenage birth itself from the effects of other risk factors that could contribute to poor outcomes. Disentangling the various factors associated with adolescent childbearing and its consequences in this way is extremely important for any policy discussion about the expected benefits of investing in pregnancy prevention and about the needs for other potential supports to overcome the challenges faced by young mothers and their children.

The Kids Having Kids Research Project was the vision of Paul Tudor Jones, founder of the Robin Hood Foundation and chair of its board of directors, and David Saltzman, executive director of the Robin Hood Foundation. They enlisted the assistance of the Catalyst Institute to commission comprehensive, scientific research on the consequences of teen childbearing and provided significant financial support for the individual studies. The original edition of *Kids Having Kids* benefited greatly from the input of an outstanding project advisory group that included Elijah Anderson, Wendy Baldwin, Douglas Besharov, Claire Brindis, Sarah Brown, Michael Carrera, Mary Elizabeth Corcoran, Sheldon H. Danziger, Joy Dryfoos, David Ellwood, Jacqueline D. Forrest, Frank Furstenberg, Irving B. Harris, Karen Hein, Evelyn Kappeler, Marianna Kastrinakis, Arleen Leibowitz, Sara S. McLanahan, Robert A. Moffitt, David Myers, Susan Newcomer, Susan Philliber, Carol Roddy, Robert St. Peter, Robert Valdez, and Terry Watkins.

This revised edition of *Kids Having Kids* entailed updating trends in teenage sexual activity, pregnancy, and childbearing through 2004 (chapter 2), reestimating the consequences of teen childbearing for mothers and children using data through the early 2000s (chapters 3 and 5 through 9), and updating the estimated costs of teen childbearing for teen mothers, taxpayers, and society based on more recent estimates of consequences (chapter 10). In addition, this edition includes a synthesis of the research estimating the effectiveness of interventions aimed at preventing teen pregnancy (chapter 11).

Our ability to update this volume depended on the willingness of many of the original study authors to update their research or to work with us to allow us to do so. The work required for us and contributing authors benefited from the generous support of the Robin Hood Foundation, the W. T. Grant Foundation, and the National Campaign to Prevent Teenage Pregnancy. Importantly, however, any opinions expressed in this book are those of us and the contributing authors. They do not necessarily reflect the views of the Robin Hood Foundation, the W. T. Grant Foundation, or the National Campaign to Prevent Teen Pregnancy.

Rebecca A. Maynard and Saul D. Hoffman

1

The Study, the Context, and the Findings in Brief

Saul D. Hoffman and Rebecca A. Maynard

Early pregnancy and childbearing remain pressing concerns in the United States. Each year, 7.5 percent of all 15- to 19-year-old women become pregnant (Alan Guttmacher Institute 2006). In 2004, these pregnancies resulted in 422,000 births among teenagers, 80 percent of which were first births (Martin et al. 2006).[1] Despite a 36 percent drop in the teen pregnancy rate between 1990 and 2002 (the most recent data available) and a 33 percent decline in the teen fertility rate between 1991 and 2004, the United States still has the highest teen pregnancy and birth rates in the industrialized world. Rates of teen pregnancy and birth in the United States are two to six times higher than those in most of western Europe, including France, Holland, Denmark, and Sweden (Singh and Darroch 2000; UNICEF 2001).

Adolescent childbearing has long been associated with adverse consequences for teen mothers, fathers, and their children. The earliest literature placed the responsibility for these adverse outcomes almost exclusively on the teenage birth itself. Arthur Campbell famously wrote, "The girl who has an illegitimate child at the age of 16 suddenly has 90 percent of her life's script written for her" (1968, 238). Two decades later, a National Research Council report, *Risking the Future* concluded, "Women who become parents as teenagers are at greater risk of social and economic disadvantage throughout their lives than those who delay childbearing" (Hayes 1987, 138). President Clinton echoed this perspective in his 1995 State of the Union address, when he declared, with some understandable political hyperbole, that teen pregnancy is "our most serious social problem."

Social scientists, while acknowledging the poor economic circumstances of teen mothers and their families, have examined the causal relationship more closely, attempting to determine to what extent the adverse outcomes are attributable to teen pregnancy itself, rather than to the wider environment in which most of these pregnancies and the subsequent childrearing take place.[2] The young women who become teen mothers often face many disadvantages arising from the families and communities in which they live. Their families often have lower average incomes, their communities may have fewer public amenities and support systems, and their public school systems may be weaker. Each disadvantage, including the early age of the mother's first birth, contributes uniquely to the poorer outcomes for these women and their children. If too much weight is assigned to giving birth as a teen, there is a very real risk of overstating what can be accomplished by a delay in the age at first birth.

In 1997, a group of researchers organized by the Robin Hood Foundation published *Kids Having Kids,* the first comprehensive effort to identify the consequences of teen births for the mothers, the fathers, and the children themselves. The researchers examined a very wide range of outcomes and took great care to distinguish as clearly as possible the causal impact of a teen birth itself from the effects of other risk factors that could contribute to poor outcomes. Unlike most previous research, which compared teenage (under age 20) mothers with those who delayed childbearing until age 20 or later, the first edition of *Kids Having Kids* focused on adolescent women who give birth at age 18 or younger. It placed primary importance on assessing the likely consequences of delaying their childbearing for an average of about four years, or until the would-be teen mothers reached age 20 to 21. The focus on young teens reflected the strong public concern about the high rate of childbearing among those under age 18, the vast majority of which resulted from unplanned pregnancies. Still school age, almost certain to be unmarried, even less likely to be prepared for parenthood, these very young mothers highlight the most visible and concerning dimensions of teenage pregnancy and parenthood. The decision to estimate the benefits for would-be teen mothers of delaying childbearing until age 20 or 21 was based on a judgment that a delay this long plausibly could be achieved and, if so, would address most of the major public concerns over teenage parenting.

This second edition of *Kids Having Kids* returns to the same central issue a decade later: What is the impact of a teen birth on outcomes for mothers, fathers, and especially the children? What would be the benefits of delaying first births? What are the costs of adolescent childbearing to the mothers, to the taxpayers, and to society as a whole? How have the impacts of a teen birth changed in the intervening decade since *Kids Having Kids* was first published?

This edition covers the same topics as the first, in the same order. In addition, a new chapter (11) reviews the teen pregnancy intervention literature. All chapters except one have been revised and updated either by the original authors (in the cases of chapters 5, 6, 7, and 10), or by other scholars (in the cases of chapters 2, 8, and 9), or by both the original authors and another scholar (3). Chapter 4, on the impacts of adolescent childbearing for fathers of children born to teen mothers, has not been updated because more recent or better data to allow improved estimates were unavailable.

Unlike the first edition of *Kids Having Kids,* this edition focuses on the consequences of all adolescent childbearing, taking care to report separately the findings pertaining to young teen mothers (defined as those who have their first child before they turn age 18) and older teen mothers (defined as those who have their first child at age 18 or 19).

Policy Context

All the analyses presented in this volume attempt to isolate the causal impact of a teen birth on the many outcomes of interest. The causal role corresponds to this thought experiment: "If we could change a young woman's age at first birth, but not change anything else about her, what impact would that have on her subsequent life outcomes and the life outcomes of her children?" The resulting impact of a teen birth is referred to as its *net* effect—that is, its effect *net* of the impact of other risk factors that are not changed. The net effect represents a *causal* impact, not just a correlation. The results reported in this volume are as close to net impacts as possible given data limitations.

In order to estimate the net effect of teenage childbearing, it is necessary to compare young women who are as similar as possible in all respects except for the age at which they first had a birth. This comparison is done using various statistical techniques that *control for* or *adjust for* all the other risk factors that contribute to the outcome being studied. The specific way in which this is done varies from study to study, depending on the data source used and the measures of family and community risk factors available in that data. The result is equivalent to finding the average difference in outcomes between young women who are identical except for the ages at which they had a first birth.

Findings in Brief

Kids Having Kids consists of a background study of trends in adolescent childbearing, seven coordinated studies that each focus on a particular dimension of the consequences of adolescent childbearing, a summative assessment of the costs of teen births based on the measured consequences, and a review of what is known about the effectiveness of pregnancy prevention intervention strategies. Each study of the consequences of adolescent childbearing uses the best available dataset to address that particular set of questions (table 1.1). Each study also uses statistical analyses to control for various non-pregnancy-related factors that might affect outcomes (table 1.2). The review of intervention effectiveness is based on a systematic review of evidence through early 2006.

Trends in Fertility and Sexual Activity (Chapter 2)

In 1997, when the first edition of *Kids Having Kids* was published, the United States had just seen a decade of unsettling changes in the teen birth rate. Between 1986 and 1991, the teen birth rate rose five years in a row, reversing three decades of steady decline and rising nearly 25 percent in the process. Then, just as suddenly, it began to fall. By 1996, the teen birth rate was down 13 percent from its 1991 peak, but it still stood more than 10 percent above its 1986 level (Martin et al. 2006).

The teen birth rate has continued to fall steadily and presently is about 33 percent below its 1991 peak. Fertility rates have fallen for all age groups and all racial and ethnic groups, with especially sharp declines for younger teenagers and non-Hispanic black teenagers. Recently published data show a 2005 fertility rate for 15- to 19-year-olds of 40.4 births per 1,000, which is the lowest rate ever recorded for U.S. teens in the 65 years for which consistent data are available (Hamilton, Martin, and Ventura 2006). This is a 2 percent decline from the 2004 rate, and, notably, the

Table 1.1. Studies and Data Sources

Study	Data source
Trends in Fertility and Sexual Activity Data reported in the 2008 edition 　(Saul D. Hoffman)	Vital Statistics; U.S. Bureau of the Census; 　various published reports through 　2005; various derivative sources
Consequences of Teen Childbearing *　for Mothers* Estimates first reported in the 1997 edition 　(V. Joseph Hotz, Susan W. McElroy, 　and Seth G. Sanders) updated in 　2008 edition	National Longitudinal Survey of Youth 　(NLSY) (females age 14–21 in 1979), 　data for 1979–93
Estimates reported in the 2008 edition 　(Saul D. Hoffman)	NLSY (females age 14–21 in 1979), data 　for 1979–2000
Costs and Consequences for the Fathers Estimates reported in the 1997 edition 　(Michael J. Brien and Robert J. Willis)	NLSY (males age 27 in one year of the 　follow-up survey); 1989 National 　Maternal and Infant Health Survey, 　linked with Vital Statistics
Outcomes for Children of Teen Mothers *　from Kindergarten through Adolescence* Estimates reported in the 2008 edition 　(Jennifer S. Manlove, Elizabeth 　Terry-Humen, Lisa A. Mincieli, and 　Kristin A. Moore)	National Longitudinal Survey of Youth, 　1997 Cohort (NLSY97) (adolescents 　age 12–16 in 1997), annual survey data 　for 1997 through 2002; Early Childhood 　Longitudinal Study, Kindergarten 　Cohort, data for children in kindergarten 　in 1998–99
Children's Health and Health Care Estimates reported in the 2008 edition 　(Barbara Wolfe and Emilie McHugh 　Rivers)	2002 Medical Expenditure Panel Survey, 　data for a sample of children under 　age 15
Consequences of Teen Childbearing for *　Child Abuse, Neglect, and* *　Foster Care Placement* Estimates reported in the 2008 edition 　(Robert M. Goerge, Allen Harden, 　and Bong Joo Lee)	Illinois Integrated Database on Children 　and Family Services; Illinois birth 　certificate data

(continued)

Table 1.1. *(Continued)*

Study	Data source
Consequences of Teen Childbearing for Incarceration among Adult Children	
Estimates first reported in the 1997 edition (Jeffrey Grogger)	NLSY97 (sample of males age 27–34 in 1991)
Estimates reported in the 2008 edition (Lauren S. Scher and Saul D. Hoffman)	NLSY97 (sample of males age 38–45 in 2002)
Children of Teen Mothers as Young Adults	
Estimates first reported in the 1997 edition (Robert Haveman, Barbara Wolfe, and Elaine Peterson)	Panel Study of Income Dynamics (persons 0–6 years old in 1968 and surveyed each year through 1988)
Estimates reported in the 2008 edition (Saul D. Hoffman and Lauren S. Scher)	NLSY, 1979 Cohort (NLSY79), Young Adult Sample, data through 2002 for children of the original NLSY79 sample

decline is concentrated entirely among 15–17-year-olds. The 2004–05 decline of .07 births per 1,000 is larger than the decrease between 2003 and 2004 (.05 births per 1,000) but about half the size of the annual changes from 2000 to 2003 (1.9 births per 1,000). This pattern may suggest that the decline in the teen birth rate is abating.[3]

The rest of the fertility picture for teenagers in the United States is much more mixed. Despite recent declines, the fertility rate among U.S. teens remains well above rates in western Europe and in other countries with a comparable level of economic development (Singh and Darroch 2000). Further, the proportion of teen births that are outside marriage, which had remained essentially unchanged between 1998 and 2001, has increased slowly but steadily since then. Presently, over 84 percent of teenage child-bearing is nonmarital (Hamilton, Martin, and Ventura 2007).

In recent years, lower proportions of teenagers have been reporting having ever had sexual intercourse than was the case in 1995 (Abma et al. 2004). While the declines have been observed among males of all ages, the same is not true for females. In recent years, most teenagers report not being sexually active, defined as having had sex within the past month or three months.

Contraceptive use is far from perfect among sexually active teenagers as a group, especially at first intercourse and among younger teens. Yet, the percentage using contraception has increased, and there have been increases in consistency of condom use and in the use of such long-acting contraceptives as DepoProvera®. Recent evidence suggests that higher rates of contraceptive use and use of more effective modes of contraception are a major factor in the declining pregnancy rates (Santelli et al. 2007). Abortion has declined by about a third from its peak in the late 1980s. Currently, about 3 in 10 teenage pregnancies (28 percent) end in abortion (Ventura et al. 2006).

Consequences for the Mothers (Chapter 3)

In the first edition of *Kids Having Kids,* V. Joseph Hotz, Susan Williams McElroy, and Seth G. Sanders examined the impact of a teenage birth on a wide range of outcomes for the mothers—education, employment, earnings, fertility, and marriage, among others. Part 1 of this chapter reports this original research with updated data through 1993. The authors use an innovative research approach that compares teenage mothers not with women who did not have teenage births, but with young women whose first teenage pregnancies ended in miscarriages. Since miscarriage is largely a random event that results in a delay of age at first birth, a comparison of outcomes for teens whose first pregnancies ended in births with outcomes for teens whose first pregnancies ended in miscarriages should, the authors argue, provide an unbiased estimate of the causal impact of a teen birth.

Using data through 1993, the authors find that a teen birth is not a negative causal factor in the outcomes they examine. Indeed, Hotz and colleagues conclude that adolescent childbearing, properly analyzed, is actually beneficial to the teen mothers over a wide range of outcomes: young women who have an early birth earn more, marry men who earn higher incomes, and receive less support from welfare through their mid-20s to early 30s than if they delay their childbearing until their early 20s. The negative impacts of adolescent childbearing are limited to high school graduation rates and to the number of years teen mothers spend as single parents.

Hotz, McElroy, and Sanders's re-analyses support the basic findings of their chapter in the first edition of *Kids Having Kids,* although most effects are slightly weaker than reported in 1997. The authors continue

Table 1.2. Control Variables Used in the Analyses

			Consequences of Teen Childbearing for:				
	Mothers (chapter 3)	Fathers (chapter 4)	Children from kindergarten through adolescence (chapter 5)	Children's health and health care (chapter 6)	Abuse, neglect, and foster care placement (chapter 7)	Incarceration among adult children (chapter 8)	Children as adults (chapter 9)
Demographic characteristics							
Marital status		✓		✓			
Race/ethnicity	✓	✓	✓	✓	✓	✓	✓
AFQT score	✓	✓					
Child's age			✓	✓		✓	
Birth order				✓	✓	✓	✓
Mother's age at birth	✓	✓	✓	✓	✓	✓	✓
Family background							
Living arrangement as teen	✓	✓	✓				✓
Mother's education	✓	✓	✓				✓
Father's education	✓	✓					✓
Mother's achievement test score	✓						✓
Family income	✓						

Years lived in poverty

Mother on welfare/family in poverty

Religion

Number of children

Home resources

Mother's nativity

Mother's language at home not English

Mother's number of siblings

Mother grew up in city, town, or rural area

Grandmother's education

Grandmother's age at first birth

Other

Region of residence

Child's health

Birth year

State per capita spending on family planning

Neighborhood unemployment rate

State maximum welfare benefits

AFQT = Armed Forces Qualifying Test

to conclude that adolescent childbearing is not an important causal factor in the poorer adult outcomes of women who were teen mothers.

In part 2 of this chapter, Hoffman further updates Hotz, McElroy, and Sanders's analysis using data through 2000, when all the young women were in their mid-30s. His analyses of data for the same period as Hotz and colleagues yields findings roughly consistent with theirs, although Hoffman's findings are typically less positive and, in the case of post-secondary schooling, quite negative.

Importantly, these conclusions are based most heavily on the experience of women in the sample who entered their teen years in the early 1970s, because only these mothers had reached their mid-30s in the time-frame included in the analyses of Hotz, McElroy, and Sanders. With the addition of the longer-term follow-up data for the sample members who entered their teens in the mid- to late 1970s, Hoffman finds weaker positive effects than Hotz and colleagues and some stronger negative effects.

Hoffman also finds some tentative evidence that the effects of a teen birth may be becoming more negative. He examines teen birth impacts separately for earlier and later cohorts of teen mothers in order to reconcile the differences in the findings between his sample and that used by Hotz, McElroy, and Sanders. Across the full range of outcomes examined, Hoffman finds evidence that the effects of an early teen birth differ for the earlier and later cohorts of teen mothers. The positive or benign effects found by Hotz and colleagues hold only for the older cohort, while the effects are far more negative for the younger cohort. However, because these estimates are based on relatively small samples and have large associated standard errors, this analysis should be interpreted conservatively.

Costs and Consequences for the Fathers (Chapter 4)

Chapter 4 focuses on two perspectives when assessing the consequences of teenage parenting for fathers. The first is the fathers' perspective: what are the consequences for men who father children when they are teenagers? The second is the mothers' perspective: what resources are potentially available from their partners, and how do these resources vary with the age at which the women become mothers?

Although men who have children as young teenagers begin their careers having higher incomes and working more hours than do those who delay parenthood, men who wait to have a child have higher levels of education, earn more, and work more hours by the time they reach their late 20s. The important question for policy is how much this difference has to do with the differences in the characteristics of those who become young fathers and those who do not, and how much is the result of the birth and whether the man assumes responsibility for the child by marrying the mother.

Michael J. Brien and Robert J. Willis find that when differences in the characteristics of the fathers are accounted for, fathering a child only modestly affects the educational achievement and earnings trajectories of fathers. There does, however, seem to be a substantial "marriage penalty" for those who choose to take responsibility for their children by marrying the mothers. After controlling for the characteristics of the fathers, those who marry the mothers of their children appear to work more in order to provide for their children they have chosen to support.

Looking at the implications for men who father children of teen mothers, the authors find evidence that, if these fathers were to have delayed childbearing, they would have had substantially higher incomes over their lifetimes. Importantly, this would result in an expectation that those who opt not to marry the mothers of their children would have greater capacity to contribute child support if they had waited until the mothers were older.

Outcomes for Children from Kindergarten through Adolescence (Chapter 5)

This chapter uses recent nationally representative data to update the portrait of the consequences of teen childbearing for the health, development, and welfare of children and adolescents. This chapter examines a broad set of outcomes in five domains: cognitive development and academic achievement, behavioral outcomes, home environment, relationship outcomes, and physical health and well-being. The analysis uses two large national datasets: the Early Childhood Longitudinal Study, Kindergarten Cohort (ECLS-K) to examine outcomes for children at kindergarten entry, and the National Longitudinal Survey of Youth, 1997 Cohort (NLSY97) to look at outcomes during adolescence.

Jennifer S. Manlove, Elizabeth Terry-Humen, Lisa A. Mincieli, and Kristin A. Moore examine outcomes for children of teen parents and compare these outcomes with those for children born to older mothers. As in the previous edition of *Kids Having Kids,* the authors find that children of teenage mothers fare poorly compared with other children. However, much of the difference is explained by factors other than adolescent child-bearing. Compared with children whose mothers begin parenting at age 20 to 21, children of teen mothers are much more likely to be low birth weight, have lower health assessment scores, have lower cognitive attainment and proficiency scores at kindergarten entry, and exhibit more behavior problems. Adolescent children have significantly lower academic achievement as measured by performance on standardized tests, and they are at higher risk of not completing high school. Generally, these differences are most pronounced for the children born to women who have their first child before age 18.

For example, compared with children whose mothers begin parenting at age 20 to 21, children of teen mothers have lower standardized test scores at kindergarten entry, and adolescent daughters of teen mothers are less likely to graduate from high school, net of controls. In addition, children of teen mothers exhibit more behavior problems, and children of the youngest teen mothers are more likely to be low birth weight. Adolescent children of teen mothers are also more likely to be married or cohabiting at a young age and are more likely to have teen births themselves.

These adverse effects for children are most pronounced for outcomes measured at kindergarten. However, unlike chapter 5 in the previous edition of *Kids Having Kids,* which found more pronounced differences for children born to women who have their first child before age 18, this chapter finds similarly poor outcomes among children of younger and older teen mothers. The authors suggest that this similarity may result, in part, from the different living situations of younger and older teen mothers. These findings suggest that it will take more than convincing teen mothers to delay childbearing for a few years to eliminate the myriad disadvantages their children face relative to children whose mothers choose to begin parenting in their 20s or later.

Children's Health and Health Care (Chapter 6)

In the first edition of *Kids Having Kids,* Barbara Wolfe and Maria Perozek examined the impact of a teenage birth on the health and health care use of children through age 14 using data on child health and medical expenditures data as of 1987. They found that young teen childbearing, in particular, significantly affected the proportion of children who were reported to be in excellent health and the proportions with acute or chronic conditions. Children of teen mothers also had higher health system use rates, and a larger fraction of their health care costs were paid by the public sector.

For this edition, Wolfe and Emilie McHugh Rivers update the analysis using 2002 child health and medical expenditure data. This newer study finds that children of young teen mothers are slightly more likely to have chronic medical conditions but less likely to have acute conditions. Their mothers are about as likely to report their children are in "excellent" health and are no more likely to report their children are in "fair or poor" health. Children of young teen mothers are less likely to see a medical provider than the children of older mothers. On average, from age 1 to 14, the children of teen mothers age 17 and younger receive less health care spending than the children of older mothers, but the difference is not particularly large. It is unclear whether the differences reflect genuine differences in health or differences in use of the health care system. Thus, it is not possible to know whether the lower health care expenditures are good or bad for the children involved.

Children of younger mothers rely more heavily on publicly provided health care than children of older mothers.[4] An estimated 60 percent of the health care of children age 1 through 14 whose mothers were under age 18 when they had their first child is provided through these sources, compared with 50 percent for children of mothers who were 20 or 21 at first birth. The average child of a young teen mother uses almost $145 more in publicly provided health care annually than the child of a woman who had her first birth at age 20 or 21.

The updated analysis also examines the health and medical expenditures of children born to older teen mothers (age 18 and 19). From birth to age 14, these children are, on average, about as healthy as the children of nonteen mothers. Like the children of young teen mothers, they are slightly more likely to report having chronic medical conditions than the children of nonteen mothers but are less likely to report acute conditions. Their mothers are also about as likely to report the children are in "excellent" health and no more likely to report the children are in "fair or poor" health.

Average total health expenditures for infants confirm this health disparity: expenditures for infants (0 to 1 year) are 75 percent higher than for infants of nonteen mothers. This expenditure pattern does not, however, persist; as a result, from age 1 to 14, these children have average annual health expenditures only slightly higher than those for the children of mothers who have a first birth at age 20 or 21. As always, health expenditure differences may reflect differences in access and use as well as differences in health.

The children of older teen mothers actually receive a larger share of their health expenditures through public programs than do the children of younger teen mothers and nonteen mothers. Sixty-three percent of their health expenditures are paid for by public programs, primarily Medicaid and the State Children's Health Insurance Program, compared with 50 percent for children of mothers who were 20 or 21 at first birth and 60 percent for the children of younger teen mothers. Eighty-four percent of health care expenses for children age 0 to 1 of older teen mothers are provided through these programs.

Child Abuse, Neglect, and Foster Care Placement (Chapter 7)

This innovative chapter uses administrative records from Illinois, where a state database links births to administrative records of incidents of abuse or neglect and foster care placement. The analysis in the first edition of *Kids Having Kids* examined the experience of children born between 1982 and 1988 using data through 1992. The updated analysis for this edition examines abuse or neglect and foster care placements through 2005 for children born between 1989 and 1998.

In 2004, 532,000 children were in foster care and nearly 5.5 million children were referred to state and local authorities for suspicion of abuse and neglect. According to an Urban Institute study of federal, state, and local spending on child welfare, total federal spending on programs to support foster care, adoption, and other activities amounted to $11.6 billion; state and local spending added another $11.6 billion (Scarcella et al. 2006). Most of this money—probably 90 percent or more—was spent on foster care, adoption, and related services.

Having a child placed in foster care is a relatively rare event. However, young teen mothers are 2.2 times more likely (3.1 percent versus 1.4 percent) to have a child placed in foster care during the first five years after a birth than women who had a first birth at age 20 to 21. Young teen mothers are also twice as likely to have a reported case of child abuse or neglect as are women who had a first birth at age 20 to 21. Almost 1 in 10 children of young teen mothers were reported for abuse or neglect, compared with 1 in 20 for children of mothers age 20 to 21. After controlling for several other risk factors that also affect these outcomes, delaying a birth from age 17 or earlier to age 20 to 21 would lower the foster care placement rate for these women by a third, while instances of abuse and neglect would fall by almost 40 percent.

Children born to mothers age 18 to 19 at first birth are 33 percent more likely to be in foster care and 39 percent more likely to have a report of abuse or neglect during the first five years after birth than children born to mothers age 20 or 21. After adjusting for various risk factors, children of mothers age 18 to 19 at first birth are 13 percent more likely to be in foster care and 24 percent more likely to be the subject of a report of abuse or neglect than otherwise similar children born to mothers age 20 to 21.

This study is unique in its ability to analyze statistically the determinants of abuse and neglect reports and of foster care placement. Yet, it also is important to appreciate the limitations of this study. It is limited to one state, albeit one whose demographic profile is fairly similar to that of the nation. Further, because the analysis is based on administrative records, it lacks detailed information on other risk factors that could be important causes of abuse, neglect, or foster care placements. The reported effects may reflect correlation, rather than causal impacts.

Incarceration among Children of Teen Mothers (Chapter 8)

In the first edition of *Kids Having Kids,* Jeffrey Grogger examined the impact of a teen birth on the probability that an adult child would be incarcerated. Grogger used data from the National Longitudinal Survey of Youth, 1979 Cohort (NLSY79) to examine this issue by following a cohort of young men age 14–21 as of 1979 until 1991, when they were age 26 to 33. These men were born between 1958 and 1965, when teenage births were far more common than today and when the great majority of such births were in two-parent families.[5] Using various empirical techniques, Grogger estimated the causal impact of a teenage birth. Based on his most rigorous and conservative technique, he estimated that a delay in age at first birth from 16 to 20.5 would reduce the probability of incarceration of the sons by 11.8 percent and, in turn, would reduce the overall incarceration rate by 3.5 percent. Grogger's analysis is included as part 1 of this chapter.

This second edition adds updated results based on data through 2002, when the men are in their late 30s and early 40s (Scher and Hoffman, part 2). This extension depicts each respondent's criminal history more completely and allows the authors to analyze the impact of a teen birth on total cumulated prison time through a larger portion of an individual's lifetime as well as on the probability of ever being in prison. The updated results are generally consistent, but slightly stronger, than those of Grogger.

The sons of young teen mothers are more than twice as likely to spend time in prison as are the sons of mothers who delay childbearing until their early 20s. Nearly 14 percent of the sons of adolescent mothers have been in prison by their late 30s, compared with 6 percent of the sons of mothers age 20–21. By that same age, the sons of teen mothers have spent an average of 0.57 years in prison, more than 2.5 times longer than the average prison time of sons of women who had a first birth at age 20–21.

Based on a very conservative estimate, delaying a teen birth to age 20 to 21 would reduce the probability of a son's incarceration by 10.6 percent and reduce the average years spent incarcerated by 13.4 percent. In turn, this would reduce the total prison population by approximately 4.0 percent.

The sons of mothers who were age 18 or 19 at their birth also have an elevated risk of spending time in prison. These men are 40 percent more likely to ever have been in prison, and they spend, on average, about 30 percent more time in prison through age 40 than the sons of mothers who delayed childbearing until their early 20s. Controlling for other risk factors, a delay in their mother's age at their birth would reduce their likelihood of incarceration by 5.8 percent and reduce their average years of incarceration by 6.7 percent.

The Life Chances of the Children of Teen Mothers (Chapter 9)

In the first edition of *Kids Having Kids*, Robert Haveman, Barbara Wolfe, and Elaine Peterson examined the impact of a teen birth on three outcomes for young adults: educational attainment, having a teen birth (for young women only), and being economically inactive at age 24. The authors' analysis was based on a sample of children born between 1962 and 1968. Teen births in those years were far more common than today and far more likely to occur among married teens. Outcomes for the children were measured as of 1988, when they were age 20–26. Haveman and colleagues' analyses found substantial impacts of a teenage birth on each outcome, even after controlling for detailed individual and neighborhood characteristics. This original chapter is included in this edition as chapter 9, part 1.

In part 2, Saul Hoffman and Lauren Sue Scher use data from the NLSY79 Young Adult Sample through 2002. These young adults were born between 1970 and 1981, 8 to 13 years later than those in the original analysis, and the outcomes, measured as of 2002, are substantially more recent. As such, the revised analysis provides far more timely information.

The updated analysis shows that the daughters of young teen mothers are far more likely to become teen mothers themselves than if their mothers had delayed childbearing. After accounting for other risk factors such as family background and academic ability, it is estimated that a daughter's risk of having a birth would fall by almost 60 percent, from 33 to just 14 percent, if a would-be teen mother delayed childbearing until her early 20s. This translates into the potential to decrease the number of teen births by more than 27,000 a year.

If these young teen mothers delayed their first births until age 20 or 21, it is estimated that their children's high school graduation rate would rise to 73 percent, an increase of 10 percent. Further, after adjusting for other risk factors, the children of young teen mothers complete an average of about a quarter-year less education, which means preventing teen births would result in an estimated 35,000 adolescents a year completing one more year of schooling than they otherwise would have.

Most of the observed difference in high school graduation rates for children of older teen mothers compared with other children is attributable to factors other than teen motherhood. The estimates in this chapter suggest that high school graduation rates for the children of older teen mothers would increase by 1 percentage point if their mothers delayed their first births to at least age 20, and the graduation rates of younger teen mothers would remain about the same.

Being the daughter of an older teen mother has a strong net effect, even after accounting for other risk factors such as family background and academic ability. If a young woman's mother delayed her own first birth to age 20–21, her daughter's risk of having a teen birth would fall by one-third, from 17 percent to 11 percent.

Adding Up the Costs (Chapter 10)

The cost analysis chapter develops from the separate component studies an overall assessment of the economic consequences of adolescent childbearing from the perspective of three interest groups: the teen parents, the taxpayers who are responsible for public policies and support programs, and society as a whole. This analysis focuses on the consequences of teen childbearing in four broad domains: (1) economic productivity of mothers, fathers, and adult children; (2) private transfers and taxes; (3) public assistance from various sources; and (4) other consequences, including children's health, welfare, and criminal behavior.

In each case, the analysis measures the consequences of adolescent childbearing by comparing observed outcomes for teen mothers (as well as their spouses, the fathers of their children, and their children) with predicted outcomes assuming that these mothers delayed childbearing until age 20 to 21. The particular consequences of teen childbearing are estimated based on the results reported in chapters 2–9 and supplemental analyses provided by those chapters' authors. Then, these individual cost components are integrated into aggregate cost estimates following an analytic framework commonly applied in benefit-cost evaluations that applies clearly defined assumptions about the period over which costs are measured, the rate of time preference or discounting, and the costs (or shadow prices) associated with various consequences of teen childbearing not measured directly in dollars.

According to the analysis, the economic costs of adolescent childbearing are borne by the taxpayers and by the rest of society, not by the teen mothers. Over their first 15 years of parenthood, women who become parents before age 18 can expect to have net incomes from all sources, including various forms of public assistance, averaging about $1,600 more a year than would be expected if they delayed childbearing until age 20 to 21. In contrast, those who become parents at age 18 or 19 have average net incomes that are just over $300 more a year than would be expected if they delayed childbearing (figure 1.1).

In a steady state with the annual number of first-time teenage mothers mirroring the current level of 336,783, the average annual cost to U.S. taxpayers of teen childbearing is an estimated $7.3 billion, or $1,445 per teenage mother a year over 15 years (figure 1.2). A major source of these costs is the forgone income and consumption taxes resulting from the lower earnings of the teen mothers and the fathers of their children ($3 billion). However, even larger costs are associated with the poor social and economic outcomes for children born to teen mothers. As a result of their lower productivity, children born to teen parents contribute an estimated $2.5 billion less annually in income and consumption taxes than if their mothers delayed childbearing. In addition, teen childbearing results in an estimated $1.58 billion more annually in taxpayer expenditures for med-

Figure 1.1. Economic Consequences of Teenage Childbearing over the First 15 Years of Parenthood (average annual economic resources, $2004)

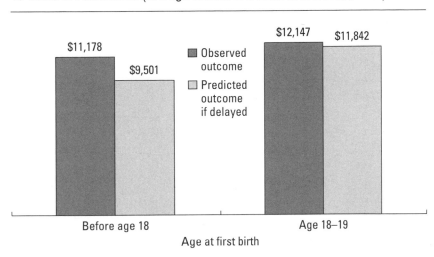

■ Observed outcome

□ Predicted outcome if delayed

$11,178 $9,501 $12,147 $11,842

Before age 18   Age 18–19

Age at first birth

Source: Authors' calculations based on data from chapters 3–9, this volume.

ical assistance of children, $2 billion more to support foster care costs, and $1.84 billion more to build and maintain prisons.

The costs to society are estimated to be nearly four times as large as those borne by taxpayers—$5,502 per teen mother a year. This means that, in a steady state, if all would-be teen mothers would delay childbearing until their early 20s, society would have nearly $28 billion annually to direct to other uses (figure 1.2). Most (about 80 percent) of this sum would derive from the higher productivity of the fathers of children born to teen mothers and the higher productivity of the children themselves. However, the mothers' productivity also would be higher, and fewer resources would be diverted for children's health care needs, foster care, and incarceration of juvenile and adult offenders.

The Effectiveness of Teenage Pregnancy Prevention Programs (Chapter 11)

While knowing the consequences of teen childbearing is an important first step, it is of limited value unless it is possible to design and implement programs that influence teens to delay the onset of sexual activity

Figure 1.2. Aggregate Annual Costs (or Benefits) of Teenage Childbearing to Taxpayers and to Society (billions, $2004)

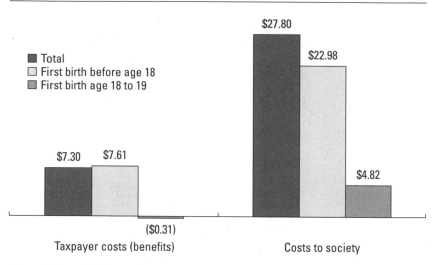

Source: Authors' calculations based on data from chapters 3–9, this volume.

or use contraception more effectively. Many programs for teens have been implemented, and some have been rigorously evaluated. Although there have been many prior reviews of the research, the reviews have applied widely different standards for searching and synthesizing the evidence and, consequently, arrive at quite different conclusions. To help resolve the inconsistencies and produce a concise, scientifically defensible summary of program evaluations, this edition of *Kids Having Kids* includes a chapter by Lauren Sue Scher on teenage intervention programs. This chapter summarizes the results of a systematic review of evidence regarding program effectiveness based on the findings from 38 randomized trials identified in published and unpublished literature. More than 37,000 teenagers and young adults participated in the studies.

The intervention programs Scher considers fall into four broad categories: clinic-based programs that provide various general reproductive services including check-ups and distribution of contraceptives; sex education programs, often called "comprehensive sex education" or "abstinence plus," that emphasize abstinence and/or contraception; multicomponent and/or youth development programs that aim to reduce various risky behaviors (for example, sexual behaviors or alcohol/drug use);

and comprehensive community-based programs that bring together multiple stakeholders across communities (for example, schools, community and faith-based institutions, housing developments) and institute multiple strategies. Outcomes that have been rigorously evaluated include sexual experience rates, consistent use of contraception among sexually active teens, and pregnancy rates.

The most promising results are for the more intensive, multicomponent youth development programs that serve higher-risk adolescents. These programs appear particularly successful in reducing pregnancy risk and pregnancy rates. Unfortunately, very few rigorous evaluations of such programs are available, and further replication and evaluation is warranted. The evidence to date is not strong enough to determine whether clinic-based, one-time consultations reduce sexual risk-taking. Only four evaluation studies are available, and none of the core outcome differences between control and treatment group are statistically significant. Similarly, rigorous evaluation of abstinence-focused sex education programs does not find evidence that these programs change the likelihood that youth will initiate having sex or that they will be more or less likely to have sex without using contraception. These programs are, however, not representative of the newer abstinence-based programs that have recently emerged, such as those funded under the Title V, Section 510 abstinence education monies (Maynard et al. 2005). None of these interventions took place within the past decade, and most used a very limited intervention.

Finally, taken as a group, there is no consistent overall evidence that sex education programs alter the likelihood that teens are sexually active, use contraception effectively, or become (or get someone) pregnant. However, some individual studies have found positive program effects, particularly related to increased contraception use. The nature of the programs included within this category varies greatly, as do the size, direction, and statistical significance of the impact estimates for the various programs.

Basic Messages

The final two chapters provide a good summary of the book's four basic messages. The first is that the economic costs for the teenage mothers are small. Rather, the consequences for mothers are nonmonetary and often not observable for several years following the birth of their first child. Kids who have kids are more likely to substitute a GED for a traditional high school diploma and are less likely to continue their education. They will have more children on average over fewer years and will spend more time as a single parent. At the same time, they work somewhat more hours than expected if they delayed childbearing.

The second message from this book is that there are myriad consequences for the children of mothers who begin parenting as teenagers. They are more likely to live in a single-parent home and a poorer-quality home, to spend more time in child care, to be the subject of abuse or neglect, and to spend time incarcerated than if their mothers had delayed childbearing.

The third message is that adolescent childbearing, particular before age 18, has significant adverse consequences for the children. These consequences cost taxpayers and society enough to merit close policy attention.

The final message is that we should look beyond the range of pregnancy prevention intervention programs commonly adopted by school districts and community-based organizations to address the incidence and associated consequences of teenage childbearing. Many factors likely have contributed to the substantial declines in teenage pregnancy and birth rates in recent years. These include the changing social norms around sex among young and unmarried individuals that have been promoted through governmental agencies and nongovernmental organizations such as the National Campaign to Prevent Teen Pregnancy with varying degrees of emphasis on reducing teen sexual activity and births, reducing nonmarital births, and preventing the spread of HIV/AIDS and other sexually transmitted infections. Improvements in contraceptive technology and expanded efforts to raise access to contraceptive services have also been important, as has the shift in welfare policy, beginning in the early 1990s, that required low-income parents to assume greater responsibility for the financial support of themselves and their children, while offering them greater assistance in doing so.[6] It seems prudent to build on these successes, while continuing efforts to develop more effective prevention services targeted at vulnerable youth.

NOTES

1. The most recent pregnancy data are for 2002, when 760,000 teenagers became pregnant (Alan Guttmacher Institute 2006). Preliminary fertility estimates for 2005 show 421,123 births to teens, of which 414,406 were to girls age 15–19 and 6,717 were to girls

age 10–14 (Hamilton et al. 2006). We focus on 2004 fertility information because it was the latest final version available when this chapter was written and when the cost estimates reported in chapter 10 were finalized.

2. Important early contributors to this literature include Furstenberg, Brooks-Gunn, and Morgan (1987); Geronimus and Korenman (1992); Grogger and Bronars (1993); Haveman and Wolfe (1994); and Hoffman, Foster, and Furstenberg (1993).

3. 2006 preliminary teen fertility data were released too late for full inclusion in this chapter. Teen fertility increased 3 percent between 2005 and 2006, the first increase reported since 1991. The 2006 teen fertility rate was 41.9 births per 1,000 women age 15 to 19 (Hamilton, Martin, and Ventura 2007).

4. Publicly provided health care includes Medicaid, the State Children's Health Insurance Program, Civilian Health and Medical Program of the Uniformed Services in the United States, and Medicare (for disabled children).

5. Between 15 and 20 percent of teen births were nonmarital during these years (Ventura and Bachrach 2000).

6. This policy shift was instituted nationally with the passage of the Personal Responsibility and Work Opportunity Reconciliation Act of 1996.

REFERENCES

Abma, Joyce C., Gladys M. Martinez, William D. Mosher, and Brittany S. Dawson. 2004. *Teenagers in the United States: Sexual Activity, Contraceptive Use, and Childbearing, 2002.* Vital and Health Statistics 23(24). Hyattsville, MD: National Center for Health Statistics.

Alan Guttmacher Institute, The. 2006. *Teenage Pregnancy Statistics: National and State Trends by Race and Ethnicity.* New York: The Alan Guttmacher Institute.

Campbell, Arthur A. 1968. "The Role of Family Planning in the Reduction of Poverty." *Journal of Marriage and the Family* 30(2): 236–45.

Furstenberg, Frank F., Jr., Jeanne Brooks-Gunn, and S. Philip Morgan. 1987. *Adolescent Mothers in Later Life.* Cambridge: Cambridge University Press.

Geronimous, Arline T., and Sanders Korenman. 1992. "The Socioeconomic Consequences of Teen Childbearing Reconsidered." *Quarterly Journal of Economics* 107(4): 1187–1214.

Grogger, Jeffrey, and Stephen Bronars. 1993. "The Socioeconomic Consequences of Teenage Childbearing: Findings from a Natural Experiment." *Family Planning Perspectives* 25(4): 156–61, 174.

Hamilton, Brady E., Joyce A. Martin, and Stephanie J. Ventura. 2006. "Births: Preliminary Data for 2005." National Vital Statistics Reports 55(11). Hyattsville, MD: National Center for Health Statistics.

———. 2007. "Births: Preliminary Data for 2006." National Vital Statistics Reports 56(7). Hyattsville, MD: National Center for Health Statistics.

Haveman, Robert, and Barbara Wolfe. 1994. *Succeeding Generations: On the Effects of Investments in Children.* New York: Russell Sage Foundation.

Hayes, Cheryl D., ed. 1987. *Risking the Future.* Vol. 1. Washington, DC: National Academy Press.

Hoffman, Saul D., E. Michael Foster, and Frank F. Furstenberg, Jr. 1993. "Reevaluating the Costs of Teenage Childbearing." *Demography* 30(1): 1–13.

Martin, Joyce A., Brady E. Hamilton, Paul D. Sutton, Stephanie J. Ventura, Fay Menacker, and Sharon Kirmeyer. 2006. "Births: Final Data for 2004." National Vital Statistics Reports 55(1). Hyattsville, MD: National Center for Health Statistics.

Maynard, Rebecca, Christopher Trenholm, Barbara Devaney, Amy Johnson, Melissa A. Clark, John Homrighausen, and Ece Kalay. 2005. *First-Year Impacts of Four Title V, Section 510 Abstinence Education Programs.* Princeton, NJ: Mathematica Policy Research, Inc.

Santelli, John S., Laura Duberstein Lindberg, Lawrence B. Finer, and Susheela Singh. 2007. "Explaining Recent Declines in Adolescent Pregnancy in the United States: The Contribution of Abstinence and Improved Contraceptive Use." *American Journal of Public Health* 97(1): 150–56.

Scarcella, Cynthia A., Roseana Bess, Erica H. Zielewski, and Rob Geen. 2006. *The Cost of Protecting Vulnerable Children V.* Washington, DC: The Urban Institute.

Singh, Susheela, and Jacqueline E. Darroch. 2000. "Adolescent Pregnancy and Child-bearing: Levels and Trends in Developed Countries." *Family Planning Perspectives* 32(1): 14–23.

UNICEF. 2001. "A League Table of Teenage Births in Rich Nations." Innocent Report Card, Issue 3. New York: UNICEF.

Ventura, Stephanie J., and Christine A. Bachrach. 2000. "Nonmarital Childbearing in the United States, 1940–99." National Vital Statistics Reports 48(16). Hyattsville, MD: National Center for Health Statistics.

Ventura, Stephanie J., Joyce C. Abma, William D. Mosher, and Stanley K. Henshaw. 2006. "Recent Trends in Teenage Pregnancy in the United States, 1990–2002." Health E Stats. Hyattsville, MD: National Center for Health Statistics. Available at http://www.cdc.gov/nchs/products/pubs/pubd/hestats/teenpreg1990-2002/teenpreg1990-2002.htm.

2

Trends in Fertility and Sexual Activity among U.S. Teenagers

Saul D. Hoffman

EDITORS' NOTE

When the first edition of Kids Having Kids *appeared in 1997, the United States had just seen a decade of startling changes in the teen birth rate. Between 1986 and 1991, the teen birth rate rose five years in a row, reversing three decades of steady decline and rising nearly 25 percent in the process. Then, just as suddenly, the teen birth rate began to fall, slowly but steadily. By 1996, the teen birth rate was down 13 percent from its 1991 peak but still stood more than 10 percent above its 1986 level. What, many observers wondered, would happen next?*

A decade later, the answer appears much clearer. Through 2004, the last year with complete information, the teen birth has now fallen an additional eight years in a row, thus making a total of 13 consecutive years with a decline. The 2004 teen birth rate is at a U.S. historic low, having fallen by one-third. Pregnancy rates and abortion rates are also down for teens.

At the same time, two troubling trends have persisted. First, teen birth rates in the United States remain very high compared with all other developed countries, even after the sharp decline. Second, more than four out of five teen births occur outside marriage, and this proportion has continued to increase in the past decade, even as the fertility rate has fallen.

Finally, substantial concerns remain about the negative consequences of teen childbearing for the parents, the children, and the public sector. Those concerns are the focus of the eight chapters in this volume.

This chapter reviews the trends in teen pregnancy, birth, abortion, sexual activity, and contraceptive use. Particular attention is paid to changes and developments since the mid-1990s. The chapter also briefly reviews recent studies that have attempted to identify the underlying causes of the decline in the teen birth rate.

Teen fertility followed the general post-World War II U.S. fertility boom, rising more than 60 percent between 1946 and 1957, the peak year of the baby boom. In that year, there were 96 births for every 1,000 teens age 15 to 19. The high teen birth rate was not much noted at that time because it was not high relative to the birth rate for women in their 20s, teen births did not account for a particularly large share of all births, and almost all the teen births were to married women. The teen fertility rate started to fall after 1957, and it fell almost every year until 1986, when it bottomed out at a rate of 50.2 births per 1,000, barely half the 1957 rate.

The falling teen fertility rate was reflected in other trends. Between 1957 and 1986, the median age at first marriage increased by almost three years, from 20.3 to 23.1.[1] Educational attainment for women also grew rapidly. The proportion of women age 25 to 29 who were high school graduates increased from 62 percent to 86 percent, and the proportion with college degrees nearly tripled from 8 percent to 22 percent.[2]

Between 1986 and 1991, however, this long-established trend of teen fertility decline reversed itself. The increase was broad based.[3] The fertility rate increased by 27 percent among 15- to 17-year-olds and by 18 percent among 18- to 19-year-olds. It increased by 25 percent for white teens and 20 percent for black teens.[4] In 1991, the peak year of the increase, more than 1 million adolescent girls became pregnant and more than 520,000 had a birth. Of every 1,000 girls age 15 to 19 in that year, 116 became pregnant and 62 had a birth. Among black teen girls, there were more than 222 pregnancies and 115 births for every 1,000 girls (Martin et al. 2006).

The teen fertility rate has now fallen every year since 1991, dropping by one-third. As of 2004, it stands at a historic low of 41.1 births per 1,000 girls age 15 to 19 (Martin et al. 2006). In 2004, there were a total of 422,043 births to young women age 19 and younger: 140,761 to girls age 17 and younger (including 6,781 to girls age 15 and younger) and 281,282 to girls age 18 or 19.[5] Of these teen births, just under 80 percent (336,783) were first births. Table 2.1 shows the 2004 teen fertility rate by age, race, and Hispanic origin.[6] While the overall fertility rate is 41.1 births per 1,000 young women age 15 to 19, it varies substantially among groups. Not surprisingly, the rate increases with age, from 22.1 births per 1,000 for girls age 15 to 17 to 70.0 births per 1,000 for 18- to 19-year-olds. Hispanics have the highest teen birth rate, followed by non-Hispanic blacks, American Indians, non-Hispanic whites, and Asians or Pacific Islanders. Rates also vary substantially within the Hispanic category: Mexicans teens have higher fertility rates (95.5 per 1,000) than Puerto Ricans (62.6), Cubans (23.5), and other Hispanics (57.7).[7]

Much like the increase in teen fertility between 1986 and 1991, the decline in fertility rates since 1991 has been broad based, including all ages, races, and ethnicities. Table 2.2 summarizes the fall in the teen fertility rates between 1991 and 2004. The fertility rate for all teens has fallen by one-third, but the decline has been greater for 15- to 17-year olds (43 percent) than for 18- to 19-year-olds (26 percent). (Between 1986 and 1991, the fertility rate rose more rapidly for younger teens than for the older teens.) Non-Hispanic black teens have had the largest decline—47 percent for 15- to 19-year-olds, 57 percent for 15- to 17-year-olds, and 36 per-

Table 2.1. Fertility Rates of Women Age 15–24 by Race and Hispanic Origin, 2004

Mother's age	All	Non-Hispanic white	Non-Hispanic black	American Indian	Asian or Pacific Islander	Hispanic[a]
15–19	41.1	26.7	63.1	52.5	17.3	82.6
15–17	22.1	12.0	37.1	30.0	8.9	49.7
18–19	70.0	48.7	103.9	87.0	29.6	133.5
20–24	101.7	81.9	126.9	109.7	59.8	165.3

Sources: Martin et al. (2006), table A (teens), tables 4 and 7 (age 20–24).

[a]Race and Hispanic origin are reported separately on birth certificates. Persons of Hispanic origin may be of any race.

Table 2.2. Decline in Fertility Rate by Age, Race, and Hispanic Origin, 1991–2004 (percent)

Mother's age	All	Non-Hispanic white	Non-Hispanic black	American Indian	Asian or Pacific Islander	Hispanic
15–19	33	38	47	38	37	21
15–17	43	49	57	42	45	28
18–19	26	31	36	35	30	14

Source: Martin et al. (2006), table A.

cent for 18- to 19-year-olds. The rate has fallen least for Hispanic teens (21 percent for all, 28 percent for 15- to 17- year-olds, and 14 percent for 18- to 19-year-olds). The decline in the fertility rate has been fairly similar for non-Hispanic whites, Native Americans, and Asians or Pacific Islanders (Martin et al. 2006).

Despite this substantial reduction in the teen birth rate, the United States' rates of adolescent pregnancy and childbearing are still conspicuously higher than other countries that share its level of income and economic development and, indeed, are often higher than countries with far lower average incomes. One study compared the United States to 45 developed countries—from Albania to Yugoslavia—as of the late 1990s (Singh and Darroch 2000). Of these 45 countries, just one had a higher teen fertility rate—Armenia, which barely nosed out the United States. In much of Europe, teen birth rates were one-quarter to one-fifth of the rate in the United States. Denmark, France, Germany, the Netherlands, Portugal, Spain, Sweden, and Switzerland are just some of the many European countries with teen birth rates a fraction of the United States'. Canada has a teen birth rate less than half the U.S. rate.

Figure 2.1 shows teen birth rates for 13 industrialized countries in 1990 and 2003. In 1990, the United States had the highest teen birth rate (59.9); most countries had rates a quarter of that or less. Thirteen years later, the United States still has the highest rate, and still by a considerable margin. Just as in 1990, the United Kingdom has the next-highest teen birth rate among these countries; its rate fell by 19 percent to 27 births per 1,000. At the opposite end of the spectrum, Japan has a teen birth rate of just 5.7 births per 1,000 women age 15 to 19.

As figure 2.1 shows, the teen birth rate fell in all these countries except Japan, where it rose from a very low level. In percentage terms, the largest

Figure 2.1. Teen Fertility Rates for Selected Industrialized Countries, 1990 and 2003

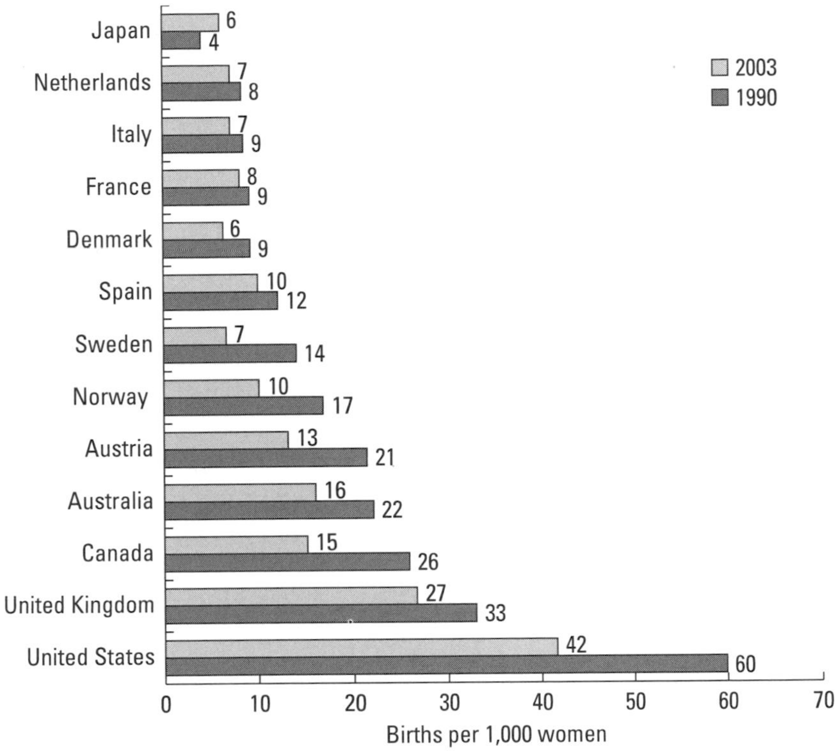

Sources: Martin et al. (2006); United Nations (2003).

decline in the teen birth rate between 1990 and 2003 occurred in Sweden, where the rate fell 53 percent. The teen birth rate also fell substantially in Denmark, Norway, Austria, and Canada. In continental Europe, teen birth rates, which were already low in 1990, fell approximately 10 to 15 percent through 2003. Although the difference between the United States and other countries is narrower than in 1990, it remains substantial.

Marriage among Teen Mothers

In 1957, when the teen fertility rate was more than twice its current rate, virtually all births occurred within marriage. The median age at first marriage for women was just a shade over 20.[8] Social pressure to legitimate premarital pregnancies was strong, and "shotgun" marriages occurring between conception and birth were common. Only one teen birth in seven was nonmarital in 1957 (Ventura and Bachrach 2000).

Since then, even as the teen fertility rate has been steadily falling, the link between teen marriage and teen motherhood has been steadily weakening. The proportion of all teen births to unmarried mothers doubled between 1960 and 1970 and then rose even more sharply, reaching nearly 50 percent by 1980. The nonmarital proportion reached 60 percent in 1986, 70 percent in 1992, and 80 percent in 2002. In 2004, 82 percent of all births to girls age 15 to 19 were nonmarital.

Figure 2.2 shows the trend in the nonmarital birth ratio beginning in 1980. The proportion rose very steadily and sharply in the 1980s and steadily but less rapidly through most of the 1990s. The trend line flattened out between 1998 and 2001, rising at a rate less than one-tenth the average over these years. But since 2001, the nonmarital birth proportion has increased again, at about 1 percentage point a year. As the figure shows, the proportion rose for both whites and blacks. (Comparable data for Hispanics are first available in 1990. Although not shown in the fig-

Figure 2.2. Percent of U.S. Teen Births to Unmarried Mothers by Race, 1980–2004

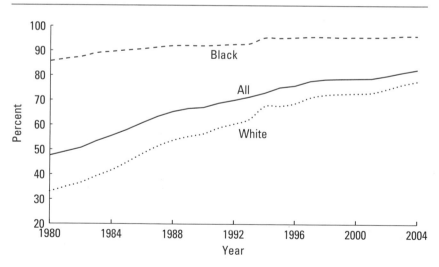

Sources: Martin et al. (2002, 2005, 2006); Ventura and Bachrach (2000).

Table 2.3. Nonmarital Birth Ratio by Age, Race, and Hispanic Origin, 2004 (percent)

Mother's age	All	Non-Hispanic white	Non-Hispanic black	American Indian	Asian or Pacific Islander	Hispanic
15–19	82.4	78.0	96.6	89.0	75.3	77.6
15–17	90.3	88.5	98.9	94.8	86.1	85.6
18–19	78.7	74.2	95.2	86.0	70.6	73.0

Source: Martin et al. (2006), table 18.

ure, the pattern for Hispanics closely follows the trend line for whites.) For black teens, the proportion already exceeded 85 percent in 1980 and has increased another 10 percentage points since then. For whites, the proportion doubled between 1980 and 1994 from one-third to two-thirds. Since then, it has increased at a more moderate rate—about 1 percentage point a year—and currently stands just short of 78 percent. The upward trend in the overall nonmarital birth proportion since 2001 has been driven by the rising nonmarital birth proportion for white teens.

Table 2.3 shows the nonmarital birth ratio for 2004 separately by age, race, and ethnicity. For every age and racial or ethnic group shown, more than 70 percent of births are nonmarital. Ninety percent of all births to 15- to 17-year-olds are nonmarital, and nearly 79 percent of births to 18- to 19-year-olds are. For non-Hispanic blacks, marriage has virtually disappeared as a realistic alternative: 99 percent of births to 15- to 17-year-olds were nonmarital, and 95 percent of births to 18- to 19-year-olds were. To put this in perspective, of the more than 97,000 births to non-Hispanic black teens, only 3,351 were to married women. Non-Hispanic whites and Hispanics have very similar proportions of births that are nonmarital, approximately 78 percent for 15- to 17-year-olds and 74 percent for 18- to 19-year-olds.

The Precursors of Fertility among Teenagers

The trend in fertility rates discussed above is a function of the extent of sexual activity, the use of effective contraception, and the use of abortion. This section summarizes what is known about those factors.

Sexual Activity

The best and most current information about sexual activity of teens comes from the National Survey of Family Growth (NSFG). The NSFG is a nationally representative survey that has been administered by the National Center for Health Statistics periodically since 1973. It originally sampled only married women age 15 to 44, but never-married women were added to the survey in 1982, and men age 15 to 44 were added in the 2002 survey. Men age 15 to 44 had previously been surveyed in the National Survey of Adolescent Males (NSAM). The most recent data are for 2002. Previous NSFG and NSAM surveys in 1988 and 1995 allow comparisons over time in sexual activity.

In 2002, about 70 percent of never-married women and 65 percent of never-married men have ever had sexual intercourse before reaching their 19th birthday (figure 2.3).[9] The trajectories for men and women are similar; men are slightly more likely than women to have had sexual intercourse by ages 14 and 15, and women are slightly more likely than men to have had sexual intercourse at ages 16 and higher. By age 15, about 14 per-

Figure 2.3. Percent of Never-Married Teens Who Have Ever Had Sexual Intercourse by Age and Gender, 2002

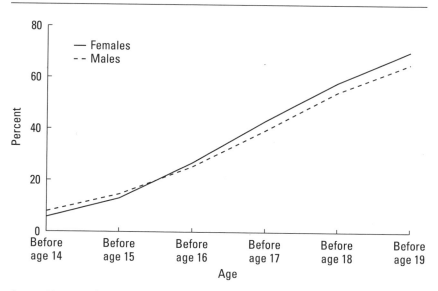

Source: Abma et al. (2004); all data from National Survey of Family Growth, various years.

cent of teens are sexually experienced, up from about 8 percent by age 14. Thereafter, the rate rises sharply and steadily to about 25 percent by age 16, about 40 percent by age 17, 56 percent by age 18, and 65 to 70 percent by age 19. The biggest increase occurs between age 16 and 17 for girls (16 percentage points) and between age 17 and 18 for boys (15 percentage points). At all ages from 14 to 19, the difference in the rates for men and women is relatively small.

Among all never-married teens in 2002, non-Hispanic blacks (both men and women) are most likely to have ever had sexual intercourse; among women, Hispanics are least likely to have ever had sexual intercourse, while among men, non-Hispanic whites are the least likely. The low rate of sexual experience for Hispanic women is recent; in 1995, Hispanic women were more likely to have had sexual intercourse than non-Hispanic white women. Indeed, the proportion of Hispanic women with sexual experience fell 15 percentage points between the 1995 and 2002 surveys, from 53 percent to 38 percent. Among men, the proportion with sexual experience for Hispanics is about 9 percentage points lower than for blacks, and the proportion for white men is another 14 percentage points lower. Teens, both male and female, whose mothers are college graduates are least likely to have had sexual intercourse, as are teens living with both biological or adoptive parents and teens whose own mothers were age 20 or older when they first had children. These latter impacts are best understood as correlations, rather than causal relationships, since other risk factors are not controlled for.

How has teen sexual activity changed over the past two decades? Figures 2.4 and 2.5 show the share of teens who are sexually experienced by ages 17 and 19 at three points in time: 1988, 1995, and 2002. For never-married women, the incidence of sexual activity increased between 1988 and 1995 for younger teens from 38 percent to 47 percent but fell for older teens from 77 percent to 70 percent. Between 1995 and 2002, just the opposite occurred: the proportion sexually experienced by age 17 fell more than 4 percentage points, while the proportion at age 19 increased 0.4 percentage points. For men, the proportion sexually experienced by age 17 was constant between 1988 and 1995, but it dropped very sharply between 1995 and 2002, from 53 percent to 39 percent (a 25 percent decline). For 19-year-olds, the rate increased sharply between 1988 and 1995 (up almost 9 percentage points) and then dropped more than 18 percentage points between 1995 and 2002.

Figure 2.4. Percent of Never-Married Females Who Have Ever Had Sexual Intercourse by Age, 1988–2002

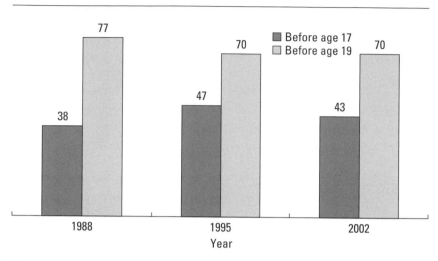

Source: Abma et al. (2004); all data from National Survey of Family Growth, various years.

Figure 2.5. Percent of Never-Married Males Who Have Ever Had Sexual Intercourse by Age, 1988–2002

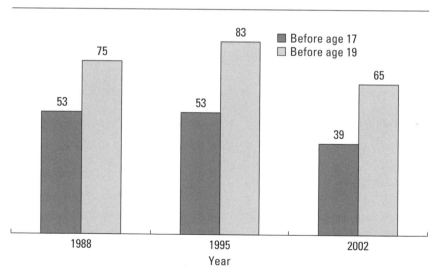

Source: Abma et al. (2004); all data from National Survey of Family Growth, various years.

The overall pattern of changes suggests a general rise in age at first sexual experience. For men, the proportions that are sexually experienced have fallen consistently for both age groups, relative to 1988 and 1995 (figure 2.5). The recent decline for older teens is particularly large. For women, the pattern is less clear, but there is some evidence, especially since 1995, of a delay in age at first sex.

Although many teens are sexually experienced (i.e., they have ever had sex), the majority are not sexually active, usually defined as having had sex within the past month or past three months.[10] In 2002, 72 percent of never-married women and 75 percent of never-married men age 15 to 19 had not had sex within the past month, and about 60 percent of both men and women had not had sex in the past three months. Since about 45 percent of both men and women age 15 to 19 have never had sex, these figures mean that among all female teens who have ever had sex, 37 percent did not have sex within the past month and 25 percent did not have sex within the past three months. Among male teens who have ever had sex, 44 percent have not had sex within the past month and 32 percent have not had sex within the past three months. Among all teens that have ever had sex, about 9 percent had sex only once.

Not all sexual activity is voluntary.[11] In 2002, 9.6 percent of women who had their first sexual experience as a teen reported that the intercourse was nonvoluntary. This figure is not much changed from the 9.0 percent figure reported for 1995. Almost 25 percent who first have sex at age 14 or younger report that the act was nonvoluntary, compared with 10 percent who first have sex at age 15 to 16 and 5 percent who first have sex at age 17 to 19. Consistent with evidence from the 1995 survey, the incidence of nonvoluntary sex is higher the greater the age difference in partners and for Hispanics and non-Hispanic blacks.

Contraceptive Use

In 2002, among women age 15 to 19 who had ever had sexual intercourse, about a quarter used no contraception at their first intercourse (figure 2.6).[12] Two-thirds used a condom, one-sixth were taking birth control pills, and one-seventh used a dual method, usually a hormonal method along with a condom. Contraceptive method varies substantially with age. More than 33 percent of teens who first had intercourse at age 14 used no method, compared with 17 percent of those who were age 17 or older at first intercourse. Failure to use contraception increases with

Figure 2.6. Contraceptive Used for First Intercourse among Females Age 15–19, 2002

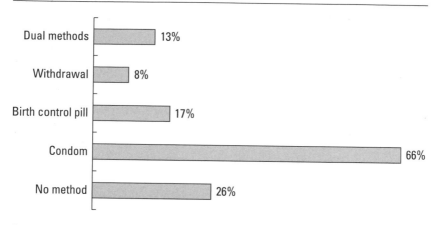

Source: Abma et al. (2004); all data from National Survey of Family Growth, various years.

the age of the male partner or if the young woman is Hispanic. The younger a girl is at first intercourse, the more likely she is to use a condom only and the less likely she is to use the pill or dual methods, both of which are more reliable.

Virtually all teen women who have ever had sexual intercourse (98 percent) have at some time used some contraception (table 2.4). Hispanic

Table 2.4. Contraceptive Use among Sexually Experienced Teens Age 15 to 19, by Race and Ethnicity, 2002 (percent)

Method ever used	Total	Non-Hispanic white	Non-Hispanic black	Hispanic
Any method	97.7	98.4	97.1	94.3
Pill	61.4	67.9	55.2	36.5
Injectable	20.7	17.9	27.0	24.3
Emergency contraception	8.1	9.1	6.0	7.3
Condom	93.7	95.9	94.6	82.8
Periodic abstinence	10.8	10.1	11.9	10.6
Withdrawal	55.0	60.7	41.1	52.1

Source: Abma et al. (2004), table 19.

women are slightly more likely to have never used contraception than non-Hispanic whites and blacks. The mode of contraception used varies by race and ethnicity. Hispanic women are far less likely to ever have used birth control pills than non-Hispanic whites and blacks—37, 68, and 55 percent, respectively. Blacks and Hispanics are more likely to have used injectable contraceptives, which are highly reliable. Emergency contraception has been used by 8 percent of all teen women who have ever had sexual intercourse;[13] non-Hispanic whites are more likely to use this method than the other two groups. Overall, more than 90 percent have ever used a condom; the proportion is substantially lower for Hispanics than for whites and blacks.

Table 2.5 compares contraceptive use in 1988, 1995, and 2002. The figures shown represent the proportions who used a particular contraceptive method at last intercourse (within the past three months) in the top section or ever in the lower section. Comparisons across the years are

Table 2.5. Reported Use of Contraception among Sexually Experienced Never-Married Teens Age 15 to 19, by Year (percent)

Method	1988	1995	2002
Used indicated contraceptive method at last intercourse:[a]			
Any method	79.9	70.7	83.2
Pill	42.7	25.0	34.2
Injectable	—	7.0	9.1
Condom	31.3	38.2	54.3
Dual methods	—	—	19.5
Ever used contraceptive method:			
Any method	—	96.2	97.7
Pill	—	51.6	61.4
Injectable	—	9.7	20.7
Condom	—	92.8	93.7
Emergency contraception	—	—	8.1
Periodic abstinence	—	13.2	10.8
Withdrawal	—	42.3	55.0

Source: Abma et al. (2004), tables 18 and 20.

[a]Refers to sexual intercourse within previous three months.

potentially sensitive to differences in the age distribution of women in the different samples.

Between 1988 and 1995, contraceptive use at last intercourse declined, with the sole exception of the condom. The proportion using any method declined more than 9 percentage points, and the proportion using the pill declined more than 17 percentage points. Condom use increased, as did injectables, which were not used in 1988.

Between 1995 and 2002, contraceptive use at last intercourse increased in all categories. Eighty-three percent of women used some method in 2002, compared with 71 percent in 1995. Use of the pill increased 9 percentage points, injectable methods increased slightly, and use of the condom increased by almost 50 percent. Nearly one in five women used a dual method, usually a hormonal method and a condom, at last intercourse.

The information on whether women have every used a particular mode of birth control is available only for 1995 and 2002. The proportion that ever used any method was over 96 percent in 1995 and increased to 98 percent in 2002. The most important changes are the increases in the proportions using the pill (up 10 percentage points), injectables (doubled to more than 20 percent), and emergency contraception (from 0 to 8 percent).

The general pattern observed here is one of better, but far from perfect, use of contraception.

Pregnancy

In 2002, the most recent year with information about teen pregnancy, just under 750,000 teens became pregnant. About a third of the pregnancies were to girls age 15 to 17, a figure that closely matched their share of all teen births. The 750,000 pregnancies translated into a teen pregnancy rate of 75.4 pregnancies for every 1,000 girls age 15 to 19. For girls age 15 to 17, the pregnancy rate was 42.3; for girls age 18 to 19, it was 125.6. The pregnancy rate is highest for black and Hispanic teens (134.2 and 131.5 per 1,000, respectively) and lowest for non-Hispanic whites (48.2 per 1,000). It is currently estimated that 30 percent of girls have a pregnancy some time between ages 14 and 19 (National Campaign to Prevent Teen Pregnancy 2006). At the recent peak of teen pregnancies in 1991, 40 percent of girls became pregnant before their 20th birthday.

Teen pregnancy rates have declined since 1990 for all age groups and all racial and ethnic groups.[14] Figure 2.7 shows the time trend by age; fig-

Figure 2.7. Pregnancy Rate of U.S. Women Age 15–19 by Age, 1990–2002

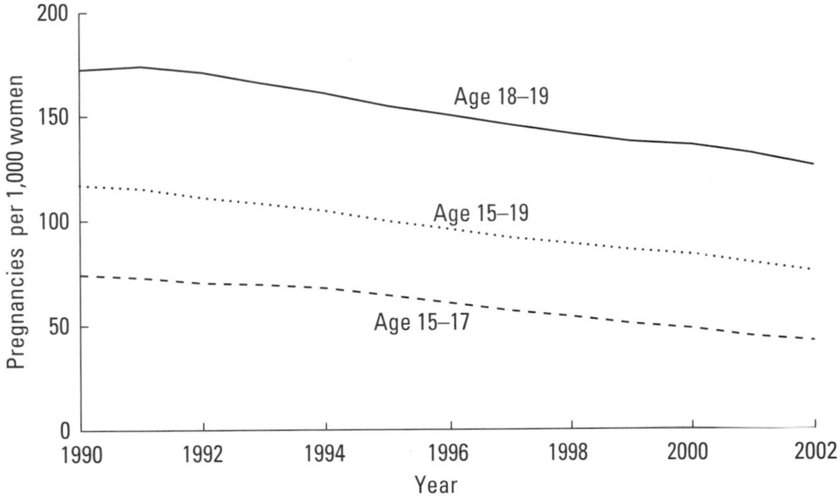

Source: Alan Guttmacher Institute (2006).

ure 2.8 shows the trend by race and Hispanic origin. In 1990, there were 115 pregnancies per 1,000 women age 15 to 19; the rate was 172 for 18- to 19-year-olds and 74 for 15- to 17-year-olds. These pregnancy rates led to birth rates of 94.0 and 38.6, respectively, for 18- to 19- and 15- to 17-year-olds. The pregnancy rate fell 27 percent for 18- to 19-year-olds and 43 percent for 15- to 17-year-olds, rates virtually identical to the declines in the birth rate for these two age groups of 26 percent and 43 percent, respectively. Since 2000, the pregnancy rate for both age groups has fallen by the largest percentage for any consecutive two-year period since 1990. The rate fell 12.2 percent for 15- to 17-year-olds and 7.4 percent for 18- to 19-year-olds.

As seen in figure 2.8, the teen pregnancy rate has fallen very sharply for black teens (down 40 percent) and much less sharply for Hispanics (18.9 percent). In 1990, the pregnancy rate for black teens was more than one-third higher than the rate for Hispanics; by 2002, that differential was all but eliminated. For whites, the teen pregnancy rate fell 34 percent. Between 2000 and 2002, the pregnancy rate fell 12.5 percent for blacks, 9 percent for whites, and less than 5 percent for Hispanics.

Figure 2.8. Pregnancy Rate of U.S. Women Age 15–19 by Race and Hispanic Origin, 1990–2002

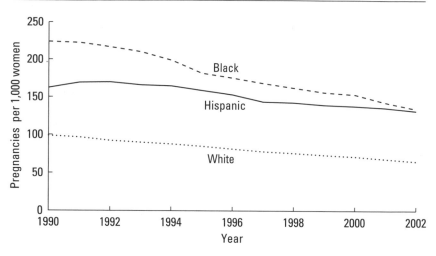

Source: Alan Guttmacher Institute (2006).

Explaining the Decline in Teen Fertility

The most natural question is why the teen birth rate spiked between 1986 and 1991 and why it has declined since then. Some research on the causes of the decline is available, but virtually none on the spike. This research has focused on the trend in pregnancies, rather than births, and has examined the impact of the two proximate behaviors of pregnancy: rates of sexual activity and use of contraception.

One study examined the trend between 1988 and 1995 (Darroch and Singh 1999), a time spanning the spike and the first part of the decline.[15] During this period, the pregnancy rate fell from 111.4 per 1,000 to 101.1 per 1,000, a decline of about 9 percent. Arithmetically, the pregnancy rate is the product of the proportion of women who have had sexual intercourse and the proportion of such women who become pregnant;[16] this latter term is referred to as the pregnancy rate among sexually experienced women. Changes in sexual activity are reflected in the first term, while changes in contraceptive behavior, including consistency of use and choice of mode, are reflected in the second term.[17] Darroch and Singh then estimate how the teen pregnancy rate would have changed if first one and then the other factor alone had changed. They conclude that approximately 25 percent of the decline in the pregnancy rate came from a smaller proportion of teens who were sexually experienced and 75 percent came from a lower pregnancy rate among sexually experienced women. They argue further that the average frequency of sexual intercourse changed little over this period and that contraceptive use did not markedly change, but that teenage contraceptive users were adopting more effective methods, primarily injectables and implants. Darroch and Singh suggest that this last factor is the primary explanation for the decline in the teen pregnancy rate.

Applying the same technique to the 1995 to 2002 period suggests a more balanced contribution of changes in the rate of sexual experience and the pregnancy rate among sexually experienced teens. Over this period, the pregnancy rate fell from 99.6 to 75.4 pregnancies per 1,000 teen girls age 15 to 19, and the proportion that had ever had sexual intercourse fell from 53 percent to 47 percent. These figures suggest that 43 percent of the decline in the pregnancy rate results from a decrease in sexual activity and 57 percent from a lower pregnancy rate among sexually experienced women.[18]

A more recent study examined the period from 1991 to 2001 (Santelli et al. 2004) but is limited to changes in pregnancy rates among 15- to 17-year-olds, a group that contributes just one-third of teen pregnancies and births and that has had a more volatile time trend than older teens, both during the spike and in the decline period.[19] This research examines the impact of contraceptive behavior directly by using contraceptive failure rates for each contraceptive mode.[20] Contraceptive failure rates vary widely across modes: 4 percent for injectables, 7 percent for the birth control pill, 15 percent for condoms, and 85 percent for no method. Over the time studied, the pregnancy rate for 15- to 17-year-olds declined 33 percent, while the proportion that had ever had sexual intercourse fell 16 percent.

Changes in use of contraceptive mode adjusted for the contraceptive failure rate for each mode suggest a 15 percent decline in the probability of becoming pregnant. On that basis, the authors attribute 53 percent of the decline in the pregnancy rate to decreased sexual experience. These results, taken together with the figures presented above for the 1995 to 2002 period, which were calculated using an entirely different approach, suggest that declines in sexual activity among teens are a more important cause of the decline in teen pregnancy than they were in the 1988 to 1995 period.

It is well understood that studies like these do not explain why contraceptive use and sexual activity have changed as they have. At this time, there are many possible candidates but no meaningful assessment of the quantitative importance of each. Typically cited causes include concerns about HIV/AIDS and sexually transmitted diseases, which may have led to more conservative sexual behavior and to more attention to contraception; welfare reform in 1996, which imposed far more restrictive rules regarding receipt of assistance, particularly for teens; changes in available contraceptives to include long-lasting injectables; and a more conservative culture generally, including more discussion of the risks and consequences of sex and more positive messages about abstinence. Additional research in this area would be extremely valuable.

Abortion

Following the legalization of abortion in 1973, the proportion of teen pregnancies ending in abortion increased sharply, just as it did for non-teens.[21] In 1972, less than 25 percent of teen pregnancies were terminated by an abortion; by 1979, 45 percent were (figure 2.9). The *abortion ratio* (abortions as a fraction of births plus abortions) remained at that level

Figure 2.9. Percent of Pregnancies Ended by Abortion among U.S. Women Age 15–19, 1972–2002

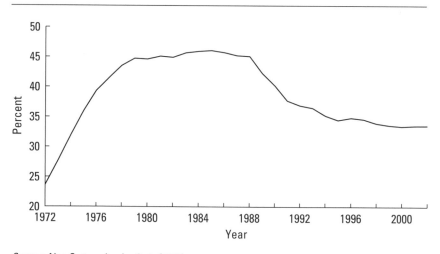

Source: Alan Guttmacher Institute (2006).

through most of the 1980s but then began a steady decline in 1989 that lasted through the mid-1990s. Between 1988 and 1995, the abortion ratio fell more than 10 percentage points, from 45.1 to 34.5 percent. Since 1995, the teen abortion ratio has stabilized at about 33 percent. The most recent data are for 2002, when the teen abortion ratio was 34 percent—approximately 215,000 abortions for 640,000 pregnancies.

In 2002, the abortion ratio varied considerably by age and race (figure 2.10). Pregnant Hispanic teens are least likely to have an abortion (26 percent), while pregnant black teens are the most likely (43 percent). Younger pregnant teens are slightly more likely to have an abortion than older ones (36 versus 32 percent).

Another measure of the prevalence of abortion is the *abortion rate,* which measures the incidence of abortions among all women age 15 to 19 rather than as a proportion of pregnancies. This measure incorporates the impact of both changes in pregnancy rates and changes in abortion, conditional on pregnancy. It is a useful measure for thinking about how common abortion is. This rate is shown in see figure 2.11. As seen there, the abortion rate followed a time trend similar to that of the abortion ratio through 1995, but it has continued to decline since then, unlike the abortion ratio. This second trend is solely a result of the recent decline in the

Figure 2.10. Abortion Ratio of U.S. Women Age 15–19, by Age, Race, and Hispanic Origin, 2002

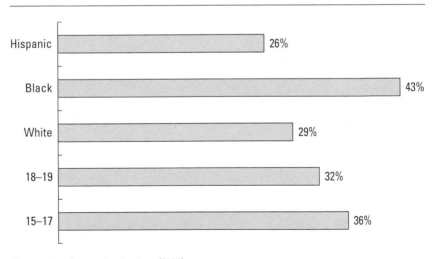

Source: Alan Guttmacher Institute (2006).

Figure 2.11. Percent of U.S. Women Age 15–19 Who Had an Abortion, 1972–2002

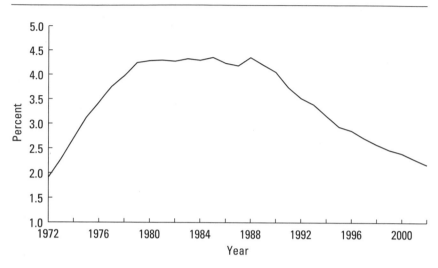

Source: Alan Guttmacher Institute (2006).

pregnancy rate, since the proportion of teen pregnancies ending in abortion has changed very little since the late 1990s. At its peak in 1988, 4 percent of teen girls had an abortion. In 2002, the most recent year with abortion data, the rate had fallen to 2 percent. Less than 2 percent of white teens had an abortion in 2002, compared with nearly 5 percent of black teens.

Conclusion

The past two decades have seen teen birth rates first break a three-decade pattern of decline by spiking 25 percent between 1986 and 1991 and then return to the historical pattern by falling 33 percent since then. The fertility decline has included all age groups, all races, and both Hispanics and non-Hispanics. Younger teens and non-Hispanic blacks have had particularly sharp declines. The rate for Hispanic teens fell least.

Nothing is certain in subjects such as this, but it seems unlikely that teen fertility rates will spike again in the next decade or so, as they did in the late 1980s. Preliminary estimates for 2005 show a 1.7 percent decline in teen fertility (from 41.1 to 40.4), entirely concentrated among 15- to 17-year-olds (Hamilton, Martin, and Ventura 2006). This decline is larger than the decrease between 2003 and 2004 but about half the size of annual changes from 2000 to 2003.

The rest of the teen fertility picture is much more mixed. Despite the recent decline, the teen fertility rate in the United States remains well above the rates in Western Europe and in other countries with a comparable level of economic development. The proportion of births to single teen mothers now exceeds 82 percent. This proportion has started to increase again after several years in the late 1990s of virtually no change. While marriage is relatively rare for all ages, races, and ethnicities, it is particularly uncommon for black teens, for whom more than 96 percent of teen births are nonmarital.

Relative to 1995, the fractions of teens who have ever had sexual intercourse has fallen for men, but not across all age groups for women. Most teens are not, however, sexually active, defined in terms of having had sex within the past month or three months. Contraceptive use is far from perfect, especially at first intercourse and among younger teens. But the percentage using contraception and the kind of contraception used has been improving, as use of condoms and injectable forms of contraception have spread. Abortion has declined about one-third from its peak in the late 1980s. Currently, nearly 33 percent of teen pregnancies end in abortion; 2 percent of teenage girls had an abortion in 2002.

Studies that attempt to explain the decline in teen fertility have focused on teen pregnancy, analyzed in terms of changes in the proportion of teens who have ever had sexual intercourse and the pregnancy rate among these sexually experienced teens. For an earlier period (1988 to 1995), one study attributes three-quarters of the decline to a falling pregnancy rate among sexually experienced teens. A study for a more recent period (1991 to 2001) for younger teens only finds a more balanced responsibility.

Table A.2.1. Births by Age and Parity of Mother, 2004

Age of mother	Number of Births			Percent of Births in Age Group		Percent of Births to Teens by Age of Mother	
	Total	First birth	Higher order birth[a]	First birth	Higher order birth[a]	First birth	Higher order birth[a]
Total under age 20	422,043	336,783	85,260	79.8	20.2	100.0	100.0
Under age 18	140,761	126,471	14,290	89.8	10.2	37.6	16.8
Under age 15	6,781	6,636	145	97.9	2.1	2.0	0.2
Age 15	18,274	17,491	783	95.7	4.3	5.2	0.9
Age 16	41,860	38,561	3,299	92.1	7.9	11.4	3.9
Age 17	73,846	63,783	10,063	86.4	13.6	18.9	11.8
Age 18–19	281,282	210,312	70,970	74.8	25.2	62.4	83.2
Age 18	117,237	93,131	24,106	79.4	20.6	27.7	28.3
Age 19	164,045	117,181	46,864	71.4	28.6	34.8	55.0
Age 20–24	1,034,454	483,752	550,702	46.8	53.2		
Older than age 24	2,655,555	810,386	1,845,169	30.5	69.5		
Total	4,112,052	1,630,921	2,481,131	39.7	60.3		

Source: Martin et al. (2006).

[a]These figures also include small numbers of births for whom birth order is not reported. In total, order is not reported for 18,633 of 4,112,042 births.

NOTES

I thank Whitney LeBoeuf for her important contributions to this chapter.

1. Data are from U.S. Census Bureau, "Table MS-2. "Estimated Median Age at First Marriage, by Sex: 1890 to the Present," http://www.census.gov/population/socdemo/hh-fam/ms2.pdf, September 21, 2006.

2. Data are from U.S. Census Bureau, "Table A-2. Percent of People 25 Years and Over Who Have Completed High School or College, by Race, Hispanic Origin and Sex: Selected Years 1940 to 2005," http://www.census.gov/population/socdemo/education/cps2005/tabA-2.xls, October 26, 2006.

3. The fertility rate for all women also rose during this period from 65.4 in 1986 to 69.3 in 1991. Rates rose for all age groups. None of the older age groups, however, had such a consistent pattern of falling fertility in the decades before 1986.

4. See Ventura et al. (2001). Teen fertility data by Hispanic origin are not available before 1989.

5. This chapter focuses on teen fertility as of 2004 because that was the latest final version of estimates available when the chapter was written. Preliminary fertility estimates for 2005 show 414,406 births to girls age 15–19, and an additional 6,717 births to girls age 10–14 (Hamilton et al. 2006). See appendix table 2A.1 for additional information about 2005 teen fertility.

6. Race and Hispanic origin are reported separately on birth certificates. Persons of Hispanic origin may be of any race.

7. The figure for Cubans is for 2000. Since 2000, the teen fertility rate for Cuban teens has not been officially reported because the sample size makes the figure unreliable.

8. Data are from U.S. Census Bureau, "Table MS-2. "Estimated Median Age at First Marriage, by Sex: 1890 to the Present," http://www.census.gov/population/socdemo/hh-fam/ms2.pdf, September 21, 2006.

9. All figures reported are from Abma et al. (2004), tables 1–3. The data refer exclusively to heterosexual intercourse.

10. All figures cited are from Abma et al. (2004), tables 4–6, or are derived from those tables.

11. All figures cited are from Abma et al. (2004), table 7.

12. All figures cited are from Abma et al. (2004), tables 15 and 17. The percentages shown may sum to more than 100; statistics for the various modes reflect use of that method regardless of whether it was used alone or with another method.

13. This is 8 percent of all who had sexual intercourse, not 8 percent of all who became pregnant.

14. All figures discussed come from the Alan Guttmacher Institute (2006), although similar statistics also are reported in Ventura and colleagues (2006). The number of pregnancies is the sum of births, abortions, and miscarriages. Abortion data come from a survey by the Alan Guttmacher Institute of abortion providers. Miscarriages are estimated as 20 percent of live births plus 10 percent of abortions.

15. Data availability limited the analysis to these years. A study using more recent data reaches qualitatively similar conclusions (Santelli et al. 2004).

16. The arithmetic relationship is the following: # Pregnancies/Population = (# Sexually Experienced/Population) × (# Pregnancies/# Sexually Experienced).

17. Neither term is perfect. The proportion of teens who are sexually experienced does not account for possible changes in the frequency of sexual activity, a term which could also affect the pregnancy rate among sexually experienced teens. The impact of contraceptive use is not measured directly but is inferred from the pregnancy rate among sexually experienced teens.

18. This figure is computed slightly differently than in Darroch and Singh (1999), whose technique, which is not truly a decomposition, does not constrain the explained portions to 100 percent. Results using their technique are qualitatively similar.

19. The analysis is limited to this age group because the data are taken from a school-based sample (Youth Risk Behavior Surveillance Survey) that is not representative of 18- to 19-year-olds.

20. The contraceptive failure rate measures the number of pregnancies that would occur among 100 women using a particular contraceptive mode over a 12-month period.

21. All abortion data cited come from the Alan Guttmacher Institute (2006) and are based on a survey of abortion providers.

REFERENCES

Abma, Joyce C., Gladys M. Martinez, William D. Mosher, and Brittany S. Dawson. 2004. *Teenagers in the United States: Sexual Activity, Contraceptive Use, and Childbearing, 2002.* Vital and Health Statistics 23(24). Hyattsville, MD: National Center for Health Statistics.

Alan Guttmacher Institute, The. 2006. *U.S. Teenage Pregnancy Statistics: National and State Trends and Trends by Race and Ethnicity.* New York: The Alan Guttmacher Institute.

Darroch, Jacqueline E., and Susheela Singh. 1999. *Why Is Teenage Pregnancy Declining? The Roles of Abstinence, Sexual Activity, and Contraceptive Use.* Occasional Report 1. New York: The Alan Guttmacher Institute.

Hamilton, Brady E., Joyce A. Martin, and Stephanie J. Ventura. 2006. "Births: Preliminary Data for 2005." National Vital Statistics Reports 55(11). Hyattsville, MD: National Center for Health Statistics.

Jones, Rachel K., Jacqueline E. Darroch, and Stanley K. Henshaw. 2002. "Contraceptive Use among U.S. Women Having Abortions in 2000–2001." *Perspectives on Sexual and Reproductive Health* 34(6): 294–303.

Martin, Joyce A., Brady E. Hamilton, Paul D. Sutton, Stephanie J. Ventura, Fay Menacker, and Sharon Kirmeyer. 2006. "Births: Final Data for 2004." National Vital Statistics Reports 55(1). Hyattsville, MD: National Center for Health Statistics.

Martin, Joyce A., Brady E. Hamilton, Paul D. Sutton, Stephanie J. Ventura, Fay Menacker, and Martha L. Munson. 2005. "Births: Final Data for 2003." National Vital Statistics Reports 54(2). Hyattsville, MD: National Center for Health Statistics.

Martin, Joyce A., Brady E. Hamilton, Stephanie J. Ventura, Fay Menacker, Melissa M. Park, and Paul D. Sutton. 2002. "Births: Final Data for 2001." National Vital Statistics Reports 51(2). Hyattsville, MD: National Center for Health Statistics.

The National Campaign to Prevent Teen Pregnancy. 2006. *Fact Sheet: How Is the 3 in 10 Statistic Calculated?* Washington, DC: National Campaign to Prevent Teen Pregnancy.

Santelli, John, Joyce Abma, Stephanie Ventura, Laura Lindberg, Brian Morrow, John Anderson, Sheryl Lyss, and Brady Hamilton. 2004. "Can Changes in Sexual Behaviors among High School Students Explain the Decline in Teen Pregnancy Rates in the 1990s?" *Journal of Adolescent Health* 35(2): 80–90.

Singh, Susheela, and Jacqueline E. Darroch 2000. "Adolescent Pregnancy and Childbearing: Levels and Trends in Developed Countries." *Family Planning Perspectives* 32(1): 14–23.

United Nations. Department of Economic and Social Development. 2003. *Demographic Yearbook 2003.* New York: United Nations

Ventura, Stephanie J., and Christine A. Bachrach. 2000. "Nonmarital Childbearing in the United States, 1940–99." National Vital Statistics Reports 48(16). Hyattsville, MD: National Center for Health Statistics.

Ventura, Stephanie J., T. J. Mathews, and Brady E. Hamilton. 2001. "Births to Teenagers in the United States, 1940–2000." National Vital Statistics Reports 49(10). Hyattsville, MD: National Center for Health Statistics.

3

Consequences of Teen Childbearing for Mothers

EDITORS' NOTE

The 1997 study of the impacts of teen childbearing by Hotz, McElroy, and Sanders was a very ambitious effort to examine the socioeconomic consequences for the mothers. In part 1 of this chapter, the authors revise their study, using data that adds another year to the outcomes (through 1993), and they adjust the analysis to improve the accuracy of their estimates. Hotz, McElroy, and Sanders use the natural experiment research methodology to compare outcomes for a nationally representative sample of teenagers who became pregnant and gave birth in the mid-1970s with outcomes for their counterparts who became pregnant and reported having had a miscarriage.

The findings and inferences drawn in this updated study are much the same as those reported in 1997. In particular, the authors find that women who have their first child before age 18 do not work less, earn less, or receive less spousal income and are not more dependent on forms of public assistance than they would have been had they delayed childbearing. Hotz, McElroy, and Sanders also indicate that the effects of teen mothers failing to delay childbearing appear relatively transitory and decline as the mother, and her children, age.

In part 2 of this chapter, Hoffman further updates the original analysis by extending the period of observation through 2000, when all sample members were at least 35 years old. The estimates of life-cycle effects based on this new analysis better represent the consequences of teenage child-bearing for younger women in the NLSY79 sample. The findings from this analysis for the study sample are qualitatively similar to those reported by Hotz, McElroy, and Sanders, although the effects are typically weaker than in their analysis. Further analysis that separates the experiences of teen mothers who gave birth in the early 1970s from those who gave birth in the late 1970s and early 1980s shows that the positive effects reported by Hotz, McElroy, and Sanders hold only for the former group. Teen birth effects are often negative for the latter group of teen mothers.

Consequences of Teen Childbearing for Mothers through 1993

V. Joseph Hotz, Susan Williams McElroy, and Seth G. Sanders

There is growing concern in the United States about the number of children born to teen mothers and the proportion of these births that occur out of wedlock. Two decades ago, the National Research Council concluded that "adolescent pregnancy and childbearing are matters of substantial national concern" (Hayes 1987, ii) and President Bill Clinton, in his 1995 State of the Union Address, asserted that teenage pregnancy is "our most serious social problem." Part of the concern centered on the plight of teen mothers. The everyday hardships of teen motherhood come into public consciousness through media attention to and the prevalence of teenage childbearing throughout the United States. Further, there is a strong statistical association between the age at which a woman has her first child and her subsequent socioeconomic well-being. For example, women who have babies during their teens tend to have low levels of education, employment, and earnings, and high levels of dependence on public assistance. They also spend more time than average as single parents.

The association with indicators of economic and social disadvantage has fueled the view that teen childbearing *causes* the poor socioeconomic outcomes endured by teen mothers. There appears to be a compelling logic behind this perception. Adolescence is an important period for a person's educational attainment, especially regarding the completion of high school and preparation for a vocation; this attainment has become even more crucial as the earnings prospects for unskilled workers has declined (Juhn, Murphy, and Pierce 1993). Adolescence is also an important period in a person's psychosocial development. A young mother—particularly a single mother—will have less time and energy than her childless counterpart to socialize, develop as an individual, and learn how to develop healthy interpersonal relationships (and, hence, a support network). All these opportunities are presumably important for her socioeconomic well-being in later life. Thus, it is no wonder that teen childbearing is perceived as a trap door that propels young mothers downward socioeconomically.

It is hard to dispute the evidence that teen mothers have tough lives and limited options. As we show in the next section, the data paint a grim picture of teen motherhood when comparing the socioeconomic attainment of teen mothers with those of women who delay their childbearing. What is at issue is the appropriateness of such standard comparisons and the validity of the conclusions about the *causal* link between adolescent childbearing and the well-being of young mothers. In this chapter, we address the following question: *What would be the adolescent mother's (behavioral) outcomes if she were to delay her childbearing until she was older but nothing else changed in the wider socioeconomic context?* This question, we argue, is the relevant one for assessing whether teen childbearing in itself is the reason young mothers appear to fare so poorly over their subsequent lives.

Obtaining reliable answers to this question is difficult. The adverse outcomes attributed to adolescent childbearing may simply reflect preexisting differences in family background, such as poverty and other factors that make teen mothers different from women who delay childbearing. As such, the apparent consequences noted above, and illustrated below, may have little to do with the timing of motherhood.

Random assignment to "treatment" and "control" groups is the standard evaluation method for dealing with the confounding influences of preexisting factors when estimating causal effects. In such evaluations, "treatments" are randomly assigned to some members of a sample and not to others. Then, estimates of the average causal effect of the treatment are obtained from the average difference in subsequent outcomes for the treatment and "control" groups.

Unfortunately, use of such experimental designs is simply not feasible in the context of teen childbearing. Rather, social scientists must resort to nonexperimental (or quasi-experimental) statistical methods to sort out these causal links. The latter methods attempt to adjust for the influence of preexisting differences between comparison groups by using such statistical techniques as regression analysis to mitigate their influence and, thus, to isolate the causal relationship between adolescent childbearing and the socioeconomic attainment of such mothers. Such techniques may not adjust completely for all the background differences between teen mothers and women who did not bear children in their teens and, as such, produce biased estimates. Many factors not measured in available datasets—or factors that cannot be measured, or even identified, directly or reliably—are likely to affect the age at which a woman has her first child. In addition, the various factors that affect when a woman has a child may exert other independent effects on her subsequent socioeconomic attainment.

To avoid obtaining biased estimates of the causal effects of the consequences and costs of early childbearing, we exploit a "natural experiment" associated with human reproduction. Drawing on our related work (Hotz, McElroy, and Sanders 2005), we compare the behavior of teen mothers with that of women who became pregnant as teens but who experienced miscarriages. As miscarriages are purely random events *and* the only way in which pregnancies do not result in births, women who experience them constitute the ideal control group that a randomized experiment would provide. While these conditions are not met in practice, use of this comparison group appears to approximate the ideal conditions that would be achieved with a randomized experimental design (Hotz, Mullin, and Sanders 1997).

Before proceeding, it is important to stress the limits of our analysis. We address but one facet of teen childbearing, namely, the effects on the teen mothers themselves and whether these particular effects are the reason that this group of women requires government subsidies. Our analysis does not consider the consequences and costs of adolescent childbearing to at least two other groups: the fathers of children born to teen mothers and, more important, the children themselves. While we find little evidence that teen childbearing in itself harms mothers, our results do not preclude the possibility that early childbearing adversely affects these other two groups. Those costs and consequences are the subject of other chapters in this book.

The Apparent Consequences of Teen Childbearing

We use the National Longitudinal Survey of Youth, 1979 Cohort (NLSY79) to portray statistically the prevalence of adolescent childbearing in the United States and its apparent consequences for teen mothers. The NLSY79 is a nationally representative sample of young men and women who were 14 to 21 years old in 1979. Thus, the teenage years of women in our study (ages 13 to 19) occurred between 1970 and 1985. Respondents have been interviewed each year since 1979; we use data through the 1993 interview in our analysis. The female respondents were asked about their pregnancy and childbearing, marital arrangements, and educational and labor force activities.

We use two samples from the NLSY79. To describe the general characteristics of young women growing up during the 1980s, we focus on the sample of women that includes a subsample drawn to be representative of the U.S. population of women age 14 to 21 as of 1979. This sample consists of 2,477 non-Hispanic white women, as well as 1,472 women in two supplemental subsamples of black women and 977 Hispanic women, for a total sample of 4,926 women.[1] We refer to this sample as our *All Women's Sample.*

We focus much of our regression analysis described below on the subset of women in the All Women's Sample who reported that they experienced their first *pregnancy* as a teenager. We refer to that subset as our *Teen Pregnancy Sample.* We describe this second sample in detail later in the chapter.

Estimates of Teen Childbearing and Its Apparent Consequences

In the All Women's Sample, 6.6 percent of white women, 21.6 percent of black women, and 13.3 percent of Hispanic women reported having their first birth before reaching the age of 18. (As elsewhere in the book, we define teen childbearing as births that women have at ages younger than 18.) In terms of the U.S. population as a whole, 9.2 percent of women who were teenagers during the 1970s and early 1980s had their first birth as teens. Using our data from the NLSY79, we briefly compare the attainment of teen mothers with women who did not experience a birth before age 18.

The differences in the childbearing and marital experiences as of age 30 between teen mothers and women who postponed their childbearing indicate that teen mothers bear 1.3 more children on average than do women who delay (figure 3.1). They also spend five times more time between ages 14 and 30 as single mothers than women who delay.

The educational attainment of teen mothers also differs substantially from that of young women who delay (figure 3.2). Only 32 percent of teen mothers have graduated from high school—that is, have received a regular high school diploma—by age 30, compared with over 84 percent of women who delay motherhood. This figure is not surprising; the presence of a young child makes it very difficult for teen mothers to continue their educations. Many of these mothers ultimately attain a high school degree by obtaining a general educational development (GED) certificate. Some 26 percent of teen mothers complete high school via this route. As we discuss below, there is a good deal of controversy about whether the GED is "equivalent" to a regular high school diploma, especially regarding an individual's ability to compete for jobs and wages in the labor market. However, regardless of the method of completing high school, only 59 percent of teen mothers attain a high school diploma or GED certificate by the time they reach age 30. In contrast, 90 percent of women who do not give birth as teens end up obtaining high school diplomas or GEDs by the same age.

Figure 3.1. Childbearing and Single Motherhood Experiences by Age 30 for Teen Mothers and Women Who Delayed Their Childbearing

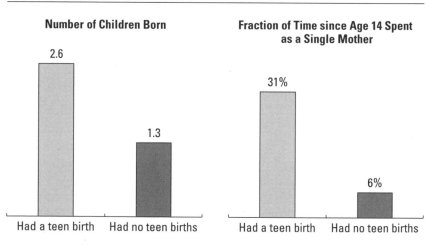

Source: National Longitudinal Survey of Youth, All Women's Sample.

Figure 3.2. Educational Attainment by Age 30 for Teen Mothers and Women Who Delayed Their Childbearing

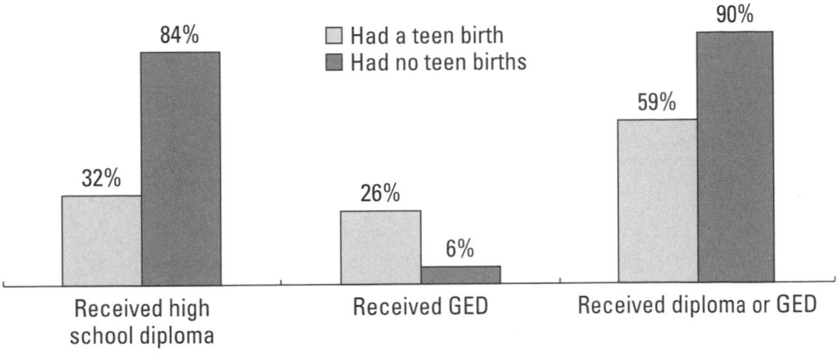

Source: National Longitudinal Survey of Youth, All Women's Sample.

Given their lower educational attainment, it is not surprising that teen mothers are less successful in the labor market than women who do not become mothers at such a young age (figure 3.3). Not only do teen mothers earn less, on average, at almost every age, but also the gap between them and women who delay grows with age. By age 30, for example, the annual earnings of teen mothers are only 57 percent of the earnings of those who delay childbearing ($11,716 versus $20,602 in 2004 dollars). Part of this gap can be accounted for by the greater number of hours women who delay childbearing work compared with teen mothers (1,419 versus 1,200 a year at age 30, not shown) as well as the substantially lower wage rates of teen mothers.

Finally, consistent with other estimates, we find that teen mothers receive substantially higher levels of public assistance than do women who delay their childbearing (figure 3.4). By age 30, teen mothers receive over four times more in public assistance benefits than do women who delay ($2,680 versus $617).

Teen Mothers and Those Observed to Delay Childbearing: An Inappropriate Comparison?

As the evidence makes clear, the *gross*, or *unadjusted*, disparities in socio-economic attainment of teen mothers and those who delay childbearing are substantial, making an apparently strong case that teen mothers impose

Figure 3.3. Annual Labor Market Earnings of Teen Mothers and Women Who Delayed Their Childbearing

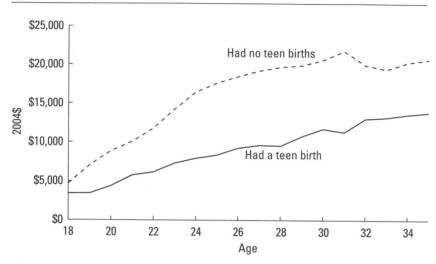

Source: National Longitudinal Survey of Youth, All Women's Sample.

Figure 3.4. Annual AFDC and Food Stamp Benefits of Teen Mothers and Women Who Delayed Their Childbearing

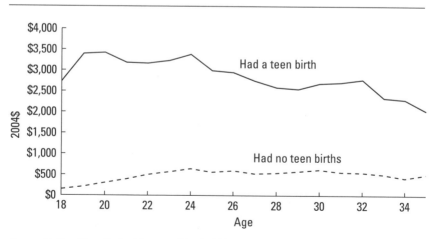

Source: National Longitudinal Survey of Youth, All Women's Sample.

substantial costs on U.S. taxpayers. It is tempting to conclude from these findings that if society could convince teen mothers to delay motherhood until they were older, they would substantially improve their material well-being and, as a result, reduce their burden on society. But does such a conclusion follow? Can we conclude that failure to delay childbearing causes these disparities?

The assertion that adolescent childbearing *causes* the poor socioeconomic outcomes presented above implies that a teen mother was on the same upwardly mobile life course as her counterpart who did not have a child as a teenager but, *by having her first birth as a teenager,* altered the remainder of her life detrimentally. For these two groups of women to be *comparable,* teen mothers and the women with whom they are being compared would have to have virtually identical socioeconomic and background characteristics before the age at which teen mothers had their first child. In fact, this is not the case.

Teen mothers come from much more disadvantaged backgrounds than do women who delay childbearing (table 3.1). Teen mothers grew

Table 3.1. Background Characteristics of Teen Mothers and Women Who Delayed Childbearing until after Age 18

Characteristic	Teen Mothers Mean	Teen Mothers Standard deviation	Not Teen Mothers Mean	Not Teen Mothers Standard deviation
Race/ethnicity (%)				
White	58	49	82	39
Black	33	47	12	33
Hispanic	9	29	6	24
Family on welfare in 1978 (%)	19	39	11	31
Family income in 1978 (2004$)	$38,916	$28,553	$64,646	$40,586
In female-headed household at age 14 (%)	20	40	12	32
In intact household at age 14 (%)	69	46	84	37
Mother's education (years)	9.88	2.86	11.67	2.76
Father's education (years)	9.94	3.37	11.91	3.56
Armed Forces Qualifying Test score	25.81	21.39	49.58	27.49

Source: 1979 National Longitudinal Survey of Youth, All Women's Sample, 1979–93.

up in poorer homes (the average annual income of the households in which women who had had teen births resided in 1978 was $38,916 in 2004 dollars versus $64,646 for their counterparts) and with less-educated parents (the fathers of women who later became teen mothers completed an average of only 9.94 years of school versus 11.91 years of schooling for the fathers of other women) than women who delay childbearing. Teen mothers were also more likely to grow up in single-parent families (20 percent versus 12 percent) and more likely to have been in families on welfare when growing up (19 percent versus 11 percent) than women who did not have a child as a teen.

One can, in principle, "adjust" for these differences in background characteristics by using statistical techniques, such as regression analysis. One then compares the adjusted estimates of socioeconomic attainment to estimate the causal effects of early childbearing. At issue is the adequacy of these adjustments for dealing with *selection bias*, namely, the possibility that selective unobserved differences remain between women who have children as teenagers and those who do not. The potential for such bias clouds the internal and external validity of many nonexperimental methods for estimating the causal effect of early childbearing.

One concern often raised when estimating the socioeconomic attainment of young women is the importance of heterogeneity in their cognitive abilities and in market-related skills not captured by educational attainment. While most data sources do not have measures of such attainment for respondents, one is available in the NLSY79—the Armed Forces Qualifying Test (AFQT). This aptitude test, which was administered in 1981 to all respondents of the NLSY79, has been a good predictor not only of the likelihood that enlistees will be successful in the military but also of initial success in the civilian labor force. The average AFQT score of teen mothers, 25.81, is almost one standard deviation below the average score of women who were not teen mothers (49.58), providing further evidence that the two groups were not comparable at the outset (see also table 3.1). While the AFQT scores enable us to control for achievement, there are likely a host of other dimensions along which teen mothers may differ from women who delay their childbearing and which are likely to affect their socioeconomic attainment, most of which are not measured in datasets like the NLSY79.[2]

Thus, one must find alternative strategies for isolating the causal effects of early childbearing on the socioeconomic attainment of teen mothers.

Exploiting a Natural Experiment

The most common strategy used in scientific evaluations of causal effects is experiments in which treatments, including a treatment that represents the status quo, are randomly assigned to a sample of subjects and their subsequent behavior monitored. When properly conducted, such experiments ensure that, on average, the group receiving the treatment of interest and the group representing the status quo are the same in all ways except for their treatment status and that the differences in average outcomes for these two groups directly measure the average effect of the treatment under consideration.

While the postponement of births cannot be investigated with controlled randomized experiments, nature provides the opportunity to conduct a very similar investigation. Many pregnancies end in spontaneous abortions, or miscarriages, which evidence from epidemiological studies of miscarriages indicates are mostly random events.[3] If so, women who miscarry as teenagers constitute an almost random sample of women who become pregnant as teenagers but are precluded from having a child at that age. While women who experience random miscarriages may be an appropriate comparison group for women who are *at risk* to have a birth, they do not constitute the appropriate comparison group for women who actually have births. This is because pregnant women can elect to have an induced abortion rather than have a birth. Further, researchers strongly suspect that women who have induced abortions are *not* a random sample of pregnant women.[4]

Under certain conditions, however, one can use an adjusted difference in average outcomes of *pregnant women who do not experience a miscarriage* and *those who do*—where the adjustment consists of weighting this difference by the proportion of nonmiscarrying women who have births—to obtain unbiased estimates of the effect of the failure of a teen mother to delay motherhood.[5] The conditions required for the validity of this method are that (a) all miscarriages are random events, (b) all women truthfully report whether they experienced a pregnancy and the way it was resolved, and (c) there is no additional "effect" of having an induced abortion beyond not experiencing a birth. Each of these conditions is potentially violated in practice. Some miscarriages appear to be induced by the excessive use of alcohol or tobacco by pregnant women. There is clear evidence that abortions—especially among young women—are underreported and that abortions can, in and of themselves, be life changing. However, relaxing each assumption (by forming conservative upper and lower bounds on the effects of adolescent childbearing for a number of the socioeconomic outcomes of mothers considered here) does not change the central conclusions drawn about the effects of adolescent childbearing based on the adjusted differences-in-means outcomes for teen women who experience miscarriages and those who do not (Hotz et al. 1997).

Thus, under the above conditions, the natural experiment of using data on teenagers who experience miscarriages allows us to address the following causal question concerning teen childbearing: "If, in the socioeconomic environment currently facing them, women who gave birth as teens had delayed their childbearing, how would their subsequent outcomes have been different?" Obtaining reliable answers to this question is central to the social and policy debates over adolescent childbearing in the United States. For example, one important issue, and a central focus of this volume, is the costs to government associated with teen childbearing. Previous analyses of this question have estimated how much government spends in welfare, food stamps, and other public assistance on women who began motherhood as teenagers (Burt and Haffner 1986; Burt 1992). While an important baseline, such costs do not necessarily represent the costs to government that are directly attributable to early childbearing (or the failure of these women to delay motherhood). By obtaining reliable estimates of the question of causality posed above for outcomes such as receipt of public assistance benefits, we can draw conclusions about what the government might save if teen mothers were all to delay their childbearing until they were older.[6]

Estimation Methods and Sample Used

The estimates of the effects of teen childbearing presented below are produced with a modified version of the design involving data on women whose first births end in a miscarriage. In particular, we use a variant of regression analysis, called the *method of instrumental variables*,[7] which further adjusts the differences in outcomes for women who do and do not experience miscarriages as teens for differences in personal and background characteristics of these women. Means and standard deviations of these characteristics are presented in table 3.2 for the Teen Pregnancy sample.[8]

In the instrumental variable regression analysis, we estimated the effects for each year of the woman's life from 18 to 35 to determine the timing and duration of the effects.

Table 3.2. Background Characteristics of Women Whose First Pregnancy Occurred before Age 18 (percent, except where noted)

Characteristic	Mean	Standard deviation
Race/ethnicity		
White	65	48
Black	27	44
Hispanic	8	28
Family on welfare in 1978	16	37
Family income in 1978 (2004$)	$47,863	$35,946
Missing family income	54	50
In female-headed household at age 14	18	38
In intact household at age 14	72	45
Mother's education (years)	10.41	2.74
Missing mother's education	9	28
Father's education (years)	10.47	3.33
Missing father's education	20	40
Armed Forces Qualifying Test score (points)	31.55	23.65
How first pregnancy ended		
In a miscarriage	7	
In a birth	75	
In an abortion	18	
Number of women	1,042	

Source: 1979 National Longitudinal Survey of Youth, Teen Pregnancy Sample, 1979–93.

Before reporting our findings, we call attention to how women in our Teen Pregnancy sample resolved their first pregnancies (see also table 3.2). While most of these pregnancies resulted in a live birth, 25 percent did not. Induced abortion, the most prevalent way in which childbearing is avoided, accounted for 18 percent of these pregnancies, while 7 percent are reported to have ended in miscarriages. According to our data (not shown), the median age at first birth among women whose first teen pregnancy results in a live birth is about age 17 while the median age at first birth among women whose first teen pregnancy ended in a miscarriage is about age 20. Looking at the average (rather than the median) age at first birth, we find that women who would have had a teen birth had they not miscarried actually had their first birth some time after their 21st birthday. On average, a miscarriage delayed a first birth for these women for at least three to four years.[9]

Therefore, our estimates of the effects of adolescent childbearing can be reliably used to infer what the levels of socioeconomic attainment would be for teen mothers if they were to delay their childbearing for at least three to four years, a length of time consistent with a realistic goal for policy interventions that might cause at-risk teenage women to postpone entry into motherhood. This delay is similar to that used for estimates elsewhere in this book.

It is important to note that the statistics on pregnancy resolutions and the incidence of pregnancies in the NLSY79 data are based on self-reports. Abortions, miscarriages, and pregnancies are likely significantly under-reported in these data. Abortions among young women, in particular, appear to be substantially underreported (Jones and Forrest 1990). Further, epidemiological clinical-based studies of spontaneous abortions (miscarriages) find that between 11 and 14 percent of pregnancies end in miscarriages (Kline et al. 1989). We explicitly investigated the implications of such underreporting for our estimates of the effects of early childbearing on the socioeconomic attainment of teen mothers, using more reliable data sources on the incidence of abortions and births to supplement our analysis of the NLSY79 data (Hotz et al. 1997). Our findings and inferences about these causal effects do not change when we account for this source of bias in the data used in our instrumental variable regression analysis.

Estimated Effects of Delaying Childbearing on Adult Outcomes among Teen Mothers

This section discusses our estimated effects of early childbearing, or, put differently, the likely effects of delaying childbearing for three to four years on a range of socioeconomic outcomes for teenage mothers.[10] Coefficient estimates and levels of statistical significance from our instrumental variable regressions are displayed in appendix table A.3.1.[11] These regression models allow the effect of teen mothers delaying their childbearing to older ages to vary over the life cycle as a polynomial function of age. We used these coefficient estimates to produce more readily interpretable estimates of what the average outcomes of teen mothers would be at various ages *if these mothers had delayed their childbearing at least three to four years.* Estimates of the age-specific effects, their corresponding levels of statistical significance, and average effects over ages 18–30 and

18–35 are presented in table A.3.2.[12] The age-specific estimated effects are formed by taking the derivative of the coefficients for the regression functions reported in table A.3.1 about the teen birth indicator variable and its interactions and then evaluating these derivatives at each age.

At the outset, several general comments are in order. It is important to distinguish between two types of effects of early childbearing on a teen mother's subsequent socioeconomic status: permanent effects and those that represent temporary substitution of behaviors over the life course. In some respects, early childbearing permanently affects mothers. For example, early childbearing permanently increases the total number of children a woman will bear and the proportion of her lifetime she will spend as a single mother. In contrast, most of, if not all, the effects of early childbearing appear to reflect differences in the *timing* of events and activities over the mother's life cycle. For example, although teen mothers have lower labor-market earnings in their late teens and early 20s than what they would have earned had they postponed their childbearing, they earn more money in their late 20s and their 30s than if they had delayed childbearing. In such cases, the ultimate effect and costs of early childbearing for the mother, or for the government, may be negligible when tallied over a mother's lifetime.

We also caution the reader about interpreting our estimated effects on outcomes measured at older ages. For most outcomes, we simply do not have much data for the older ages. The oldest women in our sample are 35 as of the 1993 interview of the NLSY79, the last wave of data from which we constructed our analysis samples. Thus, we cannot be as confident in the estimates derived for outcomes measured after women reach their early to mid-30s. One important exception to this statement is the result for birth rate patterns. We can reasonably assume that a negligible percentage of the women will bear children beyond the age of 35.[13] Thus, we believe that our estimates accurately reflect the consequences of early childbearing on the subsequent number of children a teen mother will eventually bear.

Childbearing, Marriage, and Financial Resources from Spouses

Consider first the effects of adolescent childbearing on the number of children teen mothers bear by age 30. While gross differences shown earlier in fertility between teen mothers and women who did not bear children as teens indicate that the former group of women had 1.3 more children than the latter, most of this disparity cannot be attributed to early childbearing. In fact, we estimate that only 23 percent of these differences can be attributed to the failure of teen mothers to delay childbearing. Once we account for the selective differences in the background and personal characteristics of teen mothers, we find that, by age 30, teen mothers would be expected to have one-third of a child less, on average, than if they had delayed their childbearing for at least three to four years (first two bars in figure 3.5). This difference implies that teen mothers have 13 percent more children by age 30 that they will have to support; this difference is not statistically significantly different from zero at conventional levels of significance.[14]

Once we account for selection between teen mothers and women who do not have children as teens, we also find that the failure to delay childbearing does not have a lasting effect on a teen mother's marriage prospects. While teen mothers would spend significantly less of their early years of motherhood (ages 18 through 23) as single mothers if they delayed childbearing, this effect grows smaller with age. By age 30, the cumulative time since age 14 spent as a single mother would only be 2 percentage points

Figure 3.5. Childbearing and Single Motherhood Experiences by Age 30 for Teen Mothers versus What Would Happen If Their Childbearing Were Delayed

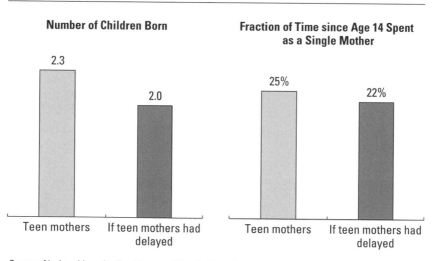

Source: National Longitudinal Survey of Youth, Teen Pregnancy Sample.

lower if the mother delayed her childbearing; this difference is not statistically significant.

Early childbearing also does not significantly reduce the amount of income available from husbands.[15] In fact, we find that through their mid-30s, teen mothers are likely to have significantly *higher* levels of income from husbands than if they had delayed childbearing (figure 3.6).[16] At age 30, the typical woman who was a teen mother can expect $15,784 a year in income (in 2004 dollars) provided by a spouse; if this same woman had delayed her childbearing, spousal income would *decline* to less than half that amount ($7,690). This difference is statistically significant. Thus, while the level of income that the typical teen mother can expect from her spouse is low at almost any stage of her early adulthood, her prospects for having this financial support for her and her children do not improve if she delays her childbearing by several years.

High School Completion

The difference between teen mothers and women who did not have births as teens also overstates the consequences of early childbearing on high

Figure 3.6. Annual Spousal Income Received by Teen Mothers versus What Would Happen If Their Childbearing Were Delayed

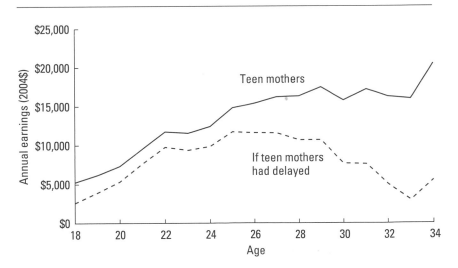

Source: National Longitudinal Survey of Youth, Teen Pregnancy Sample.

school completion. In particular, after accounting for selection, delaying childbearing among teen mothers would only reduce the likelihood of obtaining a standard high school degree by 10 percentage points (46 versus 56 percent, as shown in figure 3.7); this difference is not statistically significant.[17] For the likelihood of receiving a GED, the gross difference recorded in figure 3.2 also overstates the causal impact of teen childbearing, although less so than for obtaining a high school diploma. Teen mothers still are more likely to receive a GED (by 14 percentage points) than women who delay childbearing, regardless of how one forms the comparison group. Finally, there is no significant causal effect of early childbearing on the probability that teen mothers obtain a high school–level education, if high school diplomas and GEDs are taken as equivalent.

At issue are differences in the returns to these two forms of high school completion for these women. For men, the value of the GED in the labor market is minimal; its recipients earn no more than high school dropouts (Cameron and Heckman 1993). However, the labor-market returns to the GED are not different from those of a high school diploma for the typical woman (Cao, Stromsdorfer, and Weeks 1996). What remains undetermined is whether this equivalence in labor-market returns holds for

Figure 3.7. Educational Attainment by Age 30 for Teen Mothers versus What Would Happen If Their Childbearing Were Delayed

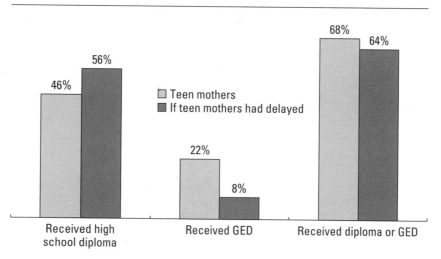

Source: National Longitudinal Survey of Youth, Teen Pregnancy Sample.

women who become teen mothers as well as for all women. We do not address this issue directly. But our findings for the effects of early childbearing on the labor-market outcomes of teen mothers, to which we now turn, are consistent with the equivalence of GED and high school graduation effects found in recent analysis for women generally.

Hours Worked and Earnings

Our natural experiment provides little evidence that early childbearing adversely affects the labor market activity of teen mothers as the unadjusted comparison suggests, although the timing of this activity varies substantially. At early ages (18 and 19), teen mothers supply fewer hours to the labor market than if they were to delay their childbearing; these differences are not statistically significant. By age 30, teen mothers are estimated to work 23 percent more hours (1,248 versus 957 hours) than if they had delayed their childbearing (figure 3.8), although the latter differential also is not statistically significant.

Studies of women's labor supply patterns typically show that women work less when their children are very young and more when the children

Figure 3.8. Annual Hours of Work for Teen Mothers versus What Would Happen If Their Childbearing Were Delayed

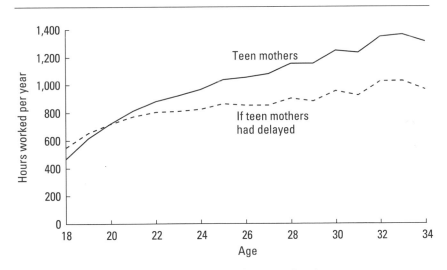

Source: National Longitudinal Survey of Youth, Teen Pregnancy Sample.

get older. Consequently, the effects we find of the failure to delay early childbearing on hours worked (and labor force participation) estimated from our natural experiment appear more consistent with life-cycle and transitory differences in the timing of childbearing between teen mothers and women who had miscarriages than with persistent lifetime, let alone negative, causal effects of teenage childbearing. While the statistical power associated with these estimates remains an issue, there is little evidence of long-term negative effects of teenage childbearing on hours worked.

Finally, the natural experiment we use for identifying the causal effect of teen mothers not delaying their childbearing indicates that the earnings of the latter are *higher at every age* from 20 on than if these women delayed their childbearing. Further, the positive effects of teen childbearing on earnings are statistically significant at the .10 or lower level from ages 25 through 30 (figure 3.9). For example, at age 30 teen mothers earn, on average, $12,816 a year in 2004 dollars; we estimate that their earnings would be 48 percent lower, or $8,640 a year, if they had delayed their childbearing.[18]

Two comments are in order about our findings on the labor market consequences of teen motherhood. First, the findings are extremely robust.

Figure 3.9. Annual Labor Market Earnings for Teen Mothers versus What Would Happen If Their Childbearing Were Delayed

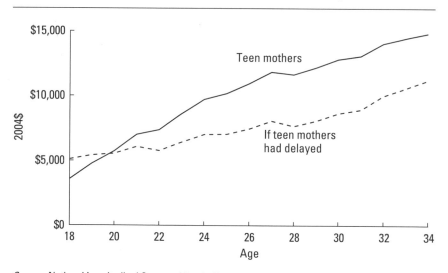

Source: National Longitudinal Survey of Youth, Teen Pregnancy Sample.

Even if we violate each condition required for our natural experiment to be valid—that miscarriages are random, that all women report truthfully, and that there is no additional "effect" of having an induced abortion other than lack of a birth—we still cannot reject that teen mothers earn *more* from their mid-20s through mid-30s than if they had delayed their births (Hotz et al. 1997). Further, our method is sufficiently powerful, in a statistical sense, to *reject* that these are *negative* at these same ages.

Second, while a definitive explanation of why teen mothers appear to benefit in the labor market from not delaying their childbearing awaits further research, we offer the following possibility. Our evidence, and that of others, documents that women who begin motherhood as teens come from less-advantaged backgrounds, are less likely to be successful in school, and, as such, are less likely to end up in occupations that require higher education than are women who postpone motherhood. Further, our evidence suggests that these women are more likely to acquire the skills on the job (rather than in school) and to work in jobs where educational credentials are less important than continuity and job-specific experience. For such women, concentrating their childbearing at early ages may prove more compatible with their likely labor-market career options than would postponing motherhood and/or spacing births more widely over their childbearing years. If this characterization is accurate, forcing teen mothers to postpone their childbearing, as miscarriages do, may "explain" why they both appear to acquire no more formal education and end up doing less well in the labor market than if they had been able to follow their preferred life-cycle plan.

Receipt of Public Assistance

As with labor-market outcomes, we find little evidence that early childbearing itself accounts for the heavy dependence of teen mothers on various forms of public assistance. Early childbearers and women who delay childbearing follow a similar trend through age 25: both groups receive increasing amounts in Aid to Families with Dependent Children (AFDC) and food stamps benefits (figure 3.10). Until age 25, teen mothers receive higher levels of such assistance on average than if they had delayed their childbearing, although this difference declines with age.[19] But, after age 25, the amounts of AFDC and food stamp benefits teen mothers receive declines, while if these mothers had delayed their childbearing, their benefits would have continued to increase slightly through age 34, although

Figure 3.10. Annual AFDC and Food Stamp Benefits for Teen Mothers versus What Would Happen If Their Childbearing Were Delayed

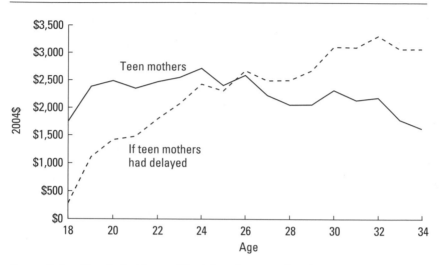

Source: National Longitudinal Survey of Youth, Teen Pregnancy Sample.

the latter differences are not statistically significant. Again, these age patterns and differentials in public assistance for teen mothers and what would have happened if they had delayed childbearing appear to reflect transitory, life-cycle effects of childbearing and rearing—that is, the receipt of public assistance benefits increases immediately after a birth but declines rather rapidly as the child ages—rather than a more persistent dependence on public assistance of teen mothers suggested by the unadjusted life-cycle patterns recorded in figure 3.4.

Are We Right? Evidence from Other Studies

No single piece of scientific evidence should be taken as proof of any proposition, whether or not the evidence is contrary to conventional wisdom. Although we are alone in approximating a controlled experiment to reduce the intrusion of selection bias, many researchers have recognized the importance of the selection bias issue in estimating the consequences of adolescent childbearing and have used various approaches to limit it.[20]

We cite three studies. Geronimus and Korenman (1992, 1993) based their studies on pairs of sisters who were raised in the same family (and therefore assumed to be of very similar background) but who differed in timing of childbearing, one sister of each pair having given birth as a teenager and the other having had her first child in adulthood.[21] The average difference in the outcomes of sisters was interpreted as the effect of adolescent childbearing. Grogger and Bronars (1993) and Bronars and Grogger (1995) compared the outcomes of women who gave birth to twins as teen and unwed mothers with those who bore single children. Because the occurrence of twins is thought to be random, the differences in the adult outcomes of the two groups of teen mothers measure the effects of adolescent childbearing (under the presumption that the effect of an extra child is the same as the effect of a first child). Ribar (1999) used statistical assumptions to reduce the mean outcomes of women who did not give birth as teenagers to what they would likely have been if these women had the same backgrounds as teen mothers. If his statistical assumptions are correct, the difference between the adult outcomes of teen mothers and his adjusted group of mothers who did not have a first birth as a teenager measures the effect of teen childbearing.

All three studies come to the same conclusion: the failure to account for selection bias vastly *overstates* the negative consequences of adolescent childbearing and certainly provides no support for the view that adolescent childbearing has large, negative consequences for the socioeconomic attainment of teen mothers. What remains uncertain is whether the effects of teen childbearing on such outcomes as labor-market attachment and earnings are slightly negative as in Bronars and Grogger (1995), negligible as in Ribar (1999), or positive as in Geronimus and Korenman (1992, 1993) and this study.[22]

Conclusion

These rather startling findings question the view that teen childbearing is one of the nation's most serious social problems, at least when one measures its severity in likely costs to taxpayers. More generally, our analysis of the costs and consequences of adolescent childbearing highlights the potential for drawing very misleading conclusions if one fails to use adequate evaluation designs when making causal inferences about the effects of selective phenomena. At the same time, we caution the reader not to overgeneralize from what we have found. As we noted at the beginning, we have considered only a few potential consequences and costs of adolescent childbearing. Further, standards of scientific inquiry dictate that further replications and scrutiny of our findings are required before one can confidently draw strong conclusions about the causal influence of teen childbearing.

We also caution against concluding from these findings that appropriately formulated public policies could not benefit young women at risk of becoming teen mothers. According to our results, programs narrowly targeted at reducing teen childbearing without addressing the social disadvantage of at-risk girls are likely to have limited success. How broader policies that raise the lifetime prospects of at-risk young women might jointly benefit them as they become adults and might incidentally reduce teen motherhood is not understood. But we believe that policies broader than those just to reduce teen childbearing stand a better chance of success, even though they are likely to be more costly.

Updated Estimates of the Consequences of Teen Childbearing for Mothers

Saul D. Hoffman

"The Impacts of Teenage Childbearing on the Mothers and the Consequences of Those Impacts for Government" by Hotz, McElroy, and Sanders (chapter 3 in *Kids Having Kids*, 1st edition) and its follow-up, chapter 3 in this volume, are very ambitious efforts to examine the causal effect of a teen birth on a wide range of socioeconomic outcomes for the mothers. The original contribution was widely recognized for its highly innovative methodology. Its findings were dramatic and controversial. It concluded, as does the revised chapter, that teen childbearing, properly analyzed, was actually beneficial to the young women who became teen mothers over diverse socioeconomic outcomes. Hotz, McElroy, and Sanders (hereafter HMS) found that young women who had an early teen birth worked more, earned more, received more income from a spouse, and received less support from welfare through their mid-30s than if they had delayed their childbearing until their early 20s.

The key to these findings was a research methodology that compared teen mothers with young women who had an early teen pregnancy that ended in a miscarriage. Since a miscarriage is usually a random event that results in a delay of age at first birth, a comparison of outcomes for teens whose first pregnancy ended in a birth with outcomes for teens whose first pregnancy ended in a miscarriage ought to provide an unbiased estimate of the causal impact of a teen birth relative to a birth at an older age. HMS described the teen birth versus miscarriage approach as a natural experiment, a research methodology that mimics a random assignment methodology and which can thereby yield more accurate estimates of causal effects. They concluded that a teen birth itself was not the source of the difficulties of the young women who became teen mothers.

In this part of chapter 3, I reanalyze the impacts of a teen birth on outcomes for the mother using the same data source as HMS and the same natural experiment research approach. This section is both an update through 2000, when all the women are at least 35 years old, and a fresh replication of a complex data analysis project. When I examine data for the same period as HMS, my findings are roughly consistent with theirs, although typically not as positive.[23] Using data through 1993 only, both HMS and I find evidence that teen childbearing generally is not an important contributor to the poor outcomes of these young women and seems to offer benefits in some areas. The one exception is postsecondary schooling, on which a teen birth has a substantial negative impact. Importantly, these conclusions are based most heavily on the women in the sample who entered their teens in the early 1970s, as only these mothers had reached their early 30s by 1993.

With the addition of the longer-term follow-up data for the younger sample members who entered their teens in the mid- to late 1970s, I find weaker positive effects than HMS and some stronger negative effects. I also examine earlier and later cohorts of teen mothers separately in order to reconcile the differences in the findings between the two samples, since the later cohorts are less fully represented in the sample analyzed by HMS. Across the range of outcomes examined, the effects of an early teen birth differ for the earlier and later cohorts of teen mothers. The positive or benign effects found by HMS hold only for the older cohorts, while the effects are far more negative for the younger cohorts.

Background and Methodological Issues

Determining the causal impact of a teen birth on adult outcomes is a daunting task, because it is inevitably impossible to measure and control for all risk factors that contribute to the outcomes of interest, especially subtle individual, family, and neighborhood characteristics that are difficult to obtain in national surveys. But it is, as the first edition of *Kids Having Kids* emphasized, a critical task: effective policy intervention must be based on causal impacts, not correlations. Young women who become teen mothers often have multiple risk factors that contribute to their life outcomes. If society wishes to design effective policies to improve these outcomes, we need to understand which risk factors are truly causal.

Basic statistical analysis tells us that if important risk factors are omitted from the analysis of outcomes for young women and if these omitted factors correlate with both the probability of a teen birth and the outcome of interest (earnings, education, etc.), then the resulting estimates do not reflect the true causal impact of a teen birth but are biased. The bias is the product of two terms, one measuring the impact of the omitted variable on the outcome of interest and the other measuring the correlation between the omitted variable and a teen birth.[24] In effect, the included variable (a teen birth) captures the correlated portion of the impact of the omitted variable. In the most likely case, estimated effects will be too large, which is precisely the point that critics of the early teen birth effects literature made.

Earlier attempts in this research literature to solve the omitted variable problem include using fuller sets of independent variables, sibling models that implicitly control for common family and neighborhood effects (Geronimus and Korenman 1992; Hoffman, Foster, and Furstenberg 1993), and a natural experiment involving twin births (Grogger and Bronars 1993). While the results vary somewhat across these studies, in general they find that teen birth effects are not as negative as in the earlier research literature but are still sufficiently large to warrant serious concern.

HMS proposed a natural experiment comparing young teen mothers with young women who became pregnant by the same age but suffered miscarriages. Since most miscarriages are, they argue, random, this approach should yield an unbiased estimate of the consequences of teen childbearing. The subsequent differences in outcomes between the two groups of women with an early pregnancy thus ought to provide an unbiased estimate of the causal effects of a teen birth.

The HMS model includes both a constant term for an early teen birth and interaction terms between a birth and a woman's age and age-squared to allow for life-cycle patterns. This is a second major methodological contribution of the HMS chapter. Previous studies typically examined impacts as of a fixed calendar year or as of a fixed age. As a result, little was known about life-cycle impacts of a teen birth, including, for example, whether teen mothers rebounded from initial disadvantages as they aged into their late 20s and mid-30s.

In practice, some complications to the miscarriage methodological design exist.[25] As HMS note, the ideal comparison group for the natural experiment is women who would have chosen to have a birth but were randomly prevented from doing so by virtue of a miscarriage. However, some women who have a miscarriage would actually have chosen to have an abortion if a miscarriage had not intervened. These women cannot be identified in the data. Thus, HMS do not quite proceed as if this were a natural experiment. Instead, they estimate an instrumental variables model, using a teen miscarriage as an instrument for a teen birth. To be a valid instrument for a teen birth, a teen miscarriage must satisfy two basic statistical requirements: it must be correlated with a teen birth and it must be uncorrelated with the outcomes of interest, conditional on the other independent variables. The former condition is clearly satisfied; the latter is plausible, but might not be valid, if, for example, a miscarriage had an independent effect on outcomes.

Data and Methods

As far as possible, I follow the research approach of HMS. Data are taken from the NLSY79 for years from 1979 to 2000 corresponding to ages 18 to 36 for the women. Like HMS, I exclude cases from the military sample and the poor white supplementary sample. I define a teen pregnancy as one that began at age 17 or earlier. The full analysis sample includes 1,013 women who had a teen pregnancy and had sufficient information in at least one year to determine the age at the beginning of the pregnancy and the outcome of the pregnancy. See the data appendix for a brief summary of the methods used to code fertility outcomes. Of these women with an early teen pregnancy, 762 had a birth, 182 had an abortion, and 69 had a miscarriage. The full person-year sample (ages 18 to 36, observed between 1978 and 2000) includes a maximum of 16,048 observations. Missing data on independent variables reduce this to 15,377. The number of available cases for particular dependent variables is typically smaller than this.[26]

Following HMS, I include as independent variables dummy variables for year of birth, race/ethnicity (whether black and whether Hispanic), family structure at age 14 (two dummy variables), parents' education, and two measures of family income (actual income and whether the family received any income from welfare, both measured as of 1978).[27] All models are estimated by two-stage least squares with a teen miscarriage used as an instrument for a teen birth, along with the corresponding age-teen birth interactions. Sample weights are used in all analyses. Incomes are reported in 2004 dollars. In these analyses, I have not adjusted standard errors for the fact that an individual may be represented many times (up to 18 years) in the data. Corrected standard errors would undoubtedly be larger. As a result, discussions of statistical significance should be interpreted conservatively.

The most significant underlying difference between my data and that used by HMS is the age range of the teen mothers included in our samples. Both analyses use data on women from the NLSY79, which includes women who were age 14–21 in 1979. The HMS sample runs from 1979 through 1993, when the maximum age of the women ranges from 28 to 35. Because of this, far fewer women are observed at older ages—only about 200 at age 35 compared with about 1,000 at ages 21 through 28. In addition, the women who are observed at older ages are exclusively from the earlier birth cohorts of the NLSY79.[28] In a closely related paper, HMS note this feature of their data and the possible effect of the smaller sample size at older ages for the reliability of their estimates of life-cycle effects (Hotz, McElroy, and Sanders 2005, footnote 25).

It is possible, however, that this sample composition issue is a more serious problem that could affect their estimates of the impact of a teen birth, especially the critical estimates of its life-cycle effects. Recall that the key HMS result is that teen mothers often do relatively poorly initially but rebound by their late 20s or early 30s and end up doing better than if they had delayed their first birth. If all birth cohorts of NLSY79 teen mothers have (or will eventually have) the same average outcome at each age, conditional on the family background variables included in the analysis, then the fact that outcomes are not observed for some women will have no impact whatsoever on the estimated causal impact of a teen birth. Had these outcomes been observed, they would have replicated the average outcome at each age for the sample actually observed and thus would leave all estimates unaffected.[29] Similarly, if the life-cycle profiles by cohort differ in level but do not differ further by age, estimates of the impacts of teen childbearing will not be affected by the sample drop-off as long as indicators (dummy variables) for each cohort are included, as they are in HMS.

A potential problem arises, however, if the cohorts have different life-cycle profiles. For example, if outcomes at older ages for the earlier cohorts of young teen mothers (who are observed into their mid-30s) are better than those that will later be observed for the later cohorts (who are observed in the HMS data only until their late 20s), this could create a distorted life-cycle profile that incorrectly suggests rebound and recovery from the early birth. The same result could also occur if outcomes at the earliest ages, which are observed only for the later cohorts, were substantially worse than for the earlier cohorts.

The early teen births in the NLSY79 occurred as early as 1970 and as late as 1983, a period that spanned substantial changes in the landscape of teen fertility. The teen fertility rate fell 22 percent between 1970 and 1976 (from 68.3 births per 1,000 women age 15–19 in 1970 to 52.8 births per 1,000) and then remained essentially steady through 1983. The proportion of teen births that were nonmarital rose from 30 percent in 1970 to 44 percent by 1978 and 53 percent by 1983. Abortion was legalized in 1973, and the proportion of teen pregnancies ending in abortion increased from 23.7 percent in 1972 to 45 percent by 1980 (see chapter 2 for more details). Births to the later cohorts of teen mothers occurred during the more punitive welfare environment of the early 1980s. Thus, experiences may have been substantially different for these teen mothers, depending on the timing of their first birth.

In most of the analyses below, I present separate estimates for two different samples, one that corresponds to the sample years included in the HMS analysis and one that follows all the women through age 35. The 1979–93 sample includes 13,988 observations, about 9 percent fewer than the 1979–2000 sample. All the additional observations, however, are for the younger cohorts at older ages. The representation of the later birth cohorts increases by 13–23 percent (two or three additional years of data)[30] and the representation of women at age 31–35 increases by 45 percent.

Table 3.3 presents information on family background and individual characteristics for the samples I use. The figures shown are weighted estimates and, thus, reflect population characteristics, rather than those of the

Table 3.3. Background Characteristics and Fertility Outcomes, Teens Pregnant at Age 17 or Earlier (percent, except where noted)

Variable	Population mean
Family background	
Black	25.9
White	65.5
Hispanic	8.6
In intact family at age 14	18.3
In female-headed family at age 14	72.3
Mother's education (years)	10.5[a]
Father's education (years)	10.6[a]
Armed Forces Qualifying Test score (points)	31.7
Family income in 1978 (2004$)	$39,339
Family income missing	22.2
Family on welfare in 1978	18.7
Teen fertility outcome	
Birth	75.2
Miscarriage	6.8
Abortion	18.0
Sample size	
Persons	1,013
Person-years 1979–2000	15,377
Person-years 1979–93	13,988

Source: Author's calculations from 1979 National Longitudinal Survey of Youth (NLSY).

Note: All means weighted using adjusted NLSY weights.

a. Adjusted for missing data.

NLSY sample.[31] The sample means presented are very similar to those present by HMS in their table 3.2. About 25 percent of the sample is black, and 9 percent is Hispanic. Less than one-fifth were in families at age 14 that included both biological parents. Average family income in 1978, converted to 2004 dollars, was more than $39,000. Just under one-fifth reported receiving income from welfare in 1978. As seen at the bottom of the table, three-quarters of the women who were pregnant at age 17 or earlier had a birth, about 7 percent had a miscarriage, and 18 percent had an abortion. These percentages are also similar to those reported by HMS.

Results

My estimates of the impact of a teen birth are reported in appendix tables A.3.3 to A.3.8. Because the empirical model is complex and much of the interest is in the life-cycle effects of a teen birth, it is far more straightforward to represent the estimates using charts that emphasize age profiles. I do this by evaluating the teen birth effect either at a specific age (educational attainment) or over the observed portion of the life cycle, typically ages 18–34. The results shown are derived directly from the estimates in the appendix by evaluating the coefficient estimates on the relevant teen birth terms at the ages of interest.

Educational Attainment

Figure 3.11 presents the estimated impact of a teen birth on educational outcomes; see table A.3.3 for the corresponding coefficient estimates and standard errors. Like HMS, I examine high school completion and obtaining a GED. I also examine an outcome not considered in their study— whether the teen mother has at least two years of postsecondary schooling. High school completion has no life-cycle pattern; young women either do

Figure 3.11. Impact of a Teen Birth on Educational Attainment of Mothers

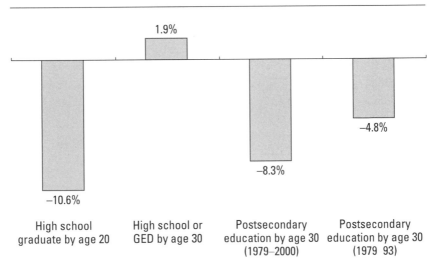

1.9%

−4.8%

−8.3%

−10.6%

| High school graduate by age 20 | High school or GED by age 30 | Postsecondary education by age 30 (1979–2000) | Postsecondary education by age 30 (1979 93) |

Source: National Longitudinal Survey of Youth, 1979–2000.

or do not complete a high school degree by age 19 or 20 at the latest. Thus, when I examine high school, I look at completion as of age 20. Because GED completion does have a life-cycle pattern, I allow for it by including an age interaction with a teen birth and by extending the age range. Life-cycle effects are minimal after age 28, which is the maximum age attained by the youngest women included in the HMS data. Thus, to simplify comparisons for this outcome, I focus just on my more restricted sample that corresponds to the one used by HMS. Finally, for postsecondary education, I present life-cycle estimates based both on the full and more limited sample to allow for effects of the younger cohorts into their mid-30s.

Both HMS and I find that a teen birth reduces the probability of completing high school by about 10 percentage points. They report a large and more than fully offsetting increase in the probability of obtaining a GED as a result of a teen birth, resulting in a 4 percentage point increase in the probability of either completing high school or obtaining a GED by age 30. I find a smaller positive effect. I find that teen mothers initially are less likely to have either a high school degree or a GED, but appear to catch up by their late 20s. By age 30, teen mothers are 1.9 percentage points more likely to have a high school degree or a GED than if they had delayed their first birth. The high school completion effect is just short of statistical significance at conventional levels, while the effect on high school or GED completion is statistically significant.

Also shown in the figure are two estimates for the impact of a teen birth on the probability of completing at least two years of postsecondary schooling by age 30.[32] Using the full sample, I find a substantial negative impact, ranging from about 7 percentage points when the women are in their early to mid-20s to 8 or 9 percentage points when they are in their early 30s. The average impact for this sample is 7.7 percentage points, a statistically significant impact. With the restricted age sample, the estimated effect is still negative, but it is about half as large and shows a strong life-cycle rebound effect not present in the full sample. These findings suggest first, that a high school degree and GED completion may not be substitutes as far as preparation for postsecondary schooling is concerned and, second, that the difference in the sample composition may be important.

Earnings

The estimated impact of an early teen birth on the mother's own earnings is shown in figure 3.12. The figure shows estimates for the full sample, for

Figure 3.12. Life-Cycle Impact of a Teen Birth on Mother's Average Annual Labor Market Earnings by Sample Years Included

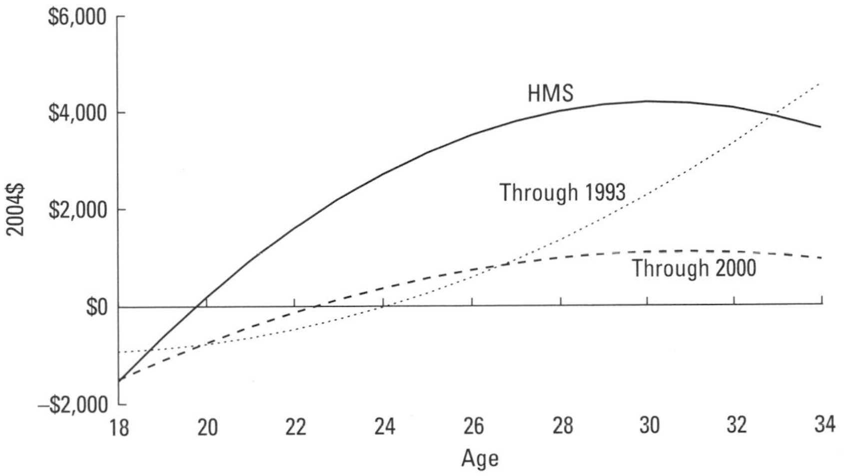

Source: National Longitudinal Survey of Youth, 1979–2000.

the sample corresponding just to the years included in HMS, and HMS's own estimates drawn from figure 3.9. Their figure shows the earnings for teen mothers and the earnings they would receive if they had delayed their first birth, based on the coefficient estimates presented in appendix table A.3.1. To simplify figure 3.12 and to make the comparison clearer, I show the *difference* in earnings for the two groups, which is the estimated causal impact of the teen birth and which is derived simply by subtracting the two earnings streams in figure 3.9 at each age. The coefficients and standard errors underlying my estimates are presented in tables A.3.4 and A.3.5.

Like HMS, I do not find negative impacts of a teen birth on a woman's labor-market earnings, although my estimates are considerably smaller than theirs. Their estimate has a very strong positive life-cycle pattern. They report that teen mothers earn somewhat less initially but much more later on than if they had delayed a first birth. The positive impact cumulates to more than $43,000 by age 34, an average of more than $2,500 annually. Using a sample similar to theirs, I find a life-cycle pattern that matches theirs at the age endpoints but has a different curvature and a smaller positive cumulative effect. My estimates suggest that the earnings impact is increasing when the women are in their 30s, rather than decreasing, as in HMS. My estimate of the total effect over these ages is about one-third of theirs. Using the full dataset, I find that the impact of a teen birth profile is positive but it is lower at all ages, much flatter, and is declining when the women are in their 30s. The cumulative earnings gain based on the full sample is $6,000, less than half the gains estimated for the restricted sample and one-seventh of HMS's estimate.[33]

Spouse Earnings

Figure 3.13 shows the effect of a teen birth on the earnings of a woman's spouse; see tables A.3.4 and A.3.5 for coefficients and standard errors. Spouse earnings are set equal to $0 for single women, so the estimate combines the impact of a teen birth on the probability of marriage with its impact on spouse earnings, conditional on marriage. I have truncated annual spouse earnings at $200,000; this affects a few very conspicuous outliers with incomes above $575,000. The HMS life-cycle pattern (see their figure 3.6) shows a very strong positive effect, beginning at about age 26. By their estimates, at age 34 the average income of the spouse of a teen

Figure 3.13. Life-Cycle Impact of a Teen Birth on Income of a Teen Mother's Spouse by Sample Years Included

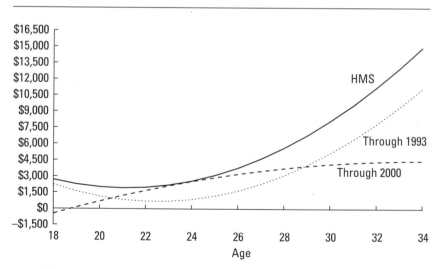

Source: National Longitudinal Survey of Youth, 1979–2000.

mother is almost $15,000 more than if she had delayed her first birth. Their estimates yield a cumulative benefit of a teen birth in higher spouse earnings of more than $96,000 through age 34.

The age profile of spouse earnings based on my restricted sample is similar to theirs. The two profiles are more or less parallel, with mine a relatively constant $2,000–$4,000 lower at most ages.[34] Both estimates suggest a rising positive impact of a teen birth on spouse earnings with the mother's age. The cumulative impact of a teen birth is more than $96,000 in the HMS estimates and about $60,000 in my estimates for the same sample. In contrast, the estimates based on the full sample are quite different. These results still show a positive effect of a teen birth, but the effect is much weaker, as is the life-cycle effect. The cumulative estimated impact of a teen birth for this sample is about half of that derived from the HMS estimates.

Welfare Assistance

All estimated impacts of a teen birth on cash welfare assistance are very similar, including those for both of the samples I examine. Extending the age range does not change the estimated impact of a teen birth at all.[35] Young teen mothers initially receive more welfare income than if they had delayed their first birth—about $1,700 more at age 18 and $1,100 more at age 20. But that the difference declines with age and becomes negative by the mid-20s. When the women are in their early to mid-30s, the teen mothers receive more than $1,200 less from welfare than if they had delayed their birth. These effects are shown in figure 3.14; the underlying estimates are in tables A.3.4 and A.3.5. For simplicity I show only the HMS estimate and mine for the full sample; the profile for the 1979–93 sample is overlapping.

I also examine the impact of a teen birth on receipt of food stamps and housing assistance through either public or subsidized housing. I focus here on just the results from the full sample, since HMS do not examine these outcomes. My findings are presented in figure 3.15, which shows the difference in the probability of food stamps use and of housing assistance as a result of a teen birth; see tables A.3.4 and A.3.5 for more information. Neither of the estimated impacts is very large, and both show a pattern of higher initial receipt that then declines steadily, more sharply for food stamps than for housing assistance. By the time the women are in their early 30s, they are approximately 13 percentage points less likely to be receiving food stamps and 1.5 percentage points less likely to be receiving

Figure 3.14. Life-Cycle Impact of a Teen Birth on Income Received from Welfare

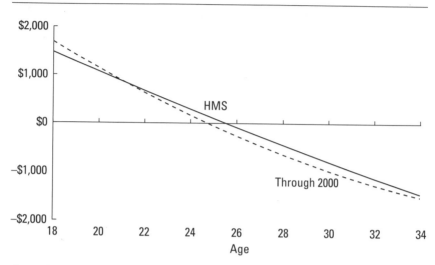

Source: National Longitudinal Survey of Youth, 1979–2000.

Figure 3.15. Life-Cycle Impact of a Teen Birth on Use of Food Stamps and Housing Assistance

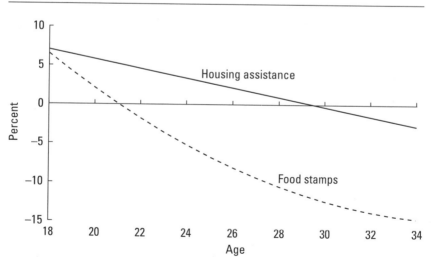

Source: National Longitudinal Survey of Youth, 1979–2000.

housing assistance than if they delayed their first birth. Cumulative impacts from age 18 to 34 are −1.1 additional year of receipt for food stamps and .44 additional years of housing assistance.

Most estimates reported in these figures are not statistically significant; in many cases, they are quite insignificant, with standard errors far larger than the estimated impacts. This also appears to be true for many estimates that HMS present in tables A.3.1 and A.3.2. This lack of significance may reflect the highly variable outcomes combined with the relatively small sample of miscarriage cases that are available to identify the teen birth effect. No ready solution to this is available in the NLSY79 data. In light of the large standard errors, one should view the results cautiously.

Cohort Differences in the Effect of a Teen Birth

The analyses presented above confirm the general propositions suggested by HMS, namely that a teen birth is not a substantial risk factor for some socioeconomic outcomes and may even have some beneficial effects, especially on own and spouse earnings. The single important exception to this pattern is the effect of a teen birth on postsecondary schooling. The estimates also suggest that the sample composition may affect the estimated impacts. For postsecondary education, own earnings, and spouse income, extending the sample period through age 35 for all women reduced positive impacts or increased negative ones. This finding suggests that the life-cycle pattern for the later cohorts, who are not observed into their 30s in the HMS sample, may differ from the pattern for the earlier cohorts.

To examine this issue more directly, I divide the sample in half and separately examine the impact of a teen birth for women in the NLSY who were born between 1957 and 1960 and ones who were born between 1961 and 1964. As I noted earlier, this period is one of substantial change in teen birth rates, in the proportion of teen births that are nonmarital, and in the economic and political environment facing teen mothers. In what follows, I am not formally testing for statistically different effects across the two cohorts. Given the smaller sample sizes and correspondingly smaller number of miscarriage cases that are used to identify the teen birth effect, it is unlikely that the observed differences are statistically different. Nonetheless, the differences are, as shown below, consistent and suggestive of an interesting cohort pattern of teen birth effects. This issue certainly needs further examination.

In figures 3.16–3.19, I show the results of estimating the impact of an early teen birth on key outcomes separately for women in the NLSY sample born between 1957 and 1960 and those born between 1961 and 1964. The impacts shown are for the same miscarriage instrumental variables approach used above. For the educational outcomes, I test for a life-cycle effect but report results from models with no age interactions. This specification fits the data far better and yields predictions similar to the models with full age-teen birth interactions.[36] For the income variables, I use the same age interactions that HMS use to make the comparison more straightforward; in some cases, the model with age interactions is not the preferred statistical model. Full estimates are shown in tables A.3.6–A.3.8.

Before looking at the outcomes separately, I want to note the general finding of the cohort analyses. As explained below, I find large differences between the two samples for most, though not all, outcomes, with the later birth cohorts consistently having more negative impacts of a teen birth. This is true for own earnings, even more so for the earnings of a spouse, and for educational attainment and, to a lesser degree, food stamp use and housing assistance. It is not true for cash assistance from welfare. This pattern is consistent with the analysis above of the impact of sample composition differences in which adding observations from the younger cohorts in their mid-30s typically yielded smaller positive impacts. It is very important to note that the number of miscarriages in the two subsamples is small and, like many of the results discussed above, is not statistically reliable. The results should be interpreted cautiously and conservatively.

Figure 3.16 shows the differential impact of an early teen birth on the probability of graduating from high school, earning a GED, or acquiring some postsecondary schooling. The results in both HMS and in my full-sample analysis showed a negative effect on high school completion but an offsetting positive effect on obtaining a GED of greater magnitude. That pattern of effects holds for the women born between 1957 and 1960: a teen birth reduces the proportion completing high school by 5.6 percentage points but increases the proportion with either a high school degree or a GED by almost 5 percentage points. For the younger cohort of women, however, the effects are more negative and not offsetting. A teen birth reduces the proportion completing high school by almost 16 percentage points and the proportion completing high school or obtaining a GED by more than 9 percentage points. Differences in the effect of a teen birth on postsecondary schooling are very large—essentially zero for the earlier cohort and −18.8 percentage points for the later cohorts.

Figure 3.16. Impact of a Teen Birth on Educational Attainment
of Teen Mothers, by Mother's Year of Birth

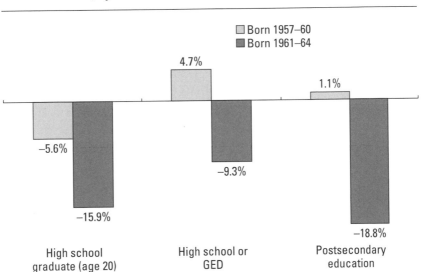

Source: National Longitudinal Survey of Youth, 1979–2000.

The life-cycle impact of a teen birth on a woman's earnings is shown in figure 3.17. For women in the older cohort, a teen birth initially decreases their earnings, but they catch up by age 22 and do better thereafter. By their mid-30s, they earn an average of about $2,100–$2,500 more a year than if they had delayed their first birth. The total cumulates to more than $13,000 from ages 18 to 34, considerably less than the total in the HMS estimates but still substantial. For the teen mothers in the later birth cohort, the impact of a birth differs. A teen birth reduces earnings by more than $1,000 at ages 18–20. The negative effect declines steadily through their mid-20s but then increases again, exceeding $1,000 at age 32 and rising to more than $1,700 at age 34. The cumulative impact on earnings is $13,000 less than if they had delayed their first birth.

The estimates of the impact of a teen birth on the earnings of a spouse are the most dramatically different by birth cohort (see figure 3.18). For teen mothers born between 1957 and 1960, I find an impact much like that found by HMS and shown in figure 3.13. The impact of a birth increases with age and exceeds $10,000 annually by the time the women are in their mid-30s. The cumulative impact is large, approximately $84,000, a figure

Figure 3.17. Life-Cycle Impact of a Teen Birth on Average Labor Market Earnings of Mothers, by Mother's Year of Birth

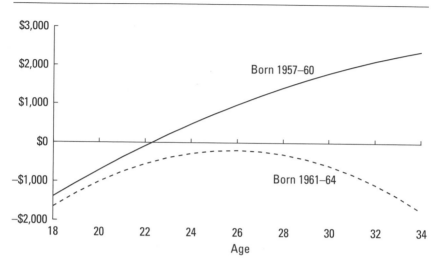

Source: National Longitudinal Survey of Youth, 1979–2000.

Figure 3.18. Life-Cycle Impact of a Teen Birth on Average Annual Income of Spouse, by Mother's Year of Birth

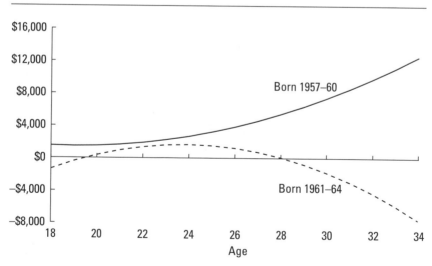

Source: National Longitudinal Survey of Youth, 1979–2000.

very similar to what they find. The teen mothers born between 1961 and 1964 do not benefit in this way. As shown in the figure, the impact of a teen birth on spouse income is much smaller for them and is negative overall. They receive slightly more income from their spouses at ages 20–28 (an average of $1,045), but then the impact turns negative, exceeding $4,000 annually by the time the women are in their mid-30s. The cumulative effect is a decrease of just under $16,000—a swing of more than $100,000 relative to the experience of the older cohorts of teen mothers. It is possible that this life-cycle pattern reflects later marriage by the women who delayed their first birth.

Differences between the two cohorts in the effect of a teen birth on welfare assistance are very small. If anything, it appears that the later birth cohort receives less in welfare assistance by the time they are in mid-20s and 30s than did the earlier cohort. This could reflect the changing welfare environment of the mid- to late 1990s. Differences by cohort in food stamp use and housing assistance are just a bit larger. The earlier birth cohort used food stamps for a total of 1.4 years less from age 18 to 34, compared with −.54 years less for the later cohort. The earlier cohort received housing assistance for .25 additional years, while the later cohort received this assistance for .59 additional years.

Summary

My estimates confirm many of the impacts of a teen birth on economic outcomes that Hotz, McElroy, and Sanders reported, especially when I use a dataset that corresponds to theirs. Like them, I find negative effects on high school completion but offsetting effects on GED completion; my offsetting effects are slightly weaker than theirs. I find positive, but weaker, effects on a woman's own earnings and on the earnings of her spouse. I find a negative impact on the probability of acquiring postsecondary schooling, an outcome not examined in HMS.

There are two major sources of the difference in findings based on the HMS analysis and this update. One is the fact that the HMS sample does not include observations through the mid-30s for the younger women in their sample. The other is possible secular trends in consequences of teen childbearing.

I find two consistent pieces of evidence that the impacts of teen childbearing may have differed for those who entered their teen years in the late

1960s and early 1970s compared with those who entered their teens in the late 1970s and early 1980s. First, when I expand the sample to allow all women in the sample to reach age 35, I find consistently weaker positive effects (earnings and spouse earnings) or stronger negative effects (post-secondary schooling); estimates of the impact on welfare income are unchanged. Second, when I examine separately the impact of a teen birth on educational attainment, earnings, and income received from a spouse for the older cohorts of women and the younger ones, I find very different impacts. For the older cohorts—the women born between 1957 and 1960 and who had first births between 1970 and 1978—a teen birth positively affects own earnings and spouse income and the probability of either completing high school or receiving a GED. These effects are consistent with the findings reported by HMS and, to a lesser extent, my full-sample findings. But for the younger cohorts—the women born between 1961 and 1965 and who had first births between 1974 and 1983—the impacts are consistently negative. They are less likely to graduate from high school, and the positive effect on completing a GED is small and not offsetting. Impacts on own earnings and the income of a spouse are also both negative and reasonably large.

Because the samples are smaller than in the full-sample analyses and, in particular, include half as many miscarriages, these results should be interpreted cautiously. Nonetheless, they do suggest a more negative impact of a teen birth, even using the miscarriage approach suggested by HMS, for more recent teen mothers.

Construction of Teen Fertility Variables in the NLSY79

Information on age at the beginning of a first pregnancy and the outcome of that pregnancy are available in the 1984–86, 1988, 1990, and 1992 interviews. From 1984 to 1990, the outcome variable is coded into four categories: birth, abortion, miscarriage, or stillbirth. In 1992, the last two categories are combined. In 1982 and 1983, information is available on the outcome of a first pregnancy (for pregnancies that did not end in a live birth) and the year and month in which that pregnancy ended. This information can be combined with information on own birth date to construct an age at first pregnancy. In most cases, the 1982–83 information is translated into and is consistent with the 1984–92 information. Some occasional inconsistency across years exists.

I code teen fertility in two steps. First, I use the 1984–92 variables to identify cases that ever report a first pregnancy at age 17 or earlier along with one of the designated fertility outcomes. I then check the 1982–83 pregnancy information and the information on the date of first birth to identify additional cases not otherwise classified that report a pregnancy that began at age 17 or earlier. I further check these cases against what I treat as the more reliable information in the 1984–92 data. Where conflicts cannot be resolved, I rely on the 1984–92 data.[37]

Table A.3.1. Coefficient Estimates from Instrumental Variables Regressions

Independent variables	Dependent Variables			
	Number of children born by age t	Fraction of time spent as single mom since age 14 at age t	Annual earnings from spouse at age t (2004$; 0 if spouse not present)	Obtained a high school diploma by age t
First pregnancy before age 18 ending in a birth	−9.8290	0.5202	36,997.1597	0.4235
Teen birth* current age	1.4607	−0.0302	−3,320.9133	−0.0454
Teen birth* current age^2	−0.0655*	0.0005	78.5829	0.0009
Teen birth* current age^3	0.0009*			
Age 18	0.8763***	−0.0031	1,949.3418	−0.1826
Age 19	1.0535***	0.0371	3,101.2436	−0.1475
Age 20	1.2457***	0.0723	4,198.9134	−0.1334
Age 21	1.4391***	0.0989	6,358.2478	−0.1248
Age 22	1.6154***	0.1215*	8,272.3094*	−0.1180
Age 23	1.7867***	0.1417**	7,855.4974	−0.1143
Age 24	1.9517***	0.1593**	8,348.9983	−0.1106
Age 25	2.0879***	0.1737**	10,106.6812*	−0.1100
Age 26	2.2304***	0.1851***	10,440.6306**	−0.1112
Age 27	2.3540***	0.1962***	10,925.3620**	−0.1156
Age 28	2.4395***	0.2049***	10,300.7667**	−0.1198
Age 29	2.4980***	0.2128***	10,627.1211**	−0.1232
Age 30	2.5209***	0.2273***	7,997.0228	−0.1237
Age 31	2.5298***	0.2370***	8,153.0130*	−0.1413
Age 32	2.4917***	0.2511***	5,607.8776	−0.1480
Age 33	2.4327***	0.2584***	3,434.7537	−0.1522
Age 34	2.2864***	0.2706***	6,494.3603	−0.1634
Age 35	2.1792***	0.2761***	−1,192.0668	−0.1373
Black	0.1627**	0.1781***	−8,258.8925***	0.1386***
Hispanic	0.1093	−0.0148	−995.0392	−0.0165
Family on welfare in 1978	0.0950	0.1001***	−2,141.3392*	0.0073
Family income in 1978	−2.66E-06**	−1.91E-07	−0.0308	2.53E-06***
Missing family income	0.1554	−0.0624**	2,492.9452	−0.0038

Obtained a GED by age t	Obtained a high school diploma or GED by age t	Annual number of hours woman worked for pay at age t	Woman's annual labor market earnings at age t (2004$)	Annual monetary value of AFDC and food stamp benefits received at age t (2004$)
−0.5578	−0.1291	−1,226.9771	−30,811.6096	9,256.9886
0.0455	−0.0004	83.2582	2,317.6478	−447.5023
−0.0007	0.0002	−1.0881	−38.3797	3.2541
−0.0606	−0.2352*	662.8880***	3,159.0816	548.6456
−0.0414	−0.1813	784.4493***	3,984.8508	1,529.6335
−0.0283	−0.1542	876.7312***	4,522.9042	1,912.0222
−0.0168	−0.1341	942.7908***	5,323.6156*	1,964.5727
−0.0106	−0.1208	989.8765***	5,299.2544*	2,267.5539*
−0.0143	−0.1207	1,008.7597****	6,137.2077**	2,446.7292*
−0.0130	−0.1156	1,032.1723***	6,872.2838**	2,998.3853**
−0.0087	−0.1105	1,079.5929***	6,879.9619**	2,759.2473**
−0.0085	−0.1115	1,079.9132***	7,544.6134**	3,060.3729**
−0.0011	−0.1087	1,085.4369***	8,353.2463***	2,989.3447**
0.0012	−0.1104	1,158.1029***	8,119.5008***	2,905.0865**
0.0120	−0.1031	1,130.3996***	8,432.2749***	3,063.6686**
0.0148	−0.1008	1,241.6135***	9,447.4251***	3,373.4780**
0.0235	−0.1097	1,216.1627***	10,012.0936***	3,434.5378**
0.0264	−0.1136	1,325.5895***	11,055.6986***	3,831.1690**
0.0240	−0.1209	1,307.3668***	11,468.8670***	3,735.2999**
0.0456	−0.1092	1,255.9788***	11,968.5256***	4,010.8824**
0.0250	−0.1035	1,295.5455***	11,357.7218**	4,087.9766**
−0.0811**	0.0577	22.7642	1,195.0996	2,181.5688***
−0.0068	−0.0231	60.4329	2,303.4359***	1,051.8640**
−0.0162	−0.0065	−159.7801**	−1,157.5256	1,450.9114***
−4.53E-07	2.08E-06***	0.0016	0.0377**	0.0016
−0.0451	−0.0516	−57.3514	567.7898	518.0340

(continued)

Table A.3.1. *(Continued)*

Independent variables	Number of children born by age *t*	Fraction of time spent as single mom since age 14 at age *t*	Annual earnings from spouse at age *t* (2004$; 0 if spouse not present)	Obtained a high school diploma by age *t*
		Dependent Variables		
In female-headed household at age 14	−0.0839	0.0738**	−2,744.4845	0.0204
In intact household at age 14	0.0081	0.0015	1,703.7833	0.1139**
Mother's education	−0.0274*	−0.0023	647.3496**	0.0281***
Missing mother's educ. (0–1)	−0.2771	0.0056	3,754.5576	0.0981
Father's education	−0.0140	−0.0005	274.8174	0.0107*
Missing father's educ. (0–1)	−0.1698	0.0256	1,153.1037	0.0376
In bottom quartile of AFQT distribution	0.2971**	0.0687***	−5,718.8481***	
In second quartile of AFQT distribution	0.2865***	0.0674***	−4,902.6898***	
In third quartile of AFQT distribution	0.0412	−0.0022	−543.1682	
Age 15 in 1979	0.0344	0.0460	−1,224.2006	0.0396
Age 16 in 1979	−0.0390	0.0287	−632.8690	0.0658
Age 17 in 1979	−0.0926	0.0202	−1,103.5287	0.0288
Age 18 in 1979	0.0314	0.0212	−2,615.9591	−0.0643
Age 19 in 1979	0.0256	0.0104	−3,084.1952	0.0417
Age 20 in 1979	−0.0468	−0.0362	−4,562.4932*	0.1460*
Age 21 or 22 in 1979	−0.0098	−0.0476	−3,219.6853	0.1874**
First pregnancy occurred before age 16	−0.2505***	−0.0420**	3,624.9554***	0.1625***
Used alcohol before first pregnancy	−0.0832	0.0116	−3,806.4996***	−0.0169
Used tobacco before first pregnancy	−0.0107	−0.0100	−2,305.3642*	−0.0881**
Number of person-years	14,096	14,096	12,665	14,737

Source: Author estimates from NLSY79.

*significant at the .10 level; **significant at the .05 level; ***significant at the .0025 level

Obtained a GED by age t	Obtained a high school diploma or GED by age t	Annual number of hours woman worked for pay at age t	Woman's annual labor market earnings at age t (2004$)	Annual monetary value of AFDC and food stamp benefits received at age t (2004$)
0.0485	0.0643	−91.0647	−406.1292	180.7888
0.0057	0.1195**	−108.2138	−878.2857	−313.8153
0.0134**	0.0416***	23.3728**	480.7057***	−70.4253
0.0257	0.1257	174.5635	3,581.1064**	−146.2049
0.0031	0.0133**	1.6125	17.8359	−64.4154
0.0811	0.1187*	−65.3181	143.9258	191.1811
		−565.7729***	−8,591.3556***	2,024.6558***
		−370.7188***	−6,345.5657***	1,742.2479***
		11.0305	−1,405.1857	−50.5426
−0.0208	0.0177	22.8480	−1,149.7029	−102.2554
0.0253	0.0913	−12.5383	453.6500	−90.2059
−0.0120	0.0170	−70.2704	−1,299.9238	124.3609
0.0366	−0.0303	−28.5731	−1,677.4227	−178.5342
0.0469	0.0770	36.2543	−1,581.3939	48.5207
0.0312	0.1804**	−47.8769	−1,533.5182	−89.2203
−0.0193	0.1714**	−40.0320	−1,521.8036	−187.9588
−0.0779***	0.0805**	19.3128	263.1737	−1,448.2615***
0.0248	0.0127	−14.7535	−201.0731	535.8166*
0.0239	−0.0677*	−105.2625*	−348.2227	740.6175**
14,737	14,737	12,907	13,573	13,563

Table A.3.2. Derived Estimated Effects of Delaying Teen Birth by Age of Mother

Independent variables	Dependent Variables			
	Number of children born by age t	Fraction of time spent as single mom since age 14 at age t	Annual earnings from spouse at age t (2004$; 0 if spouse not present)	Obtained a high school diploma by age t
Estimated impact at age:				
18	0.688***	0.123***	$2,682	−9.07%
19	0.685***	0.110***	$2,268	−10.15%
20	0.658***	0.097***	$2,012	−11.04%
21	0.612***	0.085***	$1,913	−11.74%
22	0.553***	0.074**	$1,971	−12.26%
23	0.487***	0.064*	$2,187	−12.60%
24	0.419**	0.055	$2,559	−12.74%
25	0.354*	0.047	$3,089	−12.70%
26	0.299	0.040	$3,775	−12.47%
27	0.259	0.034	$4,619	−12.05%
28	0.239	0.028	$5,621*	−11.45%
29	0.246	0.024	$6,779**	−10.66%
30	0.284	0.020	$8,094***	−9.68%
31	0.360	0.018	$9,567***	−8.52%
32	0.479	0.016	$11,197***	−7.17%
33	0.647	0.015	$12,984***	−5.63%
34	0.869*	0.015	$14,928***	−3.90%
35	1.151*	0.016	$17,029***	−1.99%
Average effect over ages 18–30	0.445	0.062	$3,659	−11.43%
Average effect over ages 18–35	0.516	0.049	$6,293	−9.77%
Number of person-years	14,096	14,096	12,665	14,737

Source: Author estimates from NLSY79.

Note: Estimated impacts at various ages are formed by taking the derivative of the coefficients for the regression functions reported in table A.3.1 about the teen birth indicator variable and its interactions, then evaluating these derivatives at each age. See endnote 12 for a description of how the statistical significance of these impacts is calculated.

*significant at the .10 level; **significant at the .05 level; ***significant at the .0025 level

Obtained a GED by age t	Obtained a high school diploma or GED by age t	Annual number of hours woman worked for pay at age t	Woman's annual labor market earnings at age t (2004$)	Annual monetary value of AFDC and food stamp benefits received at age t (2004$)
2.19%	−7.11%	−80.87	−$1,529	$2,256**
4.00%	−6.40%	−37.88	−$631	$1,929***
5.66%	−5.65%	2.95	$189	$1,609***
7.18%	−4.87%	41.59	$934	$1,294**
8.55%	−4.04%	78.06	$1,601	$987
9.77%	−3.17%	112.36	$2,191	$686
10.85%*	−2.26%	144.47	$2,705	$391
11.77%*	−1.31%	174.42	$3,142*	$103
12.55%*	−0.31%	202.18	$3,503*	−$178
13.18%**	0.72%	227.77	$3,786**	−$453
13.66%**	1.79%	251.18	$3,993**	−$722
13.99%**	2.90%	272.42	$4,123**	−$984
14.18%**	4.06%	291.48	$4,176*	−$1,239
14.21%**	5.25%	308.36	$4,153	−$1,488
14.10%**	6.48%	323.07	$4,052	−$1,731
13.84%*	7.76%	335.60	$3,875	−$1,967
13.43%	9.08%	345.96	$3,621	−$2,196
12.88%	10.43%	354.14	$3,291	−$2,419
9.81%	−1.97%	129.24	$2,168	$437
10.89%	0.74%	185.96	$2,621	−$229
14,737	14,737	12,907	13,573	13,563

Table A.3.3. Instrumental Variables Estimates of the Impact of a Teen Birth on Educational Outcomes by Sample Years Included

	Completed High School, Age 20		High school or GED, 1979–93		Postsecondary Schooling, 1979–2000		Postsecondary Schooling, 1979–93	
	Coefficient	Standard error	Coefficient	Standard error	Coefficient	Standard error	Coefficient	Standard error
Constant	−0.157	0.125	−0.957	0.131	−0.404	0.104	−0.254	0.114
Age	—	—	0.057	0.009	0.009	0.007	0.001	0.008
Age^2	—	—	−9.41E-04	1.80E-04	−3.58E-05	1.16E-04	4.53E-05	1.46E-04
Had early teen birth	−0.106	0.073	−0.211	0.108	−0.027	0.075	−0.170	0.082
Early teen birth * age	—	—	0.008	0.004	−0.002	0.003	0.004	0.003
Age 15 in 1979	−0.046	0.057	0.022	0.016	−0.009	0.010	−0.001	0.011
Age 16 in 1979	−0.011	0.054	0.026	0.014	0.009	0.010	0.003	0.010
Age 17 in 1979	0.080	0.055	0.101	0.014	−0.010	0.009	−0.005	0.010
Age 18 in 1979	−0.028	0.056	−0.021	0.014	−0.013	0.009	−0.011	0.009
Age 19 in 1979	−0.125	0.056	−0.056	0.014	0.027	0.009	0.028	0.009
Age 20 in 1979	−0.064	0.057	−0.049	0.014	−0.058	0.009	−0.053	0.009
Age 21–22 in 1979	0.031	0.054	0.076	0.013	0.041	0.009	0.042	0.009

Pregnant at age 16 or 17	0.139	0.031	0.087	0.008	0.009	0.005	0.007	0.005
Black	0.318	0.037	0.250	0.009	0.163	0.006	0.163	0.006
Hispanic	0.085	0.054	0.044	0.014	0.080	0.009	0.079	0.009
Family on welfare in 1978	-0.042	0.049	-0.022	0.012	-0.049	0.008	-0.054	0.008
Family income in 1978 ($000s)	0.007	0.002	0.0055	0.0004	0.0039	0.0003	0.0040	0.0003
Missing family income	0.030	0.040	-0.019	0.010	0.037	0.007	0.042	0.007
Mother's education	0.010	0.006	0.019	0.002	0.005	0.001	0.005	0.001
Missing mother's education	-0.029	0.083	-0.041	0.021	0.074	0.014	0.072	0.014
Father's education	0.007	0.005	0.004	0.001	0.005	0.001	0.006	0.001
Missing father's education	0.008	0.066	0.056	0.017	0.074	0.011	0.076	0.011
AFQT score	0.006	0.001	0.008	0.000	0.004	0.000	0.004	0.000
In intact household at age 14	0.138	0.051	0.147	0.013	-0.023	0.009	-0.026	0.009
In female-headed household at age 14	0.080	0.058	0.104	0.014	0.001	0.010	0.003	0.010
Sample size	970		13,145		13,932		12,543	

Source: Author estimates from NLSY79.

Table A.3.4. Instrumental Variables Estimates of the Impact of a Teen Birth on Earnings and Welfare Support, 1979–2000

	Spouse Earnings		Own Earnings		Welfare Income		Received Food Stamps		Received Housing Assistance	
	Coefficient	Standard error	Coefficient	Standard error	Coefficient	Standard error	Coefficient	Standard error	Coefficient	Standard error
Constant	−21,138.01	19,462.37	−24,285.83	11,246.36	−7,863.33	3,968.57	−0.298	0.433	−0.075	0.091
Age	1,320.88	1,483.45	1,065.20	857.21	781.14	304.37	0.062	0.034	0.021	0.006
Age^2	−15.20	27.64	−8.69	15.97	−12.70	5.71	−0.001	0.001	0.000	0.000
Had early teen birth	−17,565.88	27,258.52	−13,909.93	15,751.43	8,642.63	5,529.92	0.738	0.592	0.147	0.074
Early teen birth * age	1,291.91	2,078.27	974.29	1,200.93	−485.47	423.12	−0.050	0.046	−0.005	0.003
Early teen birth * age^2	−18.97	38.62	−15.81	22.32	5.50	7.90	0.001	0.001	—	—
Age 15 in 1979	−3,501.78	732.48	2,530.07	423.27	590.52	138.17	0.042	0.015	−0.012	0.011
Age 16 in 1979	−3,231.21	684.86	695.69	395.75	807.23	133.32	0.059	0.014	−0.003	0.010
Age 17 in 1979	−2,131.19	705.73	2,298.55	407.81	466.64	133.16	0.044	0.014	−0.030	0.010
Age 18 in 1979	−3,179.17	687.87	−61.43	397.49	620.09	131.94	0.051	0.014	−0.021	0.010
Age 19 in 1979	−3,608.96	696.48	1,275.03	402.46	71.40	131.42	0.029	0.014	0.003	0.010
Age 20 in 1979	4,381.27	694.89	−2,077.06	401.54	571.13	133.45	−0.002	0.014	−0.003	0.010
Age 21–22 in 1979	−4,251.34	679.96	2,585.01	392.91	−582.18	128.36	−0.009	0.013	−0.024	0.009
Pregnant at age 16 or 17	1,570.99	378.34	284.55	218.62	−781.80	72.48	−0.046	0.008	−0.028	0.005

Black	−8,470.11	460.47	1,563.47	266.08	1,158.44	88.20	0.130	0.009	0.129	0.007
Hispanic	−452.67	671.97	2,674.68	388.30	541.52	128.67	0.002	0.014	−0.011	0.010
Family on welfare in 1978	−7,033.26	605.74	−3,695.33	350.03	4,296.98	115.67	0.335	0.012	0.075	0.008
Family income in 1978 ($000s)	−1.57	19.91	142.32	11.51	−9.68	3.81	−0.0028	0.0004	−0.0003	0.0003
Missing family income	1,396.70	496.40	1,592.30	286.85	−194.24	94.85	−0.073	0.010	−0.026	0.007
Mother's education	856.90	79.32	445.57	45.83	1.43	15.16	−0.006	0.002	−0.004	0.001
Missing mother's education	7,003.83	1,027.33	2,902.13	593.64	627.23	196.60	−0.001	0.021	−0.056	0.015
Father's education	105.22	67.69	−53.75	39.11	−83.85	12.96	−0.007	0.001	−0.005	0.001
Missing father's education	189.88	822.34	−523.68	475.19	−442.74	157.42	−0.046	0.017	−0.046	0.012
AFQT score	77.22	9.25	142.93	5.34	−24.11	1.77	−0.003	0.000	−0.001	0.000
In intact household at age 14	1,748.36	630.45	432.53	364.30	−204.31	120.99	−0.059	0.013	−0.039	0.009
In female-headed household at age 14	−1,912.58	709.82	1,192.25	410.17	12.02	136.14	−0.043	0.014	0.008	0.010
Sample size	15,377		15,377		14,803		14,998		15,359	

Source: Author estimates from NLSY79.

Note: Spouse earnings, own earnings, and welfare income are in 2004 dollars.

Table A.3.5. Instrumental Variables Estimates of the Impact of a Teen Birth on Earnings, Spouse Earnings, and Welfare Income, 1979–93

	Spouse Earnings		Own Earnings		Welfare Income	
	Coefficient	Standard error	Coefficient	Standard error	Coefficient	Standard error
Constant	−71,590.15	21,353.40	−51,609.90	15,753.61	−7,863.33	3,968.57
Age	5,679.07	1,672.82	3,180.03	1,234.13	781.14	304.37
Age^2	−104.02	32.04	−48.90	23.64	−12.70	5.71
Had early teen birth	40,101.14	29,197.05	4,600.73	21,540.28	8,642.63	5,529.92
Early teen birth * age	−3,512.92	2,269.99	−650.49	1,674.69	−485.47	423.12
Early teen birth * age^2	78.25	43.13	19.08	31.82	5.50	7.90
Age 15 in 1979	−4,083.70	760.26	2,729.59	560.88	590.52	138.17
Age 16 in 1979	−3,739.35	705.81	1,125.71	520.72	807.23	133.32
Age 17 in 1979	−2,543.47	710.11	2,492.06	523.89	466.64	133.16
Age 18 in 1979	−3,607.98	686.84	−321.93	506.72	620.09	131.94
Age 19 in 1979	−4,028.20	680.28	1,422.58	501.88	71.40	131.42
Age 20 in 1979	4,329.53	675.83	−2,586.87	498.60	571.13	133.45
Age 21–22 in 1979	−4,354.75	650.26	3,301.67	479.74	−582.18	128.36
Pregnant at age 16 or 17	1,725.87	379.13	117.20	279.70	−781.80	72.48

Black	−8,210.28	461.21	1,933.48	340.26	1,158.44	88.20
Hispanic	−131.32	672.82	3,079.96	496.37	541.52	128.67
Family on welfare in 1978	−7,108.75	592.61	−5,014.20	437.20	4,296.98	115.67
Family income in 1978 ($000s)	−6.72	20.10	163.86	14.83	−9.68	3.81
Missing family income	1,628.34	495.35	2,010.16	365.44	−194.24	94.85
Mother's education	854.10	78.86	510.81	58.18	1.43	15.16
Missing mother's education	7,075.09	1,019.76	3,185.22	752.33	627.23	196.60
Father's education	28.72	67.51	−34.05	49.81	−83.85	12.96
Missing father's education	−961.60	820.06	−267.42	605.01	−442.74	157.42
AFQT score	71.74	9.19	173.67	6.78	−24.11	1.77
In intact household at age 14	1,419.00	632.13	814.79	466.36	−204.31	120.99
In female-headed household at age 14	−2,231.02	712.80	1,712.06	525.87	12.02	136.14
Sample size	13,988		13,988		13,779	

Source: Author estimates from NLSY79.

Note: Spouse earnings, own earnings, and welfare income are in 2004 dollars.

Table A.3.6. Instrumental Variables Estimates of the Impact of a Teen Birth on Educational Attainment by Cohort, 1979–2000

| | Completed High School (Age 20) | | | | High School or GED | |
| | Born 1957–60 | | Born 1961–64 | | Born 1957–60 | |
	Coefficient	Standard error	Coefficient	Standard error	Coefficient	Standard error
Constant	−0.272	0.160	−0.172	0.179	−0.955	0.171
Age	—	—	—	—	0.042	0.013
Age^2	—	—	—	—	−5.56E-04	2.41E-04
Had early teen birth	−0.056	0.097	−0.159	0.111	0.047	0.023
Pregnant at age 16 or 17	0.182	0.043	0.094	0.044	0.085	0.010
Black	0.307	0.052	0.341	0.052	0.241	0.012
Hispanic	0.029	0.076	0.159	0.077	0.008	0.018
Family on welfare in 1978	−0.081	0.055	0.124	0.134	−0.043	0.013
Family income in 1978 ($000s)	0.003	0.002	0.090	0.021	0.0043	0.0006
Missing family income	−0.016	0.054	0.054	0.061	−0.033	0.013
Mother's education	0.013	0.008	0.006	0.010	0.023	0.002
Missing mother's education	−0.060	0.107	0.033	0.134	−0.056	0.025
Father's education	0.011	0.007	0.000	0.008	0.006	0.002
Missing father's education	0.000	0.088	0.005	0.098	0.073	0.021
AFQT score	0.006	0.001	0.007	0.001	0.0082	0.0002
In intact household at age 14	0.051	0.077	0.203	0.067	0.100	0.018
In female-headed household at age 14	0.013	0.087	0.143	0.076	0.086	0.020
Born 1964–65	—	—	−0.002	0.059	—	—
Born 1963	—	—	0.026	0.057	—	—
Born 1962			0.106	0.055	—	—
Born 1959	0.136	0.058	—	—	0.058	0.014
Born 1958	0.148	0.060	—	—	0.128	0.014
Born 1957	0.110	0.060	—	—	0.090	0.014

Source: Author estimates from NLSY79.

Note: Sample sizes are 7,590 for 1957–60 birth cohort and 7,787 for 1961–64 cohort, except for high school completion (N = 476, 494).

	POSTSECONDARY EDUCATION					
	Born 1961–64		Born 1957–60		Born 1961–64	
	Coefficient	Standard error	Coefficient	Standard error	Coefficient	Standard error
	−1.569	0.238	−0.670	0.133	−0.052	0.123
	0.110	0.020	0.024	0.010	−0.005	0.009
	−1.94E-03	4.15E-04	−2.94E-04	1.73E-04	1.81E-04	1.59E-04
	−0.093	0.031	0.011	0.017	−0.188	0.019
	0.092	0.012	−0.019	0.007	0.040	0.008
	0.266	0.014	0.166	0.009	0.158	0.009
	0.094	0.021	0.081	0.012	0.082	0.014
	0.075	0.036	−0.074	0.009	0.034	0.023
	0.0064	0.0006	0.0028	0.0004	0.0039	0.0004
	−0.010	0.017	0.042	0.009	0.001	0.011
	0.012	0.003	0.005	0.001	0.004	0.002
	−0.028	0.037	0.049	0.018	0.089	0.023
	0.002	0.002	0.011	0.001	−0.002	0.001
	0.051	0.027	0.122	0.015	0.024	0.017
	0.0072	0.0003	0.0041	0.0002	0.0043	0.0002
	0.179	0.019	−0.021	0.013	−0.031	0.012
	0.117	0.021	0.029	0.014	−0.015	0.013
	0.043	0.017	—	—	0.017	0.010
	0.049	0.015	—	—	0.032	0.010
	0.120	0.015	—	—	0.008	0.009
	—	—	−0.022	0.010	—	—
	—	—	0.018	0.010	—	—
	—	—	−0.033	0.010	—	—

Table A.3.7. Instrumental Variables Estimates of the Impact of a Teen Birth on Own and Spouse Earnings by Cohort, 1979–2000

| | OWN EARNINGS | | | | SPOUSE EARNINGS | | | |
| | Born 1957–60 | | Born 1961–64 | | Born 1957–60 | | Born 1961–64 | |
	Coefficient	Standard error	Coefficient	Standard error	Coefficient	Standard error	Coefficient	Standard error
Constant	−15,530.07	17,298.29	−29,044.65	14,913.10	−34,552.51	31,496.51	−10,482.06	24,759.54
Age	655.96	1,304.71	1,273.21	1,148.83	2,553.92	2,375.61	−173.46	1,907.35
Age^2	−3.42	24.06	−9.85	21.58	−48.80	43.80	25.28	35.82
Had early teen birth	−10,286.53	22,324.95	−15,864.59	22,176.74	19,592.04	40,649.02	−48,774.10	3,6818.82
Early teen birth * age	631.35	1,682.88	1,210.18	1,713.53	−1,900.34	3,064.15	4,235.36	2,844.90
Early teen birth * age^2	−7.62	30.99	−23.36	32.19	49.80	56.42	−88.95	53.44
Pregnant at age 16 or 17	−343.31	297.59	1,028.88	329.14	1,895.55	541.84	1,541.92	546.46
Black	2,638.48	362.33	37.32	391.43	−8,293.13	659.73	−8,001.18	649.88
Hispanic	2,534.45	522.53	2,900.58	578.12	914.16	951.42	−1,713.81	959.83
Family on welfare in 1978	−4,197.69	383.86	−2,243.33	984.52	−7,887.65	698.94	−4,674.39	1,634.54
Family income in 1978 ($000s)	157.72	17.13	91.79	16.11	35.31	31.19	1.21	26.75

Missing family income	2,523.57	373.37	−169.27	456.85	−450.89	679.83	3,859.36	758.48
Mother's education	260.41	58.36	678.56	74.74	1,054.14	106.26	530.99	124.09
Missing mother's education	898.87	747.11	5,616.36	1,002.94	9,242.58	1,360.32	2,607.23	1,665.14
Father's education	−42.20	51.89	−127.39	60.04	110.70	94.48	185.06	99.68
Missing father's education	686.45	627.28	−2,425.29	734.59	92.68	1,142.14	921.03	1,219.59
AFQT score	143.63	6.93	149.06	8.52	94.31	12.62	52.75	14.14
In intact household at age 14	966.27	532.41	89.16	509.37	−1,109.81	969.40	3,131.85	845.67
In female-headed household at age 14	1,368.60	591.60	1,427.51	570.33	−5,407.93	1,077.17	744.48	946.89
Born 1964–65	−1,049.54	406.21	2,828.90	438.06	—	—	202.20	727.30
Born 1963	1,820.94	414.50	910.77	409.62	—	—	872.81	680.07
Born 1962	−621.97	408.15	2,718.18	403.00	—	—	1,092.46	669.08
Born 1959	−826.41	319.85	—	—	3,577.48	739.63	—	—
Born 1958	1,433.81	326.38	—	—	−1,255.48	754.72	—	—
Born 1957	−489.74	321.38	—	—	3,587.75	743.16	—	—

Source: Author estimates from NLSY79.

Notes: Sample sizes are 7,590 for 1957–60 birth cohort and 7,787 for 1961–64 cohort. Earnings are in 2004 dollars.

Table A.3.8. Instrumental Variables Estimates of the Impact of a Teen Birth on Food Stamp Use and Housing Assistance by Cohort, 1979–2000

| | Food Stamp Use | | | | Housing Assistance | | | |
| | Born 1957–60 | | Born 1961–64 | | Born 1957–60 | | Born 1961–64 | |
	Coefficient	Standard error	Coefficient	Standard error	Coefficient	Standard error	Coefficient	Standard error
Constant	−0.3160	0.5931	−0.3784	0.5393	−0.0220	0.4335	0.2010	0.3244
Age	0.0652	0.0449	0.0760	0.0422	0.0255	0.0327	−0.0120	0.0250
Age^2	−0.0012	0.0008	−0.0014	0.0008	−0.0005	0.0006	0.0004	0.0005
Had early teen birth	0.8043	0.7636	0.3752	0.8007	0.3960	0.5595	−0.4384	0.4825
Early teen birth * age	−0.0591	0.0577	−0.0164	0.0628	−0.0272	0.0422	0.0480	0.0373
Early teen birth * age^2	0.0009	0.0011	0.0000	0.0012	0.0005	0.0008	−0.0011	0.0007
Pregnant at age 16 or 17	−0.0127	0.0101	−0.0827	0.0110	−0.0190	0.0075	−0.0478	0.0072
Black	0.1348	0.0123	0.1301	0.0130	0.1041	0.0091	0.1608	0.0085
Hispanic	0.0123	0.0177	−0.0073	0.0193	−0.0370	0.0131	0.0103	0.0126
Family on welfare in 1978	0.3306	0.0130	0.2555	0.0329	0.0854	0.0096	−0.0121	0.0215
Family income in 1978 ($000s)	−0.0047	0.0006	−0.0008	0.0005	−0.0013	0.0004	0.0009	0.0004

Missing family income	-0.0941	0.0127	-0.0372	0.0152	-0.0335	0.0093	0.0002	0.0099
Mother's education	-0.0032	0.0020	-0.0090	0.0025	-0.0029	0.0015	-0.0063	0.0016
Missing mother's education	0.0086	0.0253	-0.0060	0.0335	-0.0567	0.0187	-0.0722	0.0218
Father's education	-0.0064	0.0018	-0.0089	0.0020	-0.0089	0.0013	0.0004	0.0013
Missing father's education	-0.0184	0.0212	-0.0751	0.0244	-0.0814	0.0157	-0.0006	0.0160
AFQT score	-0.0025	0.0002	-0.0029	0.0003	-0.0007	0.0002	-0.0007	0.0002
In intact household at age 14	-0.0656	0.0180	-0.0461	0.0170	-0.0489	0.0133	-0.0219	0.0111
In female-headed household at age 14	-0.0337	0.0200	-0.0459	0.0190	0.0035	0.0148	0.0123	0.0124
Born 1964–65	—	—	-0.0307	0.0145	—	—	0.0064	0.0095
Born 1963	—	—	-0.0059	0.0139	—	—	0.0179	0.0089
Born 1962	—	—	-0.0211	0.0134	—	—	-0.0116	0.0088
Born 1959	-0.0174	0.0137	—	—	0.0035	0.0102	—	—
Born 1958	-0.0328	0.0139	—	—	-0.0241	0.0104	—	—
Born 1957	-0.0282	0.0139	—	—	-0.0225	0.0102	—	—

Source: Author estimates from NLSY79.

Notes: Sample sizes are 7,590 for 1957–60 birth cohort and 7,787 for 1961–64 cohort. Earnings are in 2004 dollars.

Miscarriages and Stillbirths in the NLSY79

A comparison of the NLSY79 data to national data on stillbirths and miscarriages reported by the National Center for Health Statistics (Hoyert 1996) suggests that miscarriages are vastly underreported in the NLSY79, especially relative to stillbirths. NCHS Series 20, Number 31, "Medical and Life-Style Risk Factors Affecting Fetal Mortality, 1989–90," reports data on fetal deaths for 29 states (61 percent of all fetal deaths). Fetal deaths are defined as stillbirths or miscarriages after 20 weeks of duration. Induced abortions are not included. For women under age 30, the reported fetal death rate is 7.3 deaths per 1,000 fetal deaths plus births (see table B of that publication). I assume that this rate holds for younger teens and for the other 21 states.

During the 1980s, women who were pregnant at age 17 or earlier had approximately 285,000 births annually. This figure includes all births to adolescents age 17 and younger and three-quarters of those at age 18. Applying the 7.3/1,000 fetal death rate to the 285,000 young teen births figure yields an estimate of about 2,100 fetal deaths in pregnancies at age 17 or earlier. About half of teen pregnancies end in birth and about 13 percent in a miscarriage according to Guttmacher Institute estimates, which means approximately 74,000 early teen pregnancies ended in a miscarriage annually ($285,000 \times 2 \times .13 = 74,100$). Thus, miscarriages outnumbered fetal deaths by a factor of 35 to 1. In the NLSY sample, the ratio is closer to 7:1. Put differently, if my calculations are even close and if the NLYS79 includes 11 stillbirths from early teen pregnancies, it ought to have more than 350 miscarriages, rather than 62.

NOTES

The analysis in the updated chapter adds a year of data from the 1993 interview of the National Longitudinal Survey of Youth, 1979 Cohort. In addition, we have corrected three errors in data construction in our original data files. We have corrected a systematic error in deflating nominal dollar-valued outcome variables to constant dollar values. (We wish to thank Saul Hoffman for calling this error to our attention.) We have included a small number of observations from the low-income white component of the cross-sectional sample in the NLSY79 that were omitted from our earlier analysis files. We now use appropriate base-year weights for the particular combination of cross-sectional and supplemental samples from the NLSY79 used in our analyses. Finally, at the request of one of the volume editors, we note all dollar-valued outcome variables in 2004 dollars, rather than the 1996 dollars used in the original chapter. The details of our sample and variable construction, and the sampling weights employed in this updated study, are documented in Hotz, McElroy, and Sanders (2005).

This research was funded by a grant from the National Institute of Child Health and Human Development. Preparation of this chapter, which summarizes parts of our larger research project, was paid for by the Robin Hood Foundation. We wish to thank Sarah Gordon, Stuart Hagen, Terra McKinnish, Charles Mullin, Carl Schneider, Daniel Waldram and Juan Pantano for able and conscientious research assistance on this project. We wish to thank Robert Moffitt, Frank Furstenberg, Arlene Leibowitz, John Strauss, Susan Newcomer, Arline Geronimus, and participants in the Workshop on Low Income Populations at the Institute for Research on Poverty at the University of Wisconsin–Madison for helpful comments on an earlier draft and Charlotte Koelling, Frances Margolin, Deborah Sanders, Simon Hotz, and Gregory Kienzl for their editorial assistance in preparing this chapter. We especially wish to thank Robert Willis for numerous helpful discussions during the course of this study.

1. The NLSY79 drew random oversamples of these two minority groups to ensure adequate sample sizes for conducting separate analyses by race. For a detailed discussion of the construction of this sample, see Hotz and colleagues (2005). We use base-year sampling weights for the NLSY79 to account for the use of the minority oversamples. The NLSY79 also provides yearly updated weights to take account of nonresponse at each interview using poststratification adjustment procedures described in Frankel, McWilliams, and Spencer (1983). In an extensive evaluation of the NLSY79 data, Macurdy, Mroz, and Gritz (1998) find differences in estimating the distributions of labor market earnings and hours of work when using weighted versus unweighted data. However, they also find that it does not matter whether one weights the data with the 1979 base weights or year-by-year versions of these weights that adjust for attrition over the course of the study. We thank Jay Zagorsky of the Center for Human Resource Research at the Ohio State University for providing us with the appropriate base-year weights for our particular combination of the cross-sectional and supplemental samples. (The appropriate set of weights for this combination of subsamples is not available in the public-release versions of the NLSY79.)

2. For example, the psychological literature on teenage childbearing suggests that low self-esteem (Patten 1981; Vernor, Green, and Frothingham 1983), religiosity (Michael and Tuma 1985), and low educational aspirations and expectations (Abrahamse, Morrison, and Waite 1988) all increase the chances that a teenager will become a mother. One suspects that these factors affect a woman's educational attainment and her rates of labor force and welfare participation. None of these factors is well measured in the NLSY79 or most other data sources. That existing datasets are unlikely to allow one to convincingly adjust out background differences via ordinary regression analysis between teen mothers and women who delayed is substantiated (Hotz et al. 1997), establishing that one can reliably reject the validity of standard regression-adjustment methods when analyzing the socioeconomic outcomes of teen mothers.

3. Epidemiological studies find that while smoking and drinking during pregnancy and the use of an intrauterine device (IUD) at conception increase the likelihood that a woman miscarries, other factors such as a woman's socioeconomic status, her nutrition, or drug use do not increase miscarriage rates, although the latter factors affect birth weight. See Kline, Stein, and Susser (1989) for a summary of this evidence.

4. In Hotz and colleagues (2005), we show that the background characteristics of women who have induced abortions as teenagers differ significantly from those of women who had miscarriages (spontaneous abortions) as teens.

5. This adjustment was first noted by Bloom (1984) in the context of worker training evaluations. Also see Angrist and Imbens (1991); Heckman, Smith, and Taber (1998);

Hotz and Sanders (1994), and Heckman (1996) for further descriptions of this method. In Hotz, and colleagues (2005), we show that the background characteristics of women who have induced abortions as teenagers are significantly different from those of the women who had miscarriages (spontaneous abortions) as teens.

6. There is an important qualification to our results. We are estimating the effects of teenage births on the socioeconomic attainments of those women in the population who would likely be observed to have their first births as teenagers unless they were to experience a random denial birth by miscarrying. Because pregnancies are not random events, we do not make inferences about the causal effects of early childbearing for an individual randomly chosen from the population of all teenage women in the United States; such inferences would be meaningless for policymaking. Instead, we focus on what the data *can* identify. In general, such data, even when considered through the "natural experiment" framework of random miscarriages, will tell us very little about the likely consequences for a typical woman of having her first birth as a teen relative to delaying her childbearing. But that is not the point of this analysis. We are more interested in what portions of the mothers' apparently lowered life prospects can be considered the consequences of early childbearing. This focus is adequate for making inferences about factors like the costs to government imposed by the teenagers having babies in the United States today.

7. See Greene (1993) for a discussion of the instrumental variables method. See Hotz and colleagues (2005) for a detailed description of the implementation of this instrumental variables method to estimate the effects of teenage childbearing.

8. For a detailed discussion of how this sample was constructed, see Hotz and colleagues (2005).

9. We estimate that 12 percent of women who would have given birth as teenagers had they not miscarried (latent-birth women) had not had any children by the 1993 survey, when they were age 28 to 35. Because we do not know the age at which these women first gave birth, it is not possible to calculate exactly the mean age at first birth among all latent-birth women. If we assume that all the latent-birth women who had not given birth by the 1993 survey had a first child in 1994, then on average latent-birth women first gave birth when they were age 21. This implies that miscarriages delay the age at first birth for latent-birth women from sometime between their 17th and 18th birthdays to sometime between their 21st and 22nd birthdays, or for three to four years. Of course, not all latent-birth women who had not had a child by 1993 had a child in 1994. Therefore, a three- to four-year delay is the lower bound on the average delay from a miscarriage for this group of women.

10. In Hotz and colleagues (2005), we present results for a slightly broader and more detailed list of outcomes than that considered in this chapter.

11. The significance levels for the coefficient estimates in table A.3.1 are based on clustered standard errors in which we take account of the use of panel data on respondents, same respondent observed at different ages in order to account for potential correlation a given respondent's error terms for the regression functions being estimated at different ages. Failure to adjust tends to inflate standard errors and, thus, overstate the statistical significance of estimated coefficients. The standard errors and associated statistical tests in the second part of this chapter written by Saul Hoffman do not account for this clustering.

12. The significance levels for these age-specific effects are based on constructed t-statistics in which the standard errors for the age-specific effects were calculated taking into account the variance-covariance matrix of the coefficient estimates from the regres-

sions reported in table A.3.1 used to calculate the derivatives for the teen birth indicator variable and evaluating them at the various for which estimates are reported in table A.3.2. As noted in the preceding footnote, these standard errors are adjusted for the panel nature of our data. In analysis not reported here, we compared the standard errors on these estimated age-specific effects with and without clustering and found that failure to cluster led to standard errors that were over 50 percent higher, on average, than the clustered standard errors and led to an apparent overstating of the significance levels of the estimated age-specific effects. Again, the age-specific estimates of not delaying teen births reported by Saul Hoffman in part 2 of this chapter do not account for the panel nature of the data he used.

13. According to the Current Population Survey (CPS), for example, the birth rates (numbers of births per 1,000 women) in 1992 were 76 for women age 30–34, 38 for women age 35–39, and 9 for women age 40–44 (U.S. Bureau of the Census 1993).

14. One rejects that this delay effect is significantly different from zero at even the 0.10 level.

15. We counted the spousal-earnings variables as the annual labor-market earnings of a woman's husband if she is married and as zero if she is single.

16. The estimates of spousal earnings associated with delaying childbearing are significantly lower (at the 0.01 level) than those for teen mothers at age 29 through 34.

17. Note that the completion rates in the first four bars of figure 3.7 for teen mothers differ from those in figure 3.2. This is due to differences in the samples used to derive the estimates in these figures. In figure 3.7, the estimates are obtained from the Teen Pregnancy sample and are based on women whose *first pregnancy* that occurred *before* their 18th birthday ended in a birth, regardless of when that birth occurred. In figure 3.2 the estimates are calculated with the All Women's sample—that is, for women who experienced a *birth before* age 18, regardless of how many pregnancies she had experienced (and terminated) at earlier ages. Since most regular high school graduations occur around age 18, there is great scope for differences in the estimates of receipt of a high school diploma or a GED across the two samples.

18. In her independent assessment of the costs of teenage childbearing, Maynard (1996) calculates the likely impact of delayed childbearing among teen mothers by comparing the earnings that teen mothers receive over their first 13 years of motherhood with estimates of what women who delayed childbearing until age 21 would be expected to earn over their first 13 years of motherhood. (She uses this same approach in calculations for annual hours of work and welfare benefits received.) This approach differs from ours in how the outcomes associated with delay are calculated. In addition, using this approach does not change our basic finding that delaying teen motherhood will lower on average, rather than increase, the labor-market earnings of women who become teen mothers.

19. The differences in public assistance between teen mothers and what would have happened if they had delayed childbearing are statistically significant at ages 18 through 21.

20. If one uses the method of comparison proposed by Maynard (1996) (described in footnote 18), one reaches the same conclusion that average annual level of welfare benefits received by teen mothers would not be expected to decline if these women delayed their childbearing.

21. As noted in a summary of a National Institute of Child Health and Human Development (NICHD) conference assessing evidence on the effects of early childbearing, "the size and importance of this effect of early childbearing on a young mother's educational

and economic outcomes, and the extent to which a causal interpretation can be made, remain in dispute. Recent studies have given new emphasis to earlier concerns that traditional multivariate approaches have not adequately controlled for selectivity into early childbearing" (Bachrach and Carver 1992, 20–21).

22. This edition of *Kids Having Kids* omits a discussion of the implied costs to government associated with the impacts of teenage childbearing on outcomes for mothers that was included in the original chapter 3.

23. See Hoffman (1998) and Hoffman (2005) for a discussion of some data issues in the analyses reported in chapter 3 of the first edition of *Kids Having Kids*.

24. In a regression context, if there is an omitted variable Z, the resulting bias in the coefficient estimate equals $\beta_Z \times \lambda_{Z,T}$ where β_Z is the effect of the omitted variable on outcome Y and $\lambda_{Z,T}$ has the sign of the partial correlation between Z and T. Suppose Z is some factor that increases the probability of undesirable outcomes (i.e., $\beta_Z > 0$) and increases the probability of a teen birth ($\lambda_{Z,T} < 0$). Then, with Z omitted, T captures the correlated negative effect of Z. Omitted family and neighborhood characteristics are prime suspects.

25. Also, measuring effects at later ages inevitably means that the teen births occurred several decades ago and may not be fully representative of more recent births.

26. Not all women are observed at all ages; for example, women in the NLSY79 who were 21 in 1979 are not observed at ages 18–20. Also, beginning in 1994, the NLSY79 began conducting interviews every other year, rather than annually. Thus, outcome variables, such as earnings, are not available at every age.

27. Also included are three dummy variables indicating whether family income in 1978 and parents' education are missing.

28. Similarly, fewer women are observed at younger ages (less than age 21), and the ones who are observed are exclusively from the more recent birth cohorts.

29. Exactly as HMS suggest, the additional cases would increase the efficiency of the estimates.

30. The two or three additional years reflect every other year interviewing for four to six years, depending on the woman's age in 1993.

31. Like HMS, I use the appropriate NLSY sample weight that adjusts for year-to-year attrition and for the fact that some NLSY subsamples are not included in the analysis. The standard weights included in the NLSY data are not appropriate when some subsamples are excluded.

32. Too few of these women complete college to allow a meaningful estimate of the effect of a teen birth on this outcome.

33. The earnings impacts discussed here are not statistically significant at conventional levels. I find no statistically significant effect with simpler specifications that include either a dummy variable for an early teen birth or a dummy and a linear age term.

34. I have no explanation for why the profiles differ.

35. Welfare eligibility and benefits were restricted in the 1990s. This may affect the results.

36. *T*-statistics for age interaction effects are typically less than 0.5. I use a consistent specification across cohorts. The goal is not so much comparison with the earlier results for the full sample, but rather to identify possible differences across the cohorts.

37. Using the 1982–83 data on year of first pregnancy, I reclassified eight cases as teen miscarriages and eight others as abortions.

REFERENCES

Abrahamse, Allan F., Peter A. Morrison, and Linda J. Waite. 1988. *Beyond Stereotypes: Who Becomes a Single Teenage Mother?* Santa Monica, CA: RAND Corporation.

Angrist, Joshua, and Guido Imbens. 1991. "Sources of Identifying Information in Evaluation Models." Unpublished manuscript, Harvard University, August.

Bachrach, Christine, and Karen Carver. 1992. "Outcomes of Early Childbearing: An Appraisal of Recent Evidence." Summary of a conference. National Institute of Child Health and Human Development, May.

Bloom, Howard S. 1984. "Accounting for No-Shows in Experimental Evaluation Designs." *Evaluation Review* 8(2): 225–46.

Bronars, Stephen G., and Jeff Grogger. 1995. "The Economic Consequences of Unwed Motherhood: Using Twin Births as a Natural Experiment." *American Economic Review* 84(5): 1141–56.

Burt, Martha R. 1992. "Teenage Childbearing: How Much Does It Cost?" Washington, DC: Center for Population Options.

Burt, Martha R., and Debra W. Haffner. 1986. "Estimates of Public Costs for Teenage Childbearing: A Review of Recent Studies and Estimates of 1985 Public Costs." Washington, DC: Center for Population Options.

Cameron, Stephen V., and James J. Heckman. 1993. "The Nonequivalence of High School Equivalents." *Journal of Labor Economics* 11(1, Part 1): 1–47.

Cao, Jian, Ernst W. Stromsdorfer, and Gregory Weeks. 1996. "The Human Capital Effect of General Education Development Certificates on Low Income Women." *Journal of Human Resources* 31(1): 206–28.

Frankel, Martin, Howard McWilliams, and Bruce Spencer. 1983. *Technical Sampling Report, National Longitudinal Survey of Labor Force Behavior.* Chicago, IL: NORC, University of Chicago.

Geronimus, Arline T., and Sanders Korenman. 1992. "The Socioeconomic Consequences of Teen Childbearing Reconsidered." *Quarterly Journal of Economics* 107(4): 1187–214.

———. 1993. "The Socioeconomic Costs of Teenage Childbearing: Evidence and Interpretation." *Demography* 30(2): 281–90.

Greene, William. 1993. *Econometric Analysis.* 2nd ed. New York: Macmillan.

Grogger, Jeff, and Stephen Bronars. 1993. "The Socioeconomic Consequences of Teenage Childbearing: Findings from a Natural Experiment." *Family Planning Perspectives* 25(4): 156–61.

Hayes, Cheryl D., ed. 1987. *Risking the Future: Adolescent Sexuality, Pregnancy, and Childbearing.* Vol. I. Washington, DC: National Academy Press.

Heckman, James. 1996. "Randomization as an Instrumental Variable." *Review of Economics and Statistics* 78(2): 336–41.

Heckman, James, Jeffrey Smith, and Christopher Taber. 1998. "Accounting for Dropouts in Evaluations of Social Experiments." *Review of Economics and Statistics* 80(2): 1–14.

Hoffman, Saul D. 1998. "Teenage Childbearing Isn't So Bad After All . . . or Is It? A Review of the New Literature." *Family Planning Perspectives* 30(5): 236–39.

———. 2005. "What *Are* the Socio-Economic Effects of Teen Childbearing? A Re-Analysis of the Teen Miscarriage Natural Experiment." Mimeo, University of Delaware.

Hoffman, Saul D., E. Michael Foster, and Frank F. Furstenberg, Jr. 1993. "Reevaluating The Costs of Teenage Childbearing." *Demography* 30(1): 1–13.

Hotz, V. Joseph, and Seth Sanders. 1994. "Bounding Treatment Effects in Experimental Evaluations Subject to Post-Randomization Treatment Choice." *Bulletin of the International Statistical Institute.*

Hotz, V. Joseph, Susan Williams McElroy, and Seth G. Sanders. 2005. "Teenage Childbearing and Its Life Cycle Consequences." *Journal of Human Resources* 40(3): 683–715.

Hotz, V. Joseph, Charles Mullin, and Seth Sanders. 1997. "Bounding Causal Effects Using Contaminated Instrumental Variables: Analyzing the Effects of Teenage Childbearing Using a Natural Experiment." *Review of Economic Studies* 64:576–603.

Hoyert, Donna L. 1996. "Medical and Life-Style Risk Factors Affecting Fetal Mortality, 1989–90." Vital and Health Statistics Report 20(31). Hyattsville, MD: National Center for Health Statistics.

Jones, Elise F., and Jacqueline Darroch Forrest. 1990. "Underreporting of Abortions in Surveys of U.S. Women: 1976 to 1988." *Demography* 29(1): 113–26.

Juhn, Chinhui, Kevin M. Murphy, and Brooks Pierce. 1993. "Wage Inequality and the Rise in Returns to Skill." *Journal of Political Economy* 101(3): 410–42.

Kline, Jennie, Zena Stein, and Mervyn Susser. 1989. *Conception to Birth: Epidemiology of Prenatal Development.* New York: Oxford University Press.

Macurdy, Thomas, Thomas Mroz, and Mark Gritz. 1998. "An Evaluation of the National Longitudinal Survey on Youth." *Journal of Human Resources* 33(2): 345–436.

Maynard, Rebecca. 1996. *Kids Having Kids: A Robin Hood Foundation Special Report on the Costs of Adolescent Childbearing.* New York: Robin Hood Foundation.

Michael, Robert T., and Nancy Brandon Tuma. 1985. "Entry into Marriage and Parenthood by Young Men and Women: The Influence of Family Background." *Demography* 22(4): 515–44.

Patten, Marie 1981. "Self-Concept and Self-Esteem: Factors in Adolescent Pregnancy." *Adolescence* 16(64): 765–78.

Ribar, David. 1999. "The Socioeconomic Consequences of Young Women's Childbearing: Reconciling Disparate Evidence." *Journal of Population Economics* 12(4): 547–65.

U.S. Bureau of the Census. 1993. "Fertility of American Women 1992." Current Population Report P20-470. Washington, DC: U.S. Government Printing Office.

Vernon, Mary E. L., James A. Green, and Thomas E. Frothingham. 1983. "Teenage Pregnancy: A Prospective Study of Self-Esteem and Other Socio-Demographic Factors." *Pediatrics* 72(5): 632–35.

4

Costs and Consequences for the Fathers

Michael J. Brien and Robert J. Willis

EDITORS' NOTE

"Costs and Consequences for the Fathers" examines the impact of teen fatherhood or being the partner of a teen mother on a young man's education and earnings over the first 18 years following the birth of a child. Brien and Willis estimate that, holding marital status constant, a three-year delay in the mother's age at birth increases the present value of the father's earnings over the first 18 years by approximately $20,000–$25,000, depending on the particular race or marital status group. Building on their analysis, Maynard (1997) estimates that the fathers of the children of teen mothers earned $2,270 a year less than if the birth had been delayed to age 20 or older. These fathers also cost the public sector a total of $1.7 billion annually in lower taxes. Maynard's cost estimates in the earlier edition of Kids Having Kids *incorporated both the direct earnings effect of age delay and the indirect effect through a higher probability of marriage for older men.*

The original authors were unable to participate in the revision. Given the complexity of their analysis, it was impractical for another scholar to address this issue. As a result, this chapter has not been updated. It appears in its entirety here except for some minor text edits and the deletion of several figures that were not essential to the core argument. Further research on the economic impacts of early fatherhood, especially in the policy context of the mid-2000s, would be particularly valuable.

What are the consequences of young men entering fatherhood as teenagers or when their partners are teenagers?[1] This chapter addresses both parts of this question. Similar to the extensive literature on teen childbearing for young mothers, our first goal is to measure the impact of teen fatherhood on the father himself. In particular, we examine the role of teen childbearing on the education and skills he brings to the labor market and his subsequent earnings. Our second goal is to consider associated costs for the child and for the larger society.[2] Specifically, we measure the resources that could be provided by the fathers of children born to young mothers, constructing a profile of the potential support available to a child over his or her first 18 years of life. These two goals are interrelated since to quantify the resources available from a father, we must understand how men and their earnings, for example, are affected by the birth of a child.

Our overall aim is to determine the consequences of teen childbearing in both the short and the long term and to consider how these consequences interact with decisions about marriage and contributions of resources by both parents and by the state on behalf of the child. The first part of this chapter examines the consequences for men of having a child when they are teenagers. The second part is more from the mother's perspective and considers the resources potentially available from her partner and how these resources vary with the age a woman becomes a mother.

Consequences for Fathers

The substantive and measurement issues surrounding the implications of early fatherhood for the young man himself are analogous to those presented by Ellwood in "Teenage Unemployment: Permanent Scars or Temporary Blemishes?" (1982). In particular, he addresses a question of great importance to policymakers concerning which of two possible effects of early unemployment on the long-run economic capacities of young men is correct. The notion of permanent scars emphasizes the possibility that periods of unemployment during the critical early years in which youth accumulate large amounts of human capital may cause permanent damage to their lifetime career paths. The alternative notion of a blemish emphasizes that unemployment, however painful at the time, usually fades away and leaves no lasting effects. Consistent with the scar hypothesis, data in this area typically display a strong correlation between the current employment and earnings of men in their late 20s and their prior experience of unemployment during their teen years. However, as Ellwood correctly notes:

> The fundamental problem in capturing the long-term effects of unemployment is separating differences in employment and wages, which are causally related to early unemployment, from the differences due to unobserved personal characteristics correlated with early unemployment. (1982, p. 439)

In contrast to earlier studies, Ellwood finds that some scar effects exist but, when unobserved individual differences are controlled for, are much smaller than uncontrolled estimates would indicate.

The issues raised by Ellwood for teen unemployment can be applied to teenage fatherhood, although with some new and interesting aspects. As in teen unemployment, teen childbearing might impose either a short-term blemish or a long-term scar. Further, it is important to distinguish causal links from simple correlations between (observed and unobserved) personal characteristics and the likelihood of the event. But, unlike unemployment, which is typically temporary, the birth of a child typically has long-term, irreversible consequences for the custodial parent or parents.

"What If" Questions

To make the concept of the private costs of teen fatherhood more precise, it is useful to begin with carefully posed counterfactual questions. The first question we address is what the consequences are if a man delays the transition into fatherhood by one year. The effect of delaying fatherhood from, say, age 16 to age 21 can then be calculated as the cumulative effect of five one-year delays.

The basic idea behind this approach is illustrated in figure 4.1. The vertical axis measures the expected present discounted value of the lifetime earnings of three youth, A, B, and C, who differ in "economic potential." The horizontal axis measures the age at which a young man fathers his first child, marries the mother, and assumes the status of family breadwinner. Consider first the youth B curve, corresponding to a youth with average potential. The inverse-U shape of the curve reflects the net outcome of two countervailing forces, one associated with optimal human capital investment in education and postschool training and the other with the benefits of marriage for male earnings—the "marriage premium" found in several studies (Daniel 1993; Korenman and Neumark 1991).

Figure 4.1. Fatherhood and Human Capital

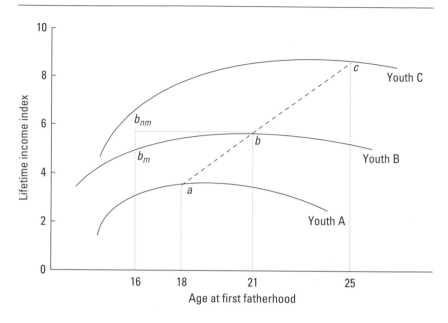

Initially, the lifetime earnings of youth B will increase by delaying marriage and fatherhood. Presumably this is because as a single person, responsible only for himself, he will be able to complete the optimal amount of schooling, participate in postschool training or apprenticeship programs, and find a job that is a good match given his skills, training, and interests. At some point, when he has completed his schooling and has found a "career job," additional delay of family responsibilities offers no further benefits to his economic prospects. Indeed, as noted above, family responsibilities are likely to provide a married man with greater incentives for economic success; additionally, his earnings potential may benefit from the household division of labor afforded by marriage. Thus, for youth B, delay of marriage and fatherhood past age 21 would be detrimental to the value of his lifetime earnings as seen by the declining portion of the curve. The other two curves represent the similarly shaped corresponding curves for youth with low and high economic potential, whose lifetime earnings are maximized when family responsibilities are delayed until age 18 and age 25, respectively.

For simplicity, assume that the optimal age of marriage and first fatherhood for a young man of a particular economic potential is given by the age at which the corresponding present value curve reaches a maximum.[3] Thus, a youth who chooses to have a child and assume family responsibilities (or has a "shotgun wedding") at an age earlier than this optimal age forgoes additional lifetime earnings, an effect analogous to Ellwood's scar effect. The magnitude of the cost of becoming a teenage father at, say, age 16 is given by the difference between the height of the lifetime earnings curve at age 16, denoted by b_m, and the height of the curve at the optimal age, denoted by b_{nm}. In addition, the marginal value of delaying fatherhood by one year is given by the difference between the height of the curve at ages 16 and 17.

The curves for youths A, B, and C are drawn under the assumption that higher long-run economic potential is correlated with higher marginal returns to delaying fatherhood. This assumption implies that if young men time marriage and fatherhood optimally, youth with higher potential will delay fatherhood longer, and that the cost of early fatherhood is higher the greater the economic potential of the youth. The empirical relationship between age of fatherhood and lifetime income in this model is given by the dashed line abc in figure 4.1, which connects the points corresponding to the optimal choices made by A, B, and C, respectively. This dashed line greatly overstates the scarring effect of early fatherhood because it fails to control for the economic potential of the youth.[4]

The theory suggests two things for our empirical work. First, controlling for differences in the economic potential of men is extremely important in isolating the impact that entering fatherhood at a nonoptimal age has on the realization of their potential. Second, factors must exist that would cause young men with a given level of economic potential to make different choices so, after controlling for potential, the observed variations in age at first fatherhood and long-run outcomes (e.g., education, occupation, midcareer earnings) trace out a given curve. A number of sources of "chance variation" in age of first fatherhood that are found among the many nonmonetary elements of the "mating game" may lead a man to become a father at an age different from the age that would maximize his net lifetime income. Examples include romantic love, sexual desire, difficulties in finding and attracting a girlfriend, and "accidental" pregnancies.

We assume that the variations in age at first fatherhood remaining after controlling for variables associated with a young man's economic potential reflect the chance outcomes of nonmonetary factors uncorrelated with his economic potential. Given this assumption, estimates of the effect that variation in age at first fatherhood has on long-run outcome variables, controlling for economic potential, identify the scarring effects of early fatherhood. However, the underlying theory itself implies that this assumption is likely to be completely correct. For example, the cost to a 16-year-old male of impregnating his girlfriend is much greater for a young man with high potential (e.g., youth C) than it is for a person with lower potential (e.g., youth A). Even though both A and C have an incentive to avoid conception, the higher cost of an "accident" to C suggests that he would be more apt to reduce the likelihood of an accident. Thus, even if all unwed conceptions were unintended, the observed relationship between age of fatherhood and outcome variables may be biased because men with higher economic potential would be less likely to have accidents. Our hope is that the observable variables we use to control for a young man's economic potential are strong enough (i.e., account for a sufficiently large portion of the true variance in the economic benefits of delaying fatherhood) to eliminate most of this bias.[5]

To this point, we have focused on the counterfactual question, "What is the consequence for a male of delaying his transition into fatherhood from age X to age X + 1?" In asking this question, we have implicitly assumed that fatherhood and marriage are inextricably linked. We now wish to relax this assumption and consider how the answer to the question may depend on marriage and child support decisions.

The theoretical framework represented in figure 4.1 can be extended to deal with marital and child support decisions associated with fatherhood. We consider two alternatives to the fatherhood/marriage case considered above. First, youth B fathers a child at age 16, but instead of marrying the mother and becoming a breadwinner, he "walks away" and provides no support for the child; indeed, his paternity is never legally established.[6] In this case, assuming that he makes no further "mistakes," he may continue on his optimal path and delay marriage and fathering additional children until the optimal age. His level of lifetime earnings is depicted by point b_{nm} if he walks away. Compared with a decision to marry, the youth benefits from higher lifetime earnings, and society benefits from the additional income taxes he will pay based on his higher earnings. However, the mother and child are deprived of the resources he would have contributed to the family. If the mother's resources (including any resources made available by the mother's family) are insufficient, society will bear the costs of providing support for the child through Aid to Families with Dependent Children (AFDC). In this scenario, an implicit transfer takes place from the rest of the society to the teen father—who bears no cost for his actions, not even a temporary blemish.

As a second case, a father whose paternity is established chooses not to marry the mother of the child. The costs to him as well as to others depend on the level of support he provides to the child. He may, for example, choose to provide an amount equivalent to the married father, although there are theoretical reasons (Weiss and Willis 1985) and much empirical evidence (e.g., Weiss and Willis 1993) to expect a nonresident father to provide considerably less. If the father pays significant child support, he may have to forgo continued schooling or training opportunities similar to those depicted for married fathers in figure 4.1.

The underlying reason for such scar effects is an imperfection in the credit market, whereby a young man who has an immediate need for cash to help support a family is prevented from borrowing against his future earnings and continuing to follow an optimal pattern of investment in schooling and training that would carry him to the peak of his present value curve in figure 4.1. Of course, if the youth comes from a prosperous background, his family may provide the needed resources so the boy "does right" by the mother and child without handicapping his own career. Additionally, if the boy's parents know they will get stuck with the bill, they have a strong incentive to exercise paternal power to reduce their chance of becoming premature grandparents. Conversely, the options of cushioning the effects of teen fatherhood and of his family's incentives to prevent it happening are both greatly reduced for youth from poor backgrounds. Of course, when they care about their son's futures, rich and poor parents alike are motivated to try to keep their teenage sons from becoming fathers if that would disrupt their careers.

The Data

The primary dataset for this analysis is the National Longitudinal Survey of Youth (NLSY). The NLSY is a nationally representative sample of 12,686 young men and women of all races who were age 14–21 in 1979.[7] Individuals were surveyed each year from 1979 until the latest wave in 1992. Overall, these data provide detailed information for a large number of respondents on various topics. Relevant to the issues examined in this chapter, the NLSY allows us to construct childbearing and marriage histories for numerous male respondents. Educational achievement, employment status, measures of labor supply and income, and a large number of background variables are also available. Also important, the NLSY includes the respondent's score on a standardized aptitude test, the Armed Forces Qualifying Test (AFQT).

Although the NLSY is one of the best available datasets for studying the impact of teenage fatherhood, it has weaknesses. Perhaps the most important drawback of any survey data on fatherhood is the strong likelihood that men will fail to report some of the children they father.[8] This problem can be severe for males who become fathers when they are young and unwed and are less likely to have contact with the child. A strength of the NLSY is, however, that starting from relatively young ages men are asked about their childbearing behavior. This feature of the data implies that we need not rely solely on retrospective fertility histories and birth reporting that might be influenced by whether the father has remained in contact with the child.

Efforts have been made to examine the validity of the male fertility reports in the NLSY. Mott (1985) compares the fertility behavior of the male respondents of the NLSY to a comparable cohort of males in the U.S. Vital Statistics.[9] His results suggest that males of all races, age 20–24 in the NLSY, underreport births by 15 percent. For black males, the underreporting grows to 23 percent. This drawback is clearly a problem in any attempt to assess the impact of having a child on the father . The men who do not report the birth are most likely those who completely walk away from the parenting responsibility and who therefore suffer little consequence of their parental status. This bias should be kept in mind in any interpretation of the results presented in this chapter. For our analysis, we use the fertility and marriage histories constructed by the Center for Human Resource Research. Technical reports suggest that the procedures used in constructing these variables greatly reduced the number of discrepancies in these histories (see, for example, Mott 1983).

In addition to marriage and fertility histories, a number of outcome and control variables are constructed (table 4.1). To capture the notion of long-run outcomes, we want to measure the outcomes as far into the future as possible. To construct a consistent measure for all NLSY respondents, the status of the individual at age 27 (the latest available age for all cohorts in the NLSY) is chosen for examination.[10] The associated value of human capital, labor supply, and earnings measures are considered at this age. The total number of years of education is used as a measure of the

Table 4.1. Outcome and Control Variables

Age 27 outcomes
Years of education
Census occupational income
Actual annual income
Hours worked in calendar year
Control variables
Marital status
Living arrangement status at age 14 (father/mother, mother only)
Mother's education
Father's education
Magazines in home at age 14
Newspapers in home at age 14
Library card in home at age 14
Lived in urban area at age 14
Race (Hispanic, black)
Armed Forces Qualifying Test score
Religion in which respondent was raised (none, Protestant, Catholic, Jewish)

Source: National Longitudinal Survey of Youth.

level of human capital; the total number of hours worked in the calendar year is constructed as a measure of labor supply.

Individual income, the closest indicator of the potential resources the father could provide to the child, is considered in two ways. The first and most basic is actual income at age 27. This measure, however, has a drawback. Although we are choosing to evaluate all individuals at one age, they may be at different points in their life cycles. Individuals who choose high levels of schooling or career paths that require considerable training may not have yet achieved the income benefits associated with their chosen occupations. For example, a plumber with a high school education may have been working in his profession for 5 to 10 years by age 27, whereas a newly graduated lawyer might be just starting his first job at age 27. Although their earnings at this age may be similar, their long-run earnings prospects are probably very different. To get around these problems, we also consider the occupations chosen at age 27. To measure long-run or permanent income, we attach to this occupation the mean income recorded, by race and education, in the 1990 U.S. Census for a cohort of men slightly older than those found in the NLSY. We refer to this measure as census income.

The control variables used in the analysis are also shown in table 4.1. Our choices are indicated by a desire to include variables that can be considered independent of the behaviors being examined. These variables are the race of the respondent, the education of the respondent's parents, the living arrangements at age 14 (residing with mother only, urban residence, and the learning environment in the home), and the religion in which the respondent was raised. Finally, as a measure of ability, we include the respondent's normalized AFQT score.[11]

To construct a sample for our analysis, we need to restrict the data. The largest restriction is exclusion of the military sample and the supplemental sample of economically disadvantaged, nonblack non-Hispanics (824 and 742 respondents, respectively). Our primary motivation for exclusion is our focus on long-run outcomes: both samples were dropped from the survey before the most recent wave of data and therefore provided insufficient long-run information.[12] Similarly, we exclude respondents who dropped out of the sample before age 27 or did not provide information in the surveys around their 27th year. We also exclude the few individuals who did not provide the appropriate data for constructing marriage and fertility histories. Finally, respondents who did not take the AFQT are also dropped (221 respondents after the other restrictions were imposed). The final analysis includes 4,231 male respondents.[13]

Basic statistics on marriage and childbearing (table 4.2) show that 64 percent of the men report having a first marriage before the 1992 survey. The average age at first marriage is 24. Clearly evident in this table are the racial differences in marriage behavior that have been found in other data. A smaller proportion of blacks reports having a first marriage, and their average age at first marriage is higher. Approximately 60 percent of the respondents have at least one birth. The average age at first birth is virtually identical to the average age at first marriage, suggesting a close relationship. The racial pattern, while still apparent in the fertility behavior, reverses. A higher percentage of blacks reports having a birth, and the difference between blacks and whites in the age at first birth is over two years.

Statistics on the relationship between marital status and fertility show that most first births occur to men who are married (table 4.3).[14] Most first pregnancies, however, are caused by men before their first marriages. Examining these numbers within races reveals large differences between blacks and the other two groups. Blacks are much more likely to have their first birth before their first marriage. Although nonmarital childbearing is

Table 4.2. Summary Statistics on Marriage and Fertility by Race

	White	Black	Hispanic	Total
Living arrangements				
Percentage reporting first marriage	72.5	48.0	68.4	64.3
Average age at first marriage (years)	23.9	24.4	23.2	23.9
Fertility				
Percentage reporting first birth	54.4	65.2	66.0	59.8
Average age at first birth (years)	25.0	22.7	23.5	24.0
Sample size	2,149	1,285	797	4,231

Source: National Longitudinal Survey of Youth.

less common for white and Hispanic men, it still composes, respectively, 13.4 percent and 30.2 percent of first births. Comparing the status at the time of each event, we see for all groups a movement to marriage when the man's partner becomes pregnant. For example, the percentage of white respondents who were never married moved from 33.9 to 13.4 in the time between conception and birth.

As an alternative way of examining the dynamic nature of these decisions, we consider the waiting time to marriage and the waiting time to the first birth, both before and after marriage. Approximately 50 percent of the white and Hispanic samples had a first marriage by age 26. At all ages, a substantially lower proportion of blacks has had a first marriage. By age 30, for example, slightly more than 50 percent of white males have

Table 4.3. Marital Status at Time of First Birth and at First Pregnancy by Race

	White	Black	Hispanic	Total
First pregnancy (percent)				
Never married	33.9	81.0	52.9	53.4
Married +	66.1	19.0	47.1	46.8
First birth (percent)				
Never married	13.4	71.5	30.2	36.1
Married +	86.6	28.5	69.8	63.9
Sample size	1,168	838	526	2,532

Source: National Longitudinal Survey of Youth.

Note: "Married +" denotes that the event occurred after the date of the first marriage.

experienced a first birth, the vast majority of which occurred within marriage. Also clearly evident are the racial differences in nonmarital childbearing, with a much higher percentage of births to blacks occurring outside marriage.

Effect of Fatherhood on a Male's Economic Well-Being

This section examines a major focus of this chapter: how the economic well-being of young men is affected by the birth of a child. We want to determine how strongly the age of entry into fatherhood and marital status at that time is associated with a young man's economic well-being.[15] We argued above that entry into fatherhood may have a scarring effect on a man if it causes him to assume responsibility for a family before he can complete his schooling and find a stable job. Conversely, if the young man can father a child outside marriage and escape the burden of marriage or child support payments, fatherhood may have no effect on his educational attainment or postschool investment in human capital. Before we discuss the long-run economic well-being of these young men, we briefly consider the evolution of education, earnings, and hours of work over their life paths.

Patterns over Men's Life Cycles

An examination of mean outcomes by age for men who had their first child before age 20, had a child after age 20 but before the end of the NLSY sample period, or were childless by the end of the survey period showed that men who wait to have a child have higher levels of education, higher incomes, and work more hours by the time they reach their late 20s (for details, see the 1997 edition of this book).[16] Except for education, however, this pattern differs across the life cycle. Men who have children at young ages appear briefly to have higher incomes and work more hours than the other fathers but then have lower earnings and hours at later ages. This evidence is consistent with the argument that childbearing has affected these men by forcing them into the labor market earlier than would have been optimal. But the age pattern is also consistent with the argument that men who are more attached to the labor market, and perhaps more prepared to have a child, begin childbearing earlier. The regression analysis presented below attempts to disentangle the direction of causation.

The same age patterns were observed for men who have had a child, broken down by whether the man was married at the time of the birth of the child. The education findings show the widest range for men who were married at the time their child was born. Married men who were teen fathers have the least schooling of all groups. Married men who delayed fatherhood until after their teen years have the most schooling of all. For men who are unmarried at the birth, the age at which they begin child-bearing has a relatively modest impact on their years of schooling. For earnings and hours worked, men who are married at the birth generally do better than fathers of the same age who are not. As with the previous analysis, this evidence is subject to several interpretations.

Impact of Age at First Fatherhood on Age 27 Outcomes

To address these and other issues more formally, we estimate a series of equations that relate four outcome variables evaluated at age 27 to variables that measure the age at which the individual transitions into fatherhood, controlling for numerous observed characteristics available in the survey. The outcomes of interest are education, census income (which is a measure of the occupational income attained in his chosen career), actual earnings, and hours worked.[17] Special attention is given to disentangling whether teen fatherhood scars a young man and hurts his economic prospects from whether men with poor long-run prospects in any case become teen fathers. The question, in other words, is which way the causation runs. The issue is especially critical in view of our theoretical expectation that the costs of teenage fatherhood will be lower for men with lower potential.[18]

We assume that, in general, most men do not make "mistakes." They choose to marry and to become fathers largely in terms of what is in their best interests. This is of course conditional on their abilities to find a mate in the marriage market, their returns from investments in education and postschool training, and the constraints that marriage and fatherhood may impose on their capacity to make human capital investments. On this assumption, the statistical relationship between the age of first fatherhood and the age 27 outcomes can be depicted in a series of figures.[19] We generally see a positive relationship between the age at first fatherhood and each of the four outcome variables. This pattern reflects the age-specific means for several broad groups of age-at-fatherhood categories.

We still need to address the counterfactual question posed earlier: "What effect would assuming the responsibilities of fatherhood at age x have on a young man's long-run well-being, relative to delaying fatherhood to age x^*, where x^* is the optimal age at first fatherhood?" The reason is that, since these regressions approximate the relationship between economic well-being and x^*, the slope of the relationship may only reflect the correlation between a man's potential returns from human capital and x^*. The positive relationship between age at first birth and various outcomes may show only that men with high potential have an incentive to delay fatherhood.

If so, controlling for variables that influence this age (such as ability) should reduce the strength of the relationship between outcomes at age 27 and age at first conception. We examine this possibility by controlling for the person's age-standardized AFQT score and family background measures listed in table 4.1.[20] As expected, the controls flatten the age profiles described above—a result that holds true for each outcome considered and for each racial group. Consider, for example, the regression results for education at age 27. For a typical nonblack male, delaying fatherhood from age 17 to age 21 would, without controls, result in a 0.8 year increase in years of schooling. With controls, this gap is cut by more than half, dropping to about 0.3 years. For blacks, a comparable delay in fatherhood is estimated to be 0.2 years without controls and is virtually eliminated when controls are added.

If a young man fathers a child but is able to escape responsibility for support of that child, theory and common sense both suggest that he will be able to carry out his optimal human capital investment program just as he would if he had not become a father. Conversely, if society (or his own conscience) forces the young man to assume responsibility, either by marrying the mother or by providing child support payments to her, his optimal program will be interrupted and he will incur the cost of lower attainment. We investigate these issues by adding controls for whether the man was married at the time of the conception.[21] The analysis allows for an interaction between the male's age and marital status at conception to capture whether the consequences of assuming responsibility are greater at younger ages (e.g., dropping out of school) than at older ages.

The difference in outcomes between men who were married and unmarried at the time of first conception is given by the entries labeled "no controls" in figures 4.2 through 4.5; the net effect after controlling for background characteristics are represented by the entries labeled "all

Figure 4.2. Effect of Marriage and Parenthood on Educational Attainment at Age 27 by First Fatherhood

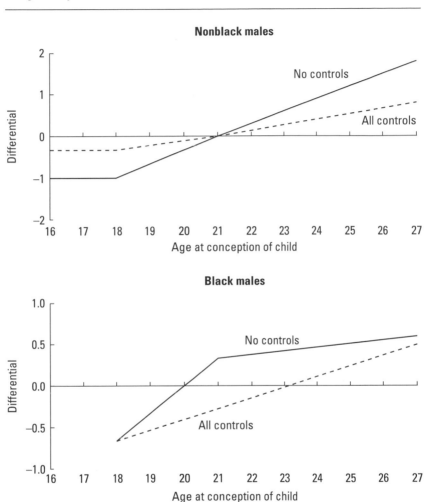

controls." For education, we see that unmarried men who become fathers before age 18 have substantially more education at age 27 than those who are married at the time they become fathers (figure 4.2). At later ages, however, education is not at all sensitive to marital status, as seen by the convergence of the values for married and unmarried men. This evidence is consistent with the hypothesis that young fathers who conceive a child outside marriage escape a rather substantial penalty for a forced marriage.

Figure 4.3. Effect of Marriage and Parenthood on Occupational Status
(Census Earnings) at Age 27 by First Fatherhood

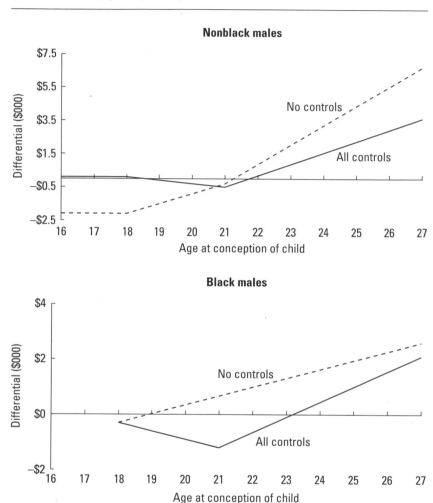

Results for the other outcome variables are less clear cut but basically
consistent with this interpretation. On the census earnings measure, the
same pattern occurs as for education, but it is less pronounced (figure
4.3). For actual earnings at age 27, men who are married at the time their
first child is conceived always earn more than men who are not married
at the same age (figure 4.4). In part, this may result from the greater

Figure 4.4. Effect of Marriage and Parenthood on Own Earnings at Age 27 by First Fatherhood

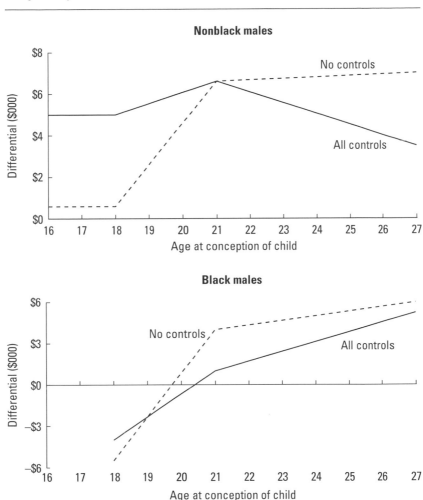

number of hours worked at age 27 by men who were married before age 18 (figure 4.5). But few men fall into this category.

One could object to the above interpretation on the grounds that a man's decision to marry is not independent of his own characteristics and depends, rather, on the magnitude of the loss the man would incur if he were forced to bear responsibility for the child. Thus, as discussed

Figure 4.5. Effect of Marriage and Parenthood on Annual Hours of Work at Age 27 by First Fatherhood

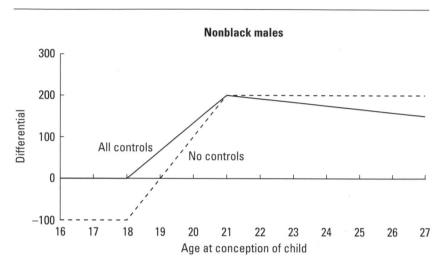

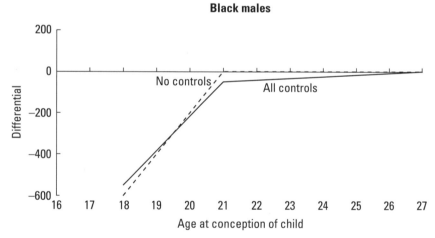

above, the optimal age of first fatherhood for the men who choose to marry and father children at an early age may be lower than for those who father children early and fail to marry. If this is true, the results described above may overstate the magnitude of the penalty for a marriage at time of the conception.

We gauge the likely severity of this problem by using the same control variables described above (i.e., AFQT and background variables).[22] The difference in predicted attainment by marital status of fathers of a given age, holding these controls constant, is given by the curves marked "all controls" in figures 4.2–4.5. In general, we see that perhaps half the estimated effect of early fatherhood on education and census earnings remains after these controls are entered. The actual earnings at age 27 of men who were married when their first child was conceived are still substantially larger than earnings of men who were not married. Indeed, the pattern becomes less irregular when the controls are imposed. This is partly explained by higher hours worked by married fathers. A more complete explanation might be the existence of a "marriage premium," although the fact that the effect of marriage is larger on actual hours at age 27 than on census earnings suggests that the higher earnings of married men may simply reflect greater effort.

To assess the effect of being married at the time of the pregnancy and the impact of the controls used, we examine whether the outcomes for the married and the unmarried groups are statistically different at ages 18, 21, and 27.[23] Outcomes reported in table 4.4 can be used to judge whether the predicted plots in figures 4.2–4.5 differ significantly.[24] For nonblacks and without controls, the effect of marital status is occasionally significant for each outcome at some ages. Adding the controls dampens the significance of the effect. For blacks, marital status appears generally insignificant.

Costs to the Child and Society

The most fundamental problem in calculating the cost of adolescent childbearing to the youth and to society is finding the fathers of the children born to teen mothers. Databases containing information on fathers provide little information on the mother if the father and mother do not live together (or later split up). Similarly, databases on teen motherhood with female respondents generally have no information about the potential resources of the father if the mother and father do not live together. Using data on the mothers and fathers available in the National Maternal and Infant Health Survey (NMIHS) we develop a "statistical matching" procedure. This enables us to estimate components of the costs of teenage parenthood for highly policy-relevant cases in which the mother and father never live with one another or split up some time following the birth of their child.

As an example of this procedure, consider a single mother who bears a child and never lives with the father. Although we do not know the

Table 4.4. Significance of Marital Status at Various Ages
of First Conception

	Age 18	Age 21	Age 27
Nonblack			
Education at age 27			
No controls	**	n.s.	***
Controls	n.s.	n.s.*	***
Census earnings at age 27			
No controls	n.s.	n.s.	***
Controls	n.s.	n.s.	**
Actual earnings at age 27			
No controls	n.s.	***	**
Controls	n.s.	***	n.s.
Annual hours at age 27			
No controls	n.s.	**	n.s.
Controls	n.s.	n.s.	n.s.
Black			
Education at age 27			
No controls		n.s.	n.s.
Controls		n.s.	n.s.
Census earnings at age 27			
No controls		n.s.	n.s.
Controls		n.s.	n.s.
Actual earnings at age 27			
No controls		n.s.	**
Controls		n.s.	*
Annual hours at age 27			
No controls		n.s.	n.s.
Controls		n.s.	n.s.

Source: National Longitudinal Survey of Youth.

Note: Full regression results are available from the authors.

n.s. = nonsignificant

*significant at the .10 level; **significant at the .05 level; ***significant at the .01 level

father's age, education, or income, we may use information from the NMIHS to calculate probabilities that the father was of a given age and educational attainment.[25] From the NLSY, we predict the expected earnings and number of children for fathers in each age and education class in each year of the child's life. We also estimate the number of children a man may have, since child support formulas are based on the number of dependents. Multiplying these estimates by the associated probability that the father was in a given class yields an estimate of the expected earnings potential of the child's father. Application of the relevant child support formula to each earnings projection yields an estimate of the expected child support payments that would be forthcoming under an ideal system of paternity establishment and child support enforcement.[26]

Policy Considerations

Implementation of the Family Support Act of 1988 has strong and interesting policy implications for the costs of teen fatherhood and their distribution among the father, the mother and child, and the rest of society. Specifically, the act mandates that each state develop a child support formula to determine the minimum support a father must pay as a function of his own income and, in some states, the income of the custodial mother. These formulas apply to fathers of children born out of wedlock as well as to divorced fathers. In addition, the act emphasizes the importance of establishing paternity for all children, regardless of the marital status of the parents at the time of the child's birth, and provides extensive (and potentially expensive) enforcement machinery to ensure that the father pays child support until the child reaches age 18. Beginning in 1994, the enforcement provisions mandate wage withholding for all child support orders.

As a concrete example of the implication of the new laws if perfectly enforced, consider a high school senior living in Wisconsin who becomes an unwed father. If the state establishes his legal paternity and applies the Wisconsin child support formula to him, he will be required to pay 17 percent of his income to the mother as child support. As long as he remains in school and has zero income, the boy owes nothing. During this period, if the mother has no family or personal resources to draw upon, the state will support the child by giving the mother AFDC transfers. Since fatherhood does not require the youth to come up with immediate cash, he will be able to continue on his optimal career path just as if paternity was never established. When he completes his education and begins earning income, however, he must begin paying child support.

We are now in a position to assess both the social and private costs of teenage fatherhood under the Wisconsin law, assuming a 10 percent interest rate. If the youth dropped out of school to earn cash when he became a father and earned $10,000 a year for the rest of his life, he would pay child support of $1,700 a year for the next 18 years. Wisconsin taxpayers, in turn, would pay $1,700 a year less in AFDC than they would if the father did not pay child support. But if the youth remained in school one more year and graduated, he could earn, say, $12,000 a year for the rest of his life—a marginal rate of return to school completion of 20 percent.[27] In this case, upon graduation, Wisconsin law would require him to pay $2,040 a year for the next 17 years. Thus, the state would pay $1,700 more in the first year of the child's life and $340 (= $2,040 − $1,700) less in the next 17 years than if the father had dropped out. The child support formula in combination with the AFDC program implicitly gives the state an "equity position" in the youth's human capital that provides the state with a rate of return approximately equal to the marginal rate of return on investment in the youth's human capital. If this rate of return exceeds the rate of interest faced by the state, the taxpayers will benefit by this policy, as will the youth. The next section describes the data and procedures used to build the statistical match of teen mothers and the fathers of the children involved. Readers interested in the findings more than the procedures used for the analysis may skip the next section.

Building a Statistical Match

The data used to provide the matching probabilities come from the NMIHS. This survey was administered to a sample of 9,953 women who gave birth in 1988, and it provides additional information to the data provided in basic vital statistics records. In general, what is needed for the analysis are data on the characteristics of both the mother and father, regardless of their marital status and living arrangement. Basic *Vital Statistics* data are not sufficient for our purpose because they underreport male characteristics. The NMIHS provides a chance to fill in data missing from the original birth certificate.

We first use the NLSY to examine the age distribution of the partners of mothers. As mentioned above, many partners of teen mothers are not teenagers themselves (table 4.5). For example, 3.4 percent of nonblack women who have a child when they are 16 years old or younger have a partner in the same age category. Many of these very young mothers, almost 40 percent, have a partner between the ages of 17 and 19; 31 percent have a partner between ages 20 and 21, and 26 percent have a partner age 22 or older. The data suggest a wider age distribution for nonblack

Table 4.5. Age Distribution of Fathers by Age of Mother

Father's race and age	Mother's Age			
	≤16	17–19	20–21	≥22
Nonblack				
≤16	0.034	0.000	0.000	0.000
17–19	0.392	0.177	0.038	0.000
20–21	0.312	0.248	0.164	0.000
≥22	0.262	0.575	0.797	1.000
Black				
<16	0.069	0.016	0.000	0.000
17–19	0.503	0.285	0.045	0.003
20–21	0.244	0.281	0.180	0.026
≥22	0.184	0.419	0.775	0.971

Source: National Longitudinal Survey of Youth.

women as evidenced by a larger fraction of partners in the highest age category. Very few women of either racial group have children with younger men.

For the statistical matching procedure, we break down the mother and father characteristics further. For women of a particular race and marital status that give birth at a given age, we calculate the probability that their partner will be in a particular age and education class.[28] These probabilities allow us to know the age, education, race, and marital status of the men with whom women, including teenage women, are having children. To calculate the potential child support payments that these men may be able to provide, we need information on both the income and the additional number of children the men will have over the life of the index child. For this information, we return to the NLSY. The primary advantage of the NLSY is that we are able to use the actual earnings of men who have had a child; this incorporates any effects that childbearing may have on the income of men.

For the purpose of the child support calculation, we assume that the man is responsible for the first 18 years of the child's life. The NLSY, however, is only a 14-year panel and cannot cover all years in which support would be necessary. This shortfall is true for both income and the number of children born to the men. We circumvent this problem by estimating predicting equations for both variables for all 18 years of the child's life.[29]

The coefficients on which the income and number of children predictions are based are presented in appendix tables B.4.1 and B.4.2, respectively.

These results indicate that the earnings of young, poorly educated fathers are extremely low at the time the child is born, but those at the median or above will experience considerable earnings growth during the next 18 years. The predicted earnings of men in the bottom quartile of the earnings distribution hover near zero for all men with less than high school educations, no matter how old they were when they became fathers.[30]

In addition to his earnings, a noncustodial father's child support obligation for his first child, as determined by the child support formula in his state of residence, generally depends on the number of other children he has fathered. For example, a young man of either racial group who is age 16 or younger when he fathers his first child is, on average, predicted to have more than one additional child by the time his first child reaches age 6 and almost two additional children before his first child reaches age 18. In contrast, a high school dropout in either racial group who delays entry into fatherhood until he is older than 21 is predicted, on average, to have less than 0.5 additional children by the time his first child reaches age 6. By the time the child is age 18, black men will have added about another 0.5 children and nonblacks only about 0.25 children. Although age at first fatherhood has a much stronger effect than educational attainment, the racial differential showing higher fertility for black than white males among the less educated is reversed among groups with some college or more education.

The next step is to calculate how much of the father's income will be devoted to child support. This will clearly vary by both personal preferences and state statutes. As a benchmark, we use the relatively straightforward child support formula mandated in Wisconsin. As described above, this standard requires that a father pay 17 percent of his income as child support for his first child. If the man has an additional child, the obligation to the first child drops to 12.5 percent of his income; with three children, this obligation is 9.7 percent; and with four children, it becomes 7.75 percent.[31] The amount a man would be obligated to pay in child support for his first child will grow as the child ages, largely because of growth in the man's earnings capacity. Nonblack fathers will typically owe more support for their first child than do black fathers. For less-educated men, these racial differences in child support obligations largely reflect racial differences in fertility. For better-educated men, the reduction in obligation to their first child caused by the higher fertility of nonblack men is more than offset by the increase in the obligation caused by their higher predicted earnings.

The final component of the calculation is to estimate the amount of child support owed by a man who fathers a child by a woman of a given age. As described above, since we do not know the characteristics of the fathers of children born out of wedlock, we must use a statistical matching procedure for our estimates. Thus, we multiply the predicted child support obligations of men of each age, race, education, and marital status by the probability that a man of each type fathered a child by a woman of a given age, and we sum these products across all types of men.

Potential Child Support

The findings from our child support analysis are presented in table 4.6. This table first shows, for women who begin childbearing at different ages, the discounted present value of the predicted partner's income over the first 18 years of the child's life. All the calculations in this table are repeated for male earnings evaluated at the 25th, 50th, and 75th percentiles and are done separately by marital status and race. For a single nonblack woman who has a child at 16 years old, for example, the estimates of the discounted present value of her partner's income over 18 years range from $81,624 for a partner in the 25th percentile to $294,231 for a partner in the 75th percentile.

Let us look in detail at the possibilities for a single nonblack woman who has a child at 17 years old by a man with income at the median (50th percentile). Her partner's predicted income over 18 years is $199,990. As a result of her delaying the birth one year, her partner's income increases 2.2 percent. If the woman delays childbearing until after she is 22 years old, that income increases 13 percent, to $221,943. Consistent with the evidence presented earlier, for each age of the mother, the predicted partner's income is higher for nonblack than for black and for married than for single women.

The potential child support payment the partner could provide under the Wisconsin standards for the predicted number of children (see previous section) appears directly below the predicted income in table 4.6. A 16-year-old single nonblack woman, for example, can look forward to $25,942 in child support. In comparison, her black counterpart would be owed $21,362. If the birth is delayed by a year, the predicted discounted

Table 4.6. Estimated Present Value of Father's Total Earnings and Child Support Over 18 Years, by Age of the Woman (dollars)

				Age of the Woman			
	≤15	16	17	18	19	20–21	≥22
				Single at Time of Birth			
Nonblack							
25th percentile							
Estimated income		81,624	86,095	93,268	95,876	100,885	106,700
Child support		10,773	11,417	12,406	12,798	13,479	14,193
Monthly child support		77	81	88	91	96	101
Median							
Estimated income		195,659	199,990	207,209	209,997	215,308	221,943
Child support		25,942	26,652	27,703	28,190	28,956	29,876
Monthly child support		185	190	197	201	206	213
75th percentile							
Estimated income		294,231	299,807	308,913	312,831	320,375	332,033
Child support		39,301	40,238	41,574	42,261	43,339	44,920
Monthly child support		280	287	296	301	309	320
Black							
25th percentile							
Estimated income	58,148	65,492	69,294	72,287	75,079	83,965	76,058
Child support	7,868	8,952	9,578	10,102	10,603	12,054	10,989
Monthly child support	56	64	68	72	76	86	78

Median							
Estimated income	147,164	156,078	162,099	166,987	171,987	182,721	179,907
Child support	19,887	21,362	22,440	23,358	24,186	26,244	26,075
Monthly child support	142	152	160	167	172	187	186
75th percentile							
Estimated income	247,979	257,001	264,851	271,279	276,405	289,217	288,545
Child support	33,557	35,196	36,680	37,946	39,008	41,513	41,827
Monthly child support	239	251	261	271	278	296	298

Married at Time of Birth

Nonblack							
25th percentile							
Estimated income		158,033	178,951	189,491	189,222	191,331	171,532
Child support		22,618	23,897	25,167	25,153	25,423	23,086
Monthly child support		161	170	179	179	181	165
Median							
Estimated income		265,340	275,587	286,248	286,300	288,840	269,443
Child support		35,816	36,899	38,114	38,160	38,500	36,402
Monthly child support		255	263	272	272	274	260
75th percentile							
Estimated income		358,396	370,788	38,110	384,362	388,039	365,729
Child support		48,547	49,796	51,271	51,359	51,843	49,546
Monthly child support		346	355	366	366	370	353

(continued)

Table 4.6. *(Continued)*

				Age of the Woman			
	≤15	16	17	18	19	20–21	≥22
Black							
25th percentile							
Estimated income	140,415	128,798	163,131	152,569	167,535	167,038	140,843
Child support	20,044	17,846	23,639	21,951	24,393	24,375	20,786
Monthly child support	143	127	169	156	174	174	148
Median							
Estimated income	229,578	211,420	252,949	242,633	257,770	257,885	239,155
Child support	32,475	28,993	36,483	34,700	37,373	37,471	35,040
Monthly child support	232	207	260	247	266	267	250
75th percentile							
Estimated income	315,180	290,967	336,931	327,819	341,549	341,773	326,713
Child support	44,642	39,998	48,655	46,949	49,584	49,729	47,986
Monthly child support	318	285	347	335	353	355	342

Source: National Longitudinal Survey of Youth.

Note: All values are in 1994 dollars.

present value of support payments increases by approximately 2.7 percent for a nonblack woman and by 5.0 percent for a black woman. In general, the value of the support always increases with the age of the woman and is, again, higher for nonblack than black and for married than single women.[32]

We next consider the impact of early childbearing on society as a whole. Would the predicted child support be enough to offset public expenditures on behalf of the child? Expressing the child support payment as a monthly flow is convenient for this purpose. This is shown immediately below the child support totals.[33] The child support potentially available to the single nonblack woman who has a child at age 16 is equivalent to a monthly payment of $185. Similarly, the $21,362 child support obligation for a single, black 16-year-old is equivalent to a monthly payment of $152. The monthly payment, of course, varies with maternal characteristics in the same way as the lump-sum payment.

How do these estimates compare with the government transfers received by a comparable woman? As an illustration, consider a woman with one child in Wisconsin. In 1994, the maximum AFDC benefit available in this state to a woman with one child was $440 a month. The predicted child support obligation of the partner of a hypothetical single 16-year-old mother represents 42 percent or 35 percent of the welfare benefit value, respectively, for a nonblack or black woman. By law, additional payments by the father can only increase the mother's income by $50 a month, with the remaining payments going to reduce AFDC payments received by the mother. In this case, if child support laws were perfectly enforced, the taxpayers' burden would decrease from $440 a month to $305 a month, a 30 percent reduction. Wisconsin has relatively generous welfare benefits; in other states, the offset of public versus private expenditure might be even greater.

In reality, of course, perfect enforcement of the child support law is not possible. Enforcement is costly, and the revenue yields will never be as high as the perfect-enforcement results shown here. Considering the net effect on taxpayers' obligations is clearly one element in determining how strictly child support laws should be enforced. However, other factors should also be considered in developing child enforcement policies. One concerns whether society should force fathers to acknowledge paternity and bear economic responsibility for their children. On the negative side, strict enforcement may reduce the development of a young man's economic potential, although (as argued earlier) the combination of AFDC and a child support obligation proportional to the father's income may be less disruptive to his investment in human capital than a forced marriage. On the positive side, strict child support enforcement may change the perceptions of young men and young women concerning the costs of becoming parents and the benefits of doing so within marriage.[34]

Conclusion

Our research addresses the costs and consequences associated with young men entering fatherhood either when they are teenagers or when their partners are teenagers. Specifically, we examine the relationship between the age at which a man first becomes a father and his subsequent education, occupational status, earnings, and work effort. In general, early entry into fatherhood is associated with lower levels of schooling, lower actual occupational income, and fewer hours worked in the labor market. The impact of early fatherhood is dampened once the analysis includes control variables thought to be associated with these outcomes. One plausible explanation is that the impact of early childbearing is tied to the issue of whether the man takes responsibility for the child. As with Ellwood's (1982) study of early unemployment, we find little evidence of a lasting scar from this behavior.

We also address the issue of whether early childbearing implies lower levels of support for the female partner and the child. In terms of potential support for the child, the evidence indicates that there are gains to delayed childbearing. For a society as a whole, the support provided by men could amount to 40–50 percent of current AFDC benefits. While the partners of the women who become teen mothers may have little to provide in their early years, the evidence does suggest growth in their income and potential child support payments throughout the life of the child. This indicates that more rigorous paternity establishment and child support enforcement could provide gains to the child as well as to society.

Table A.4.1. Education at Age 27: Selected Regression Results

	Model 1	Model 2	Model 3	Model 4
	Nonblack			
Marital status				
Married at first pregnancy		−18.595		−16.930
		(−2.69)		(−2.366)
Age at first pregnancy (spline)				
Age < 18	0.065	0.039	−0.023	0.096
	(0.33)	(0.19)	(0.17)	(0.67)
18 ≤ age < 21	0.237	0.208	0.095	0.123
	(3.53)	(2.41)	(1.73)	(1.72)
Age ≥ 21	0.307	0.048	0.133	−0.006
	(8.94)	(0.70)	(5.00)	(−.13)
No child by age 27	−0.233	1.481	0.037	0.920
	(−1.23)	(3.87)	(0.26)	(3.25)
Marriage and age spline interactions				
Married * (age < 18)		0.990		0.936
		(2.51)		(2.32)
Married * (18 ≤ age < 21)		0.250		−0.006
		(1.65)		(−.05)
Married * (age ≥ 21)		0.292		0.167
		(3.71)		(2.76)
	Black			
Marital status				
Married at first pregnancy		−0.725		−0.660
		(−.89)		(−1.00)
Age at first pregnancy (spline)				
Age < 18	0.132	0.147	0.065	0.072
	(1.40)	(1.54)	(0.79)	(0.87)
18 ≤ age < 21	0.034	0.011	−0.034	−0.014
	(0.44)	(0.13)	(−.52)	(−.20)
Age ≥ 21	0.227	0.181	0.165	0.125
	(4.47)	(2.99)	(3.79)	(2.40)
No child by age 27	−0.617	−0.262	−0.436	−0.232
	(−2.19)	(−.76)	(−1.82)	(−.81)
Marriage and age spline interactions				
Married * (18 ≤ age < 21)		0.35		0.12
		(1.17)		(0.47)
Married * (age ≥ 21)		0.059		0.122
		(0.530)		(1.280)

Notes: The dependent variable is years of school at age 27. Models 3 and 4 also include a large number of other control variables. These variables are listed in table 4.1. Full estimates are available from the authors upon request. Regressions are based on 2.946 and 1.285 observations for nonblacks and blacks, respectively. Sample weights were used in the estimation and robust standard errors were obtained using Huber's formula: *t*-statistics in parentheses. See Huber (1967).

Table A.4.2. Census Earnings at Age 27: Selected Regression Results

	Model 1	Model 2	Model 3	Model 4
	Nonblack			
Marital status				
Married at first pregnancy		−21,559.650		−24,031.380
		(−1.00)		(−1.07)
Age at first pregnancy (spline)				
Age < 18	621.897	587.484	394.948	200.092
	(1.45)	(1.27)	(1.03)	(0.49)
18 ≤ age < 21	821.942	896.825	289.275	521.080
	(3.25)	(2.54)	(1.24)	(1.61)
Age ≥ 21	987.456	83.436	441.580	−0.877
	(5.47)	(0.28)	(2.79)	0.00
No child by age 27	−1,823.529	3,989.238	−1,119.857	1,529.068
	(−1.85)	(2.49)	(−1.29)	(1.18)
Marriage and age spline interactions				
Married * (age < 18)		1,112.936		1,374.643
		(0.91)		(1.08)
Married * (18 ≤ age < 21)		368.720		−451.617
		(0.68)		(−.87)
Married * (age ≥ 21)		1,042.181		551.720
		(2.85)		(1.77)
	Black			
Marital status				
Married at first pregnancy		−477.476		−768.523
		(−.17)		(−.37)
Age at first pregnancy (spline)				
Age < 18	503.172	505.852	252.386	243.989
	(1.95)	(1.96)	(0.98)	(0.93)
18 ≤ age < 21	60.187	65.162	−115.802	−18.059
	(0.27)	(0.27)	(−.53)	(−.08)
Age ≥ 21	455.765	292.723	265.526	103.258
	(2.93)	(1.54)	(1.96)	(0.63)
No child by age 27	−995.964	124.238	−671.896	188.254
	(−1.05)	(0.11)	(−.87)	(0.20)
Marriage and age spline interactions				
Married * (18 ≤ age < 21)		258.593		−127.390
		(0.23)		(−.15)
Married * (age ≥ 21)		343.438		506.381
		(1.01)		(1.71)

Notes: The dependent variable is census income at age 27. Models 3 and 4 also include a large number of other control variables. These variables are listed in table 4.1. Full estimates are available from the authors upon request. Regressions are based on 2.820 and 1.167 observations for nonblacks and blacks, respectively. Sample weights were used in the estimation and robust standard errors were obtained using Huber's formula: *t*-statistics in parentheses. See Huber (1967). Income is expressed in 1989 dollars. Coefficients can be converted to 1994 dollars by multiplying by 1.189.

Table A.4.3. Actual Income at Age 27: Selected Regression Results

	Model 1	Model 2	Model 3	Model 4
		Nonblack		
Marital status				
Married at first pregnancy		19,078.640		−6,478.391
		(0.41)		(−.15)
Age at first pregnancy (spline)				
Age < 18	2,204.551	2,374.723	2,088.098	1,872.698
	(1.96)	(1.98)	(1.99)	(1.68)
18 ≤ age < 21	646.660	−412.112	−60.724	−890.097
	(1.07)	(−.51)	(−.11)	(−1.18)
Age ≥ 21	427.693	87.333	−15.726	98.643
	(1.51)	(0.17)	(−.06)	(0.20)
No child by age 27	−2,741.079	2,697.334	−2,026.438	425.548
	(−2.14)	(1.05)	(−1.63)	(0.18)
Marriage and age spline interactions				
Married * (age < 18)		−1,037.208		595.275
		(−.38)		(0.23)
Married * (18 ≤ age < 21)		1,736.606		442.644
		(1.22)		(0.32)
Married * (age ≥ 21)		20.299		−465.640
		(0.03)		(−.79)
		Black		
Marital status				
Married at first pregnancy		−4,315.03		−3,525.62
		(−0.87)		(−0.73)
Age at first pregnancy (spline)				
Age < 18	595.223	697.873	291.673	350.993
	(0.80)	(0.94)	(0.42)	(0.50)
18 ≤ age < 21	443.770	210.342	186.966	146.495
	(0.93)	(0.41)	(0.39)	(0.29)
Age ≥ 21	674.211	346.591	438.007	129.531
	(1.99)	(0.83)	(1.32)	(0.31)
No child by age 27	−5,026.925	−2,268.286	−4,513.675	−2,346.787
	(−2.89)	(−1.04)	(−2.67)	(−1.09)
Marriage and age spline interactions				
Married * (18 ≤ age < 21)		2,625.642		1,472.658
		(1.33)		(0.75)
Married * (age ≥ 21)		296.854		577.849
		(0.40)		(0.77)

Notes: The dependent variable is actual income at age 27. Models 3 and 4 also include a large number of other control variables. These variables are listed in table 4.1. Full estimates are available from the authors upon request. Regressions are based on 2.915 and 1.276 observations for nonblack and black, respectively. Sample weights were used in the estimation and robust standard errors were obtained using Huber's formula: *t*-statistics in parentheses. See Huber (1957). Income is expressed in 1989 dollars. Coefficients can be converted to 1994 dollars by multiplying by 1.189.

Table A.4.4. Annual Hours Worked at Age 27: Selected Regression Results

	Model 1	Model 2	Model 3	Model 4
	Nonblack			
Constant	−233.628	−1,066.456	−192.919	−822.123
	(−0.14)	(−0.59)	(−0.12)	(−0.46)
Marital status				
Married at first pregnancy		7,010.816		5,854.366
		(1.49)		(1.15)
Age at first pregnancy (spline)				
Age < 18	128.620	177.783	123.873	160.317
	(1.33)	(1.72)	(1.30)	(1.57)
18 ≤ age < 21	−14.903	−66.255	−36.151	−75.426
	(−0.42)	(−1.47)	(−1.01)	(1.66)
Age ≥ 21	23.438	15.569	16.410	17.113
	(1.71)	(0.59)	(1.20)	(0.62)
No child by age 27	−201.627	−44.609	−184.972	−100.119
	(−3.16)	(−0.31)	(−2.91)	(−0.07)
Marriage and age spline interactions				
Married * (age < 18)		−400.712		−331.365
		(−1.51)		(−1.16)
Married * (18 ≤ age < 21)		132.254		91.172
		(1.73)		(1.17)
Married * (age ≥ 21)		−5.337		−12.228
		(−0.17)		(−0.38)
	Black			
Marital status				
Married at first pregnancy		−695.468		−605.687
		(−1.59)		(−1.45)
Age at first pregnancy (spline)				
Age < 18	78.265	90.922	57.271	67.588
	(1.22)	(1.41)	(0.90)	(1.06)
18 ≤ age < 21	7.880	−0.129	4.153	2.310
	(0.19)	(0.00)	(0.10)	(0.05)
Age ≥ 21	53.050	52.078	47.200	45.627
	(2.20)	(1.80)	(1.98)	(1.61)
No child by age 27	−380.080	−378.254	−365.606	−374.121
	(−3.05)	(−2.50)	(−3.00)	(2.57)
Marriage and age spline interactions				
Married * (18 ≤ age < 21)		234.833		178.173
		(1.39)		(1.07)
Married * (age ≥ 21)		−2.806		7.362
		(−0.05)		(0.14)

Notes: The dependent variable is actual income at age 27. Models 3 and 4 also include a large number of other control variables. These variables are listed in table 4.1. Full estimates are available from the authors upon request. Regressions are based on 2.923 and 1.281 observations for nonblacks and blacks, respectively. Sample weights were used in the estimation and robust standard errors were obtained using Huber's formula: *t*-statistics in parentheses. See Huber (1967).

Table B.4.1. Quantile Regressions on Actual Income

	Percentile		
	25th	50th	75th
	Nonblack		
Constant	−958.528	4,230.852	9,665.610
	(−0.64)	(2.98)	(5.11)
Age at first birth category (≤16 omitted)			
17–18 years	1,080.903	−1,152.605	−1,589.325
	(0.81)	(−0.93)	(−0.96)
19–21 years	1,764.431	556.763	880.624
	(1.35)	(0.46)	(0.54)
≥22 years	4,681.170	4,422.390	6,206.340
	(3.53)	(3.60)	(3.76)
Age of index child (spline)			
Age < 5	479.264	960.576	988.779
	(2.92)	(6.37)	(4.90)
5 ≤ age < 10	346.057	781.254	1,133.057
	(2.27)	(5.57)	(6.08)
Age ≥ 10	9.484	888.994	1,176.474
	(0.04)	(4.28)	(4.18)
Marital status			
Married at birth	6,272.695	7,874.055	8,879.320
	(8.65)	(11.86)	(10.26)
Married * age of child	−84.764	−433.597	−638.036
	(−0.80)	(−4.43)	(−4.88)
Education category (≤ high school omitted)			
High school	3,137.032	2,254.538	1,938.799
	(4.94)	(3.79)	(2.40)
Some college	5,092.462	5,872.028	4,321.340
	(5.43)	(7.00)	(3.87)
≥ college graduate	8,935.014	14,158.730	11,996.400
	(8.07)	(13.88)	(8.50)
Education and child age interactions			
(High school) * child age	418.523	512.092	606.623
	(4.30)	(5.65)	(4.99)
(Some college)* child age	501.173	437.196	1,030.257
	(2.90)	(2.95)	(5.34)
(≥ college graduate) * child age	1,547.378	911.014	2,197.360
	(6.55)	(4.22)	(7.20)
Pseudo R^2	0.1105	0.1201	0.1224

(continued)

Table B.4.1. *(Continued)*

	Percentile		
	25th	50th	75th
	Black		
Constant	−365.435	−121.420	5,697.708
	(−0.62)	(−0.14)	(4.96)
Age at first birth category (≤16 omitted)			
17–18 years	−3.396	652.634	−807.230
	(−0.01)	(0.99)	(−0.90)
19–21 years	−597.373	1,043.062	1,627.410
	(−1.36)	(1.58)	(1.82)
≥22 years	1,143.589	3,798.522	4,237.352
	(2.39)	(5.37)	(4.49)
Age of index child (spline)			
Age < 5	368.830	1,060.652	1,316.897
	(3.92)	(7.10)	(6.63)
5 ≤ age < 10	−64.581	810.727	1,131.259
	(−0.81)	(6.62)	(6.77)
Age ≥ 10	10.037	286.614	460.873
	(0.10)	(1.84)	(2.19)
Marital status			
Married at birth	7,057.966	5,606.883	6,522.895
	(15.18)	(7.82)	(6.48)
Married * age of child	−340.934	−240.673	−545.874
	(−4.69)	(−2.10)	(−3.29)
Education category (≤ high school omitted)			
High school	2,756.513	6,132.514	4,512.678
	(6.60)	(9.34)	(4.89)
Some college	2,928.226	4,933.793	4,446.274
	(4.79)	(5.27)	(3.49)
≥ college graduate	11,875.290	19,103.870	25,010.590
	(12.21)	(11.88)	(11.57)
Education and child age interactions			
(High school) * child age	327.425	−219.328	−137.702
	(5.51)	(−2.37)	(−1.08)
(Some college) * child age	696.040	262.185	224.595
	(7.53)	(1.84)	(1.18)
(≥ college graduate) * child age	962.018	−382.814	−1,239.564
	(5.05)	(−1.19)	(−3.14)
Pseudo R^2	0.1176	0.1247	0.1132

Notes: The dependent variable is actual annual income. Regressions are based on 11,643 person/year observations. *T*-statistics are in parentheses.

Table B.4.2. Ordered Probit for the Additional Number of Children Born

	Nonblacks	Blacks
Age at first birth category (≤16 omitted)		
17–18 years	−0.546	−0.197
	(−6.43)	(−4.15)
19–21 years	−0.747	−0.320
	(−9.14)	(−7.12)
≥22 years	−1.361	−0.800
	(−16.70)	(−17.66)
Age of index child (spline)		
Age < 5	0.468	0.380
	(40.48)	(26.09)
5 ≤ age < 10	0.058	0.085
	(8.91)	(11.18)
Age ≥ 10	0.023	0.018
	(4.43)	(3.45)
Marital status		
Married at birth	0.323	0.323
	(6.63)	(6.26)
Married * age of child	−0.016	−0.025
	(−3.90)	(−5.49)
Education category (≤ high school omitted)		
High school	0.399	−0.001
	(9.72)	(−0.25)
Some college	0.441	−0.002
	(8.29)	(−.36)
≥ college graduate	0.673	−0.013
	(11.73)	(−1.24)
Education and child age interactions		
(High school) * child age	−0.004	0.070
	(−1.27)	(1.37)
(Some college) * child age	−0.013	0.073
	(−2.76)	(1.01)
(≥ college graduate) * child age	−0.005	−0.050
	(−1.09)	(−0.42)
Ancillary parameters		
Cut point 1	1.588	1.533
	(0.10)	(0.07)
Cut point 2	2.842	2.504
	(0.10)	(0.07)
Cut point 3	3.703	3.258
	(0.10)	(0.08)
Cut point 4	4.347	4.053
	(0.10)	(0.08)
Log likelihood	−29,164.691	−16,237.688

Notes: The dependent variable is number of children born beyond the index child. The nonblack and black samples contain 30,492 and 15,084 person/year observations, respectively. *Z*-statistics are in parentheses for main parameter estimate; standard errors are shown for the ancillary parameters.

NOTES

Support for this research was provided by the Robin Hood Foundation. We wish to acknowledge comments and suggestions by Frank Furstenberg, V. Joseph Hotz, Arlene Leibowitz, Robert Moffitt, Susan Philliber, and Seth Sanders. We also want to thank Charles Mullin and, especially, Honggao Cao for very able research assistance.

1. Evidence from birth certificate data suggests that most births to teen mothers were with male partners who were already past the teen years. Among nonblacks, for example, 57.4 percent of the births to young teenage women (age 16 or younger) in 1988 were fathered by men age 20 and older; the corresponding number for blacks is 42.8 percent. Similarly, for older teen mothers (age 17–19) the proportion of fathers who were age 20 or older is 82.3 percent for nonblacks and 70.0 percent for blacks (see table 4.5).

2. Though not considered in this chapter, the mothers of the children are also clearly affected by this behavior. In particular, lack of adequate support by an absent father or a lower level of support from a partner who experiences a disrupted career path requires that the woman make choices that are equally disruptive to her life.

3. A more complete analysis would consider the youth's (and mate's) utility functions (e.g., direct preferences for sexual activity, the pleasures of living with the partner, the joys of having a child, the costs of marital search) that would cause the optimal age to be somewhat earlier or later than this point. In particular, even if no marriage premium exists, so delay of fatherhood and other family responsibilities always increases the man's lifetime earnings (i.e., the curves for each youth shown in the figure are always positively sloped), at some point it is reasonable to assume that the marginal monetary benefits of delay become smaller than the marginal nonmonetary disutility, so the man will wish to begin family life.

4. Ideally, we would like to estimate the curves themselves, but sorting associated with optimizing behavior by youth induces a positive correlation between economic potential and age at first fatherhood that confounds movements along a given curve with movements across curves.

5. Alternative statistical approaches using instrumental variables do not appear promising because, in our opinion, the dataset we use does not contain plausible valid instruments with significant predictive power.

6. Although paternity is not legally established in a large number of out-of-wedlock births to AFDC-eligible mothers (see Nichols-Casebolt and Garfinkel 1991), studies suggest that many fathers voluntarily admit paternity when contacted by child support authorities (Meyer 1992). The father not knowing about the child is a topic that must be addressed in assessing the validity of the data used in our study.

7. The survey actually contains three distinct samples that can be used separately or combined. First, there is a cross-sectional sample that is representative of all young men and women in the relevant age category. Second, there is a supplemental sample that includes an oversample of youth identified as Hispanic, black, or economically disadvantaged non-Hispanic nonblacks. Finally, there is a sample that consists of individuals who, as of September 30, 1978, were serving in the military. As will be discussed below, our study only uses the cross-sectional sample.

8. An alternative approach to this problem is to use information on the sexual and reproductive behavior of males to help understand how often teenage men place themselves at the risk of fatherhood by engaging in sexual activity. This would include the

number of partners they have and their own and/or partner's use of contraception. See Ku, Sonenstein, and Pleck (1993) for a study of this type.

9. Even this relatively straightforward comparison can be complicated due to an underreporting of father's characteristics in the *Vital Statistics* data. This is particularly a problem for births to young unmarried couples.

10. To reduce the amount of nonreporting due to item nonresponse and missed surveys in the construction of the age 27 outcomes, we used an algorithm that also considered outcomes around age 27. We first used the outcomes at age 27. If that was missing, we took values first from age 26 if that was available, then age 28. We did not drift farther than one year in either direction to fill the outcome measures.

11. The AFQT was administered to approximately 93 percent of the male NLSY respondents in 1980. The raw AFQT score was constructed using the sum of Armed Services Vocational Aptitude Battery sections 2–5. To construct a normalized measure, we used the residual from a weighted regression of the raw score on cohort dummy variables. This regression controlled for the different ages at which the test had been administered. We then normalized the residual by the weighted standard deviation for each cohort.

12. The majority of the military sample was dropped after the 1984 eave, and the poor white sample was completely discontinued after the 1990 survey. The respondents used in the analysis, therefore, are solely from the cross-sectional sample. This sample, as noted above, is representative of all young men and women.

13. Due to item nonresponse, additional respondents will be dropped in the analysis presented below. The exact number of observations used in each analysis is given in each model presented. The 1979 sample weight was also used in the regression analysis presented.

14. The data for males permit only the analysis of pregnancies that lead to a live birth. This implies that a man may have impregnated a woman before this point but it did not result in a live birth. The pregnancy date is calculated as nine months before the birth date.

15. This issue has also been considered by Lerman (1993) and Pirog-Good (1993).

16. Census income is not considered since it is specifically tied to the occupation chosen at age 27. Earlier occupations are more transitory and would not be as meaningful for this portion of the analysis.

17. As previously defined, census income is the average income associated with the occupation chosen at age 27 based on the 1990 U.S. Census. It is designed to capture long-run differences in economic status.

18. Willis also shows that the rate of out-of-wedlock fatherhood tends to depend on the overall ratio of females to males in the marriage market and on the capacity of females to rear children without the contributions of the father, either through their own labor or with welfare payments. Willis shows that under conditions in which females outnumber males and are capable of economic independence, a marriage market equilibrium exists in which males and females in the lower part of the income distribution will tend to have children out of wedlock and those in the upper part of the income distribution will tend to marry. The lower the absolute income of males, the higher will be the fraction of men who become out-of-wedlock fathers. (Robert J. Willis, "A Theory of Out-of-Wedlock Childbearing," unpublished paper, Ann Arbor, Michigan, 1994.)

19. Specifically, we describe this relationship by estimating regression equations of the form $y = a + b_1\text{age}_1 + b_2\text{age}_2 + b_3\text{age}_3$, where the age variables are splines of the male's

age at conception of his first child with nodes at ages 18 and 21. For the interested reader, regression results of this specification for each of the four outcome variables being considered are presented in model 1 of appendix tables A.4.1–A.4.4. Each model presented in this section has been estimated separately for black and nonblack respondents and has been weighted using the 1979 sample weights. The means and standard deviations of the variables used in the regressions are available from the authors upon request.

20. Selected results for this regression are presented in model 3 of appendix tables A.4.1–A.4.4. The impact of these controls can be seen by examining across models 1 and 3 in the appendix tables.

21. We estimate the following regression model:

$$y = a + b_1 \text{AGE}_1 + b_2 \text{AGE}_2 + b_3 \text{AGE}_3 + c_0 M + c_1 \text{AGE}_1 M + c_2 \text{AGE}_2 M + c_3 \text{AGE}_3 M$$

where M is a dummy variable equal to 1 if the individual was married at the time of the conception of his first child and 0 otherwise. The "c" coefficients measure the difference in the level and age profile of men who are married or unmarried. These results can be found in model 2 of tables A.4.1–A.4.4.

22. This specification is labeled as model 4 in tables A.4.1–A.4.4.

23. There were no black respondents married at the time of the pregnancy in the less than 18 years old category.

24. Specifically, F-tests were conducted on the joint significance of the marriage and age interactions in models 2 and 4. See tables A.4.1–A.4.4.

25. The characteristics on which the match is made are limited by the data available on the NMIHS.

26. For an example of other research in this area, see Garfinkel and Oellerich (1989).

27. For simplicity, assume that the optimal level of education for this youth is high school graduation. Remember that the rate of return to high school graduation varies across individuals, as illustrated by the different curves in figure 4.1.

28. In constructing matching probabilities for both the mother and father, we use four age categories (<16 years, 17–18 years, 19–21 years, and >22 years), four education categories (<high school, high school graduate, some college, and college graduate and beyond), two race categories (black and nonblack), and two marital status categories (married and not married).

29. The income equations are based on quantile regressions for the 25th, 50th, and 75th percentiles. The predicted number of children is based on an ordered probit specification.

30. For more detail on predicted values based on these analytic results, see Brien and Willis (1997).

31. We assume that the number of children born to men does not exceed four. Also, these percentage obligations assume that the man fathers all subsequent children with the same mother. Alternatively, if he fathers a second child by a different woman, his obligation to the first child would be 17 percent of his income, net of his obligation to his second child, yielding an obligation of 14.1 percent [$.17 \times (1 - .17)$] rather than 12.5 percent, and so on for additional births by different women. Our data do not permit us to determine whether a given man's children are by the same or different mothers. We choose to make our calculations of potential obligations using the lower percentage obligations listed in the

text. In this sense, our estimates of a man's potential child support payments are slightly conservative.

32. The support payment is not directly proportional to the predicted income because of the potential presence of future children.

33. The flow value, p, is determined with the following formula:

$$p = \frac{\left[(rV) \div 12\right]}{\left[1 - \left(1 \div (1+r)^{18}\right)\right]}$$

where r denotes the interest rate (.05) and V denotes the discounted present value of child support payments.

34. Willis (1994) proposes a theoretical model in which child support enforcement would reduce the incidence of out-of-wedlock childbearing, but little empirical work has been done on this problem. (Robert J. Willis, "A Theory of Out-of-Wedlock Childbearing.")

In one of the few empirical papers dealing with this issue, Sonenstein, Pleck, and Ku (1994) find little evidence of an effect of the strength of child support enforcement on a young male's pregnancy risk behavior (i.e., unprotected sex), but it does appear to affect their perception of the cost of the behavior.

REFERENCES

Brien, Michael J., and Robert J. Willis. 1997. "Costs and Consequences for the Father." In *Kids Having Kids,* edited by Rebecca A. Maynard (95–144). Washington, DC: Urban Institute Press.

Daniel, Kermit E. 1993. "Does Marriage Make Workers More Productive?" Ph.D. dissertation, University of Chicago.

Ellwood, David T. 1982. "Teenage Unemployment: Permanent Scars or Temporary Blemishes?" In *The Youth Labor Market Problem: Its Nature, Causes, and Consequences,* edited by Richard B. Freeman and David A. Wise (349–90). Chicago, IL: University of Chicago Press.

Garfinkel, Irwin, and Donald Oellerich. 1989. "Noncustodial Fathers' Ability to Pay Child Support." *Demography* 26(2): 219–33.

Huber, Peter J. 1967. "The Behavior of Maximum Likelihood Estimates under Nonstandard Conditions." *Proceedings of the Fifth Berkeley Symposium on Mathematical Statistics and Probability* 1:221–33.

Korenman, Sanders, and David Neumark. 1991. "Does Marriage Really Make Men More Productive?" *Journal of Human Resources* 26(2): 282–307.

Ku, Leighton, Freya L. Sonenstein, and Joseph H. Pleck. 1993. "Factors Influencing First Intercourse for Teenage Men." *Public Health Reports* 108(6): 680–94.

Lerman, Robert I. 1993. "Employment Patterns of Unwed Fathers and Public Policy." In *Young Unwed Fathers: Changing Roles and Emerging Policies,* edited by Robert I. Lerman and Theodora J. Ooms (316–34). Philadelphia, PA: Temple University Press.

Maynard, Rebecca A. 1997. "The Costs of Adolescent Childbearing." In *Kids Having Kids: Economic Costs and Social Consequences of Teen Pregnancy,* edited by Rebecca A. Maynard (285–338). Washington, DC: Urban Institute Press.

Meyer, Daniel R. 1992. "Paternity and Public Policy." *Focus* 14(2): 1–11.

Mott, Frank L. 1983. "Fertility-Related Data in the 1982 National Longitudinal Surveys of Youth: An Evaluation of Data Quality and Some Preliminary Analytical Results." Columbus: Center for Human Resource Research, Ohio State University.

———. 1985. "Evaluation of Fertility Data and Preliminary Analytic Results from the 1983 (5th Round) Survey of the National Longitudinal Surveys of Work Experience of Youth." Columbus: Center for Human Resource Research, Ohio State University.

Nichols-Casebolt, Ann, and Irwin Garfinkel. 1991. "Trends in Paternity Adjudications and Child Support Awards." *Social Science Quarterly* 72:83–97.

Pirog-Good, Maureen A. 1993. "The Education and Labor Market Outcomes of Adolescent Fathers." Discussion Paper 1014-93. Madison: Institute for Research on Poverty, University of Wisconsin–Madison.

Sonenstein, Freya L., Joseph H. Pleck, and Leighton Ku. 1994. "Child Support Obligations and Young Men's Contraceptive Behavior: What Do Young Men Know? Does It Matter?" Paper presented at the annual meeting of the Population Association of America.

Weiss, Yoram, and Robert J. Willis. 1985. "Children as Collective Goods and Divorce Settlements." *Journal of Labor Economics* 3(3): 268–92.

———. 1993. "Transfers among Divorced Couples: Evidence and Interpretation." *Journal of Labor Economics* 11(4): 629–79.

5

Outcomes for Children of Teen Mothers from Kindergarten through Adolescence

Jennifer S. Manlove, Elizabeth Terry-Humen,
Lisa A. Mincieli, and Kristin A. Moore

Researchers have found that many negative outcomes among teen mothers are the result of their disadvantaged social and economic background *before* they had a baby. However, a study conducted in the mid-1990s by a consortium of scientists on the effects of adolescent childbearing found that the costs of teenage motherhood were borne primarily by the children and only secondarily by the mothers (Maynard 1997). This chapter provides updated information assessing the association between maternal age at first birth and child outcomes in multiple domains with two recent cohorts of young children and adolescent children of teen mothers.

Except for a recent increase in 2006, the U.S. teen birth rate has declined every year since 1991 (Ventura et al. 2006). As the teen birth rate has declined, the proportion of all births that occur to teens also has declined, from 16 percent in 1980 to 10.2 percent in 2004 (Martin et al. 2007; National Center for Health Statistics 1984), reflecting the reduced likelihood that children are born to teen mothers. Meanwhile, the median age at marriage has risen steadily from 24.7 for males and 22.0 for females in 1980 to 27.1 for males and 25.3 for females in 2005,[1] and the proportion of teen births that occur within marriage has declined from 52 percent in 1980 to 17 percent in 2005 (Martin et al. 2007).

Thus, as the birth rate has fallen and the proportion of married mothers giving birth during their teen years has declined over time, these unmarried mothers who do have a teen birth may be more disadvantaged than were the primarily married teen mothers in previous generations. The reasons for this relative disadvantage, as suggested by other research, include the greater likelihood that today's teen mothers will be unmarried, as well as their more limited educational attainment and financial prospects (Furstenberg, Levine, and Brooks-Gunn 1990). However, previous studies were based on data on teen mothers and their children from an earlier cohort, before recent declines in the teen birth rate. Recent data on outcomes among children of teen mothers will help researchers understand how maternal age is associated with child outcomes.

About This Study

This chapter uses recent nationally representative data to update the portrait of children of teen mothers. The chapter extends previous research on outcomes among children of teen mothers and addresses four gaps in the research on this topic: the limited outcome domains studied, the choice of appropriate comparison groups, the differences between older and more recent cohorts of teen mothers, and the differences (if any) for the children at different stages of their life course.

Limited Outcome Domains

Most research on the outcomes of children born to teenage mothers has focused on cognitive and academic outcomes, with some additional studies examining behavioral problems. Researchers have conducted limited research, however, on broader child and adolescent outcomes, including family environments, relationships, and health outcomes. This chapter examines a broad set of outcomes among children of teen mothers and how these outcomes compare with those of children of older mothers.

Research assessing multiple outcomes among children of teen mothers compared with outcomes of children of mothers age 20–21 suggests that teen motherhood primarily affects children's cognitive and educational performance (Moore, Morrison, and Greene 1997). Studies that control for family background characteristics and maternal characteristics measured before the birth of the child find that children of teen mothers have lower math, reading, and/or vocabulary test scores than do children of older mothers, although comparison groups vary across studies (Levine, Pollack, and Comfort 2001; Moore et al. 1997; Moore and Snyder 1991).

Adolescent children of teen mothers have lower odds of completing high school than children of mothers age 22 and older (Haveman, Wolfe, and Peterson 1997) but not children of mothers age 20–21 (Moore et al. 1997). Approaches that control for historical period (Hofferth and Reid 2002), or that compare outcomes among children born to sisters (in which one had a birth during her teen years and another had a birth in her twenties) (Geronimus, Korenman, and Hillemeier 1994; Turley 2003), suggest that the association between maternal age and child cognitive outcomes diminish, although some differences remain in some studies. Note, however, that sibling fixed-effects models are limited because only mothers with sisters in the database are included in estimates, which reduces sample size and influences sample characteristics (Hoffman 1998).

Research examining the effects of maternal age on children's behavioral outcomes and health status has shown mixed results. Some studies find, net of controls, that children of teen mothers have more behavioral problems and higher levels of fighting, skipping school, delinquency, running away, and/or early sexual experience than do children of older mothers (Hofferth and Reid 2002; Levine et al. 2001; Moore et al. 1997; Pogarsky, Lizotte, and Thornberry 2003; Pogarsky, Thornberry, and Lizotte 2006; Turley 2003). But other studies find no effects of maternal age on children's behavioral problems (Moore et al. 1997). Some studies also find that daughters of teen mothers have a greater risk of a teen birth, even after controlling for background characteristics (Haveman, Wolfe, and Pence 2001; Kahn and Anderson 1992; Manlove 1997). Studies examining health outcomes likewise have mixed findings, with one study showing that children of teen mothers have poorer health outcomes than do children of older mothers (Wolfe and Perozek 1997) and another finding no association between maternal age and child health outcomes (Moore et al. 1997).

Researchers have suggested several reasons that children of teen mothers may fare worse than other children: that teen mothers have greater family instability and lower incomes; that they provide less cognitive stimulation and emotional support within the home environment; and that because they have more children than do older mothers, fewer resources are available for each child (Levine et al. 2001; Moore et al. 1997; Pogarsky et al. 2003).

Identifying Appropriate Comparison Groups

The choice of comparison group in analyses has posed another limitation in some previous research on children of teen mothers. Many researchers have compared children of teen mothers to a heterogeneous group of children born to mothers age 20 and older. However, based on the modest success of intervention efforts, delaying first births by a decade or more may be an unrealistic goal. (The Abecedarian early childhood program achieved the largest identified delay in childbearing—1.4 years. See Campbell et al. 2002).

This chapter follows some previous research on this topic by choosing mothers age 20–21 as a reference group (Maynard 1997), which may be a more realistic goal for pregnancy prevention efforts. Note, however, that because of increases in the median age at marriage, women in their early 20s (age 20–24) currently have the highest rates of nonmarital childbearing (Martin et al. 2007; Ventura et al. 2004). Delays in marriage, combined with a growing percentage of women completing college, may mean that a more appropriate goal for pregnancy prevention efforts would be to delay childbearing until the mid-20s.[2] To address the implications of these major social changes, this chapter also contrasts outcomes for children of delayed childbearers with outcomes for children whose mothers were 20–21 when they had their first child.

Older Cohorts of Teen Mothers and Nonrepresentative Samples

A large body of research on outcomes among children of teen mothers has incorporated analyses of the Child Supplement of the 1979 National Longitudinal Survey of Youth, a nationally representative sample of mothers (not children). Relying on this source may introduce bias into findings about outcomes among children of teen mothers. Specifically, children born to teen mothers were born in an earlier decade than were children born to older mothers in the Child Supplement. In fact, one study finds that controlling for the period of birth and its interaction with the child's age accounts for most of the variance in child cognitive outcomes between children of teen mothers and children of older mothers (Hofferth and Reid 2002).

This chapter will contribute to previous research by analyzing data from nationally representative samples of children and adolescents. This work builds on previous research with earlier cohorts of teen mothers by analyzing data on a recent cohort of adolescents, born between 1981 and 1985, and of kindergarten students born in 1998 or 1999.

Life-Course Stages

Extending previous research (Moore et al. 1997), we examine the effects of early motherhood on outcomes of very young children and adolescents to test, for example, whether there are more significant effects in early childhood than in adolescence. Specifically, using data from the Early Childhood Longitudinal Study, Kindergarten Cohort (ECLS-K) and from the National Longitudinal Survey of Youth, 1997 Cohort (NLSY97), we address the following five research questions:

- *On average, do children of teen mothers differ from those whose mothers first gave birth in their early twenties?* We hypothesize that children of teen mothers will score lower on cognitive and academic outcomes and higher on behavioral problems than will children of older mothers.
- *Do differences in child outcomes by maternal age remain after controlling for family background characteristics?* We hypothesize that some differences will remain between children of teen mothers and children of mothers age 20–21, primarily in cognitive and academic outcomes, as well as in behavioral outcomes.
- *Do the negative consequences of being born to a teen mother vary by maternal age or across the stages of the child's life cycle?* Some research had shown more negative child outcomes among children of very young mothers compared with children of mothers in their later teens (Goerge and Lee 1997; Maynard 1997; Moore et al. 1997; Wolfe and Perozek 1997). Previous research also suggests effects of maternal age on both early childhood and adolescent outcomes (Haveman et al. 1997; Hofferth and Reid 2002; Levine et al. 2001; Moore et al. 1997; Moore and Snyder 1991; Pogarsky et al. 2003, 2006; Terry-Humen, Manlove, and Moore 2005; Turley 2003). We update this research by examining whether the effects are stronger in early childhood than they are in adolescence.
- *Do the associations between maternal age and child or adolescent outcomes differ by child gender?* Because there are gender differences in behavioral outcomes and sexual relationships, we hypothesize that maternal age might have a stronger effect on behavioral problems for boys and on sexual activity and pregnancy for girls.
- *Is delaying childbearing associated with especially positive outcomes?* We hypothesize that delaying first parenthood until the mid- to late 20s and 30s will be associated with more positive outcomes than

will delaying first parenthood from the teen years until the early 20s.

Data

We use two datasets to examine various outcomes occurring in early childhood and adolescence among firstborn children of teenage mothers compared with children born to older mothers. The Early Childhood Longitudinal Study, Kindergarten Cohort provides information on outcomes among children at kindergarten entry, while the National Longitudinal Survey of Youth, 1997 Cohort, allows us to focus on outcomes occurring during adolescence.

The ECLS-K is a nationally representative longitudinal study, directed by the National Center for Education Statistics, of 21,399 children in the United States who were in kindergarten during the 1998–99 school year (Westat et al. 2001). The study includes various school readiness measures collected at kindergarten entry, including measures of cognition, knowledge, and academic achievement; behavior and delinquency; home environment and family integration; relationship and interpersonal skills; and physical health and well-being. In addition to the kindergartners' direct assessments, the ECLS-K includes data from the kindergartners' parents, teachers, and school administrators on the children's school readiness outcomes and the characteristics of their families, schools, and communities. The first survey was conducted in the fall of the kindergarten year, with follow-up interviews conducted in the spring of kindergarten, and in 1st, 3rd, and 5th grades. The present analysis draws upon assessments for children in the fall of their kindergarten year.

Our sample excludes 14,884 respondents who were not firstborns, 257 respondents who had attended kindergarten previously, and 30 children who were not living in households with their biological mothers.[3] Thus, the final sample includes 6,228 firstborn kindergartners (to allow for comparisons between children of the same parity) who were living in households with their biological mothers.[4] Individual model sample sizes may vary because certain outcomes were limited to specific age groups or populations. In cases where the mother's first birth was a multiple birth, both twins were included in the analyses if they met the other sample criteria.

The NLSY97 is a nationally representative longitudinal study, directed by the Bureau of Labor Statistics, of 8,984 adolescents born in the United States between 1980 and 1984 (age 12–16 in 1997) (Bureau of Labor Statistics 2005). Adolescents were initially surveyed in 1997, with annual follow-ups between 1998 and 2002. The survey provides a rich source of information on many cognitive, behavioral, and health measures. In addition, one parent of the adolescent—usually the biological mother—was interviewed in the first year of the study. The parent survey provides detailed information about the background of the adolescent's parent, including information on the responding parent's age at first birth and family of origin.

From the full NLSY97 sample, we excluded 5,011 adolescents who were not first born, 395 additional respondents who did not live with their biological mothers, and 681 additional adolescents whose biological mothers did not complete the parent survey.[5] Our final sample includes 2,897 first-born respondents living with their biological mothers who answered the Round 1 parent survey.[6] Because the sample excludes high-risk families without a biological mother in the household or adolescents whose biological mother did not complete the parent survey, our findings with this survey should provide a conservative estimate of the association between teen motherhood and adolescent outcomes. Individual model sample sizes may vary because certain outcomes were limited to specific age groups or populations.

Methods

This chapter reports on bivariate and multivariate analyses of age-appropriate outcomes within the areas of cognition, behavior problems, family environments, relationships, and health across the two datasets. For example, for the ECLS-K children who are all approximately 5 to 6 years old, we examine scores on tests of reading and math that are appropriate for kindergartners; for the NLSY97 sample of older youth and young adults, we examine achievement test scores, such as the Armed Services Vocational Aptitude Battery, and high school graduation. For a detailed description of each outcome we examine, please see appendix A.5.

In both datasets, we present six age groupings of mothers at the birth of their first child: 17 or younger, 18–19, 20–21, 22–24, 25–29, and 30 or older. Our critical comparisons of interest are between children of mothers age 17 or younger and age 20–21, and between children of mothers age 18–19 and age 20–21. We present outcomes among children born to older mothers compared with children born to mothers age 20–21 years old as well, but we focus primarily on the consequences of *teenage* childbearing.

We present two types of analyses. We first use bivariate chi-square and general linear models analyses, for categorical and continuous measures, respectively, to show unadjusted differences between children born to teen mothers and children born to mothers age 20–21. These analyses, which do not control for any background characteristics of the child or his or her mother, also show the differences between children born to mothers age 22 and older and children born to mothers age 20–21. We then use multivariate ordinary least squares regression models and logistic regression models, in conjunction with predicted probabilities, to provide estimates of outcomes among children of younger and older mothers compared with children born to mothers age 20–21. The predicted probabilities provide adjusted estimates of the child and adolescent outcomes by holding all background characteristics constant and thus only reflect differences caused by mother's age at birth.

All multivariate models control for child and mother background characteristics, which we chose based on previous research, availability, and potential associations with the mother's age at first birth and the outcome variables. We include controls for the child's age, gender, and race/ethnicity, in addition to the mother's educational attainment, marital status at birth, language spoken in the home, and the highest educational attainment of the child's maternal grandmother. ECLS-K analyses further control for whether the kindergartner was part of a multiple birth. NLSY97 analyses take into account additional characteristics of the adolescent's mother, including the number of siblings she has; whether she was born in the United States; whether she grew up in a city, suburb, town, or rural area; and whether the maternal grandmother was a teen when the mother was born. Analyses are weighted and run in SUDAAN and Stata to account for the complex sampling design of the ECLS-K (StataCorp 2001).

While researchers have developed many and varied strategies to address the endogeneity of maternal age and outcomes among teen mothers (Geronimus et al. 1994; Geronimus and Moore 1992; Moore et al. 1993), these issues may not be as important for models examining the babies and children of young mothers. (Indeed, many policymakers only care about bivariate differences because these differences occur in their jurisdictions, not outcomes net of social, demographic, and economic controls.)

Thus, we have estimated bivariate and multivariate models with critical child and mother controls in this chapter. However, we recommend that future analyses address the potential endogeneity of parent age and child well-being.

Results

Tables 5.1 and 5.2 provide child, mother, and grandparent characteristics for each sample by age of mother at first birth. For the ECLS-K kindergarten sample (table 5.1), characteristics that differ between teen mothers and mothers age 20–21 at first birth include race/ethnicity, parent's marital status at birth, and maternal education. On average, children of mothers age 17 and younger and age 18–19 at first birth were more likely to be black or Hispanic than were children of mothers age 20–21. Only 12 percent of children of mothers age 17 and younger at birth were born to mothers married at the time of their birth, followed by 32 percent of mothers age 18–19; both percentages were lower than the 49 percent of children born to mothers age 20–21 at birth. On average, mothers who had first births during their teen years had lower educational attainment than did mothers age 20–21 at first birth.

Among the NLSY97 adolescent sample (table 5.2), children of teen mothers were also more likely to be racial or ethnic minorities, to have mothers with lower educational attainment, and to have mothers who were unmarried at their first birth than were children of mothers age 20–21. In addition, the background characteristics of teen mothers differed from those of mothers who were 20–21 when they first had a child. Teen mothers were themselves less likely to grow up with two biological parents and had, on average, a greater number of siblings than did women who gave birth at 20–21. These findings demonstrate that most women who became teen mothers had more disadvantaged family and individual characteristics than did mothers who delayed childbearing until their early 20s.

Tables 5.3–5.7 report outcomes for teen mothers compared with older mothers, before and after controls, in five outcome areas: cognitive development and academic achievement, behavior, family and home environment, relationship quality, and physical health and well-being. Each table first presents the unadjusted average for each outcome by age of mother

text continues on page 182

Table 5.1. Mother, Child, and Grandparent Characteristics of Kindergartners in Round 1, by Age of Mother at Birth of First Child (percent, except where noted)

	17 and under	18–19	20–21	22–24	25–29	30+
Total kindergartners	525	741	815	1,000	1,743	1,404
	9.29	13.20	13.96	15.94	26.68	20.93
Child characteristics						
Age (years)	5.69	5.69	5.68	5.67	5.68	5.67
Male	49.46	50.70	52.45	48.89	51.47	48.09+
Race/ethnicity						
Black	28.37***	20.63***	15.56***	13.91***	7.54***	7.25***
Hispanic	27.01***	26.53***	25.41***	20.82***	12.57***	11.01***
Other	6.58***	7.73***	7.41***	6.74***	6.81***	8.49***
Non-Hispanic white	38.03***	45.10***	51.62***	58.54***	73.07***	73.25***
Child part of a multiple birth	1.32	1.24	0.83	2.26+	3.17**	3.63**
Mother characteristics						
Speaks language other than English at home	13.76	16.06	16.45	17.77	12.14**	10.61**
Married at birth of focal child	11.66***	32.44***	49.07	60.27***	84.47***	87.44***
Highest grade completed						
Less than high school	35.92***	23.14***	13.92***	7.12***	4.27***	3.27***
High school or GED	41.57***	45.15***	40.44***	32.22***	21.83***	17.04***
Vocational degree	21.09***	28.69***	39.98***	45.21***	36.16***	29.43***
College graduate	1.42***	3.03***	5.65***	15.45***	37.74***	50.26***
Grandparent characteristics						
Highest grade completed by maternal grandparent (1–22)	12.25	12.38	12.51	13.13**	13.28**	13.81***

Source: ECLS-K.

+$p < .10$; * $p < .05$; ** $p < .01$; *** $p < .001$

Table 5.2. Mother, Child, and Grandparent Characteristics of Adolescents in Round 1, by Age of Mother at Birth of First Child (percent, except where noted)

	17 and under	18–19	20–21	22–24	25–29	30+
Total adolescents	221	403	461	638	793	381
	5.86	12.17	15.33	22.31	30.35	13.98
Child characteristics						
Age	14.16	14.08	14.00	14.02*	14.11	13.87
Male	46.7	48.5	48.7	50.0	51.2	50.0
Race/ethnicity						
Black	32.2***	20.5***	19.4***	14.7***	8.7***	9.9***
Hispanic	17.9***	14.1***	12.2***	11.5***	8.3***	7.5***
Non-Hispanic mixed	0.0***	0.4***	1.2***	1.6***	1.2***	0.2***
Nonblack/Non-Hispanic	49.9***	65.0***	67.2***	72.2***	81.8***	82.5***
Mother characteristics						
Born in the United States	91.3	91.0	90.9	88.2	90.7	89.0
Speaks language other than English at home	15.4	13.5	11.4	13.0	11.7	9.4
Lived with both biological parents until age 14	45.5***	57.3***	68.4	78.4***	82.9***	84.0***
Number of siblings	4.5*	4.3	4.0	3.8	3.6***	3.2*
Grew up in a city, town, or rural area						
Central city	27.8***	23.2***	17.0***	18.1***	19.3***	20.3***
Suburb	12.7***	11.6***	16.2***	21.8***	26.5***	22.6***
Town or other	59.5***	65.1***	66.8***	60.1***	54.2***	57.1***
Married at birth of focal child	29.7***	52.7***	65.1	81.3***	89.5***	87.5***
Highest grade completed (1–20)	11.2***	11.9**	12.4	13.0***	14.1***	14.5***
Grandparent characteristics						
Highest grade completed by maternal grandmother (1–7)	2.5	2.6	2.6	2.7	3.0***	2.9**
Grandmother a teen at mom's birth	24.5+	18.5	19.0	13.6*	8.4***	9.9***

Source: NLSY97.

+*p* < .10; **p* < .05; ***p* < .01; ****p* < .001

Table 5.3. Cognitive Outcomes and Academic Achievement among Kindergartners and Adolescents by Maternal Age at First Birth, before and after Controls

	Age of Mother when Her First Child Was Born						Estimated Consequence of Teen Childbearing Relative to Delaying to Age 20–21	
	17 and under	18–19	20–21	22–24	25–29	30+	17 and under	18–19
Kindergarten Outcomes[a]								
IRT reading scores								
Unadjusted mean outcomes	18.78***	19.59***	21.05	23.10***	25.62***	27.26***	2.83***	1.48***
Adjusted outcomes after controls	21.60*	21.59*	22.35	23.52**	24.71***	25.86***	0.75*	0.76*
IRT math scores								
Unadjusted mean outcomes	16.11***	16.50***	17.77	19.23***	21.82***	22.88**	1.70***	1.36***
Adjusted outcomes after controls	18.56	18.23*	18.91	19.63*	20.97***	21.57***	0.35	0.74*
IRT general knowledge scores								
Unadjusted mean outcomes	18.36***	19.54***	21.06	22.53***	25.17***	26.60***	2.70***	1.55***
Adjusted outcomes after controls	21.15**	21.32**	22.04	22.80*	24.10***	25.30***	0.87**	0.72**
Approaches to learning								
Unadjusted mean outcomes	3.15	3.13	3.13	3.14	3.14	3.18*	−0.02	0.01
Adjusted outcomes after controls	3.23*	3.18	3.17	3.14	3.11*	3.13	−0.06*	−0.02
Letter recognition								
Unadjusted mean outcomes	0.50***	0.55**	0.62	0.71***	0.82***	0.86***	0.11***	0.08**
Adjusted outcomes after controls	0.62+	0.63	0.66	0.72*	0.78***	0.81***	0.04+	0.03

Beginning sounds							
Unadjusted mean outcomes	0.15***	0.19**	0.24	0.34***	0.44***	0.51***	0.08***	0.05**
Adjusted outcomes after controls	0.27+	0.27	0.30	0.36**	0.40***	0.44***	0.03+	0.03
Ending sounds							
Unadjusted mean outcomes	.07***	.09**	0.13	.20***	.27***	.32***	0.05***	0.03**
Adjusted outcomes after controls	0.16	0.15	0.17	0.21**	0.24***	0.28***	0.01	0.02

Adolescent Outcomes

PIAT math scores							
Unadjusted mean outcomes	32.09***	40.74*	47.69	54.54**	62.87***	64.84***	15.60***	6.95*
Adjusted outcomes after controls	43.81	43.74	47.96	50.57	53.11*	52.64	4.15	4.22
ASVAB score							
Unadjusted mean outcomes	34.56***	40.88*	45.98	55.32***	62.85***	66.28***	11.42***	5.10*
Adjusted outcomes after controls	44.18	43.66	46.37	52.05**	53.83***	55.70***	2.19	2.71
Received high school diploma by age 19							
Unadjusted mean outcomes	0.57***	0.64*	0.71	0.80***	0.87***	0.88***	0.14***	0.07*
Adjusted outcomes after controls	0.68	0.69	0.72	0.78+	0.82***	0.83**	0.04	0.03
Enrolled in four-year college at age 19							
Unadjusted mean outcomes	0.14	0.15	0.18	0.30***	0.48***	0.46***	0.04	0.03
Adjusted outcomes after controls	0.23	0.20	0.20	0.29**	0.38***	0.35***	−0.03	0.00

Sources: ECLS-K (kindergarten outcomes) and NLSY97 (adolescent outcomes).

Note: Significance indicates difference between children born to mothers age 20–21 and all other groups.

a. Adjusted outcome models control for maternal and child factors listed in tables 5.1 and 5.2.

+p < .10; *p < .05; **p < .01; ***p < .001

Table 5.4. Behavior Outcomes among Kindergartners and Adolescents by Maternal Age at First Birth, before and after Controls

	Age of Mother when Her First Child Was Born						Estimated Consequence of Teen Childbearing Relative to Delaying to Age 20–21	
	17 and under	18–19	20–21	22–24	25–29	30+	17 and under	18–19
Kindergarten Outcomes[a]								
Internalizing problem behaviors								
Unadjusted mean outcomes	1.59*	1.59*	1.52	1.54	1.50	1.53	−0.07*	−0.07*
Adjusted outcomes after controls	1.53	1.56+	1.50	1.54	1.51	1.55*	−0.03	−0.06+
Externalizing problem behaviors								
Unadjusted mean outcomes	1.76	1.74	1.70	1.63*	1.58***	1.63*	−0.06	−0.04
Adjusted outcomes after controls	1.67	1.68	1.66	1.62	1.60*	1.67	−0.01	−0.02
Self-control								
Unadjusted mean outcomes	2.95**	2.95**	3.06	3.07	3.16***	3.11	0.11**	0.11**
Adjusted outcomes after controls	3.06	3.01*	3.09	3.07	3.13	3.06	0.03	0.08*
Adolescent Outcomes								
Sexually experienced by age 18								
Unadjusted mean outcomes	0.89	0.89+	0.83	0.78*	0.71***	0.71***	−0.06	−0.06+
Adjusted outcomes after controls	0.85	0.87	0.82	0.79	0.75*	0.76+	−0.03	−0.05

Teen birth by age 18							
Unadjusted mean outcomes	0.20***	0.17***	0.09	0.05*	0.04**	0.04**	-0.11***	-0.08***
Adjusted outcomes after controls	0.13+	0.15*	0.09	0.06	0.07	0.06	-0.04+	-0.06*
Ever used alcohol by round 3							
Unadjusted mean outcomes	0.65	0.72	0.72	0.73	0.71	0.71	0.07	0.00
Adjusted outcomes after controls	0.63*	0.70	0.72	0.71	0.69	0.71	0.09*	0.02
Ever smoked by round 3							
Unadjusted mean outcomes	0.59	0.60	0.56	0.55	0.53	0.53	-0.03	-0.04
Adjusted outcomes after controls	0.56	0.57	0.55	0.53	0.52	0.54	-0.01	-0.02
Ever used marijuana by round 3							
Unadjusted mean outcomes	0.38	0.40	0.39	0.37	0.35	0.36	0.01	-0.01
Adjusted outcomes after controls	0.33	0.37	0.38	0.36	0.35	0.38	0.05	0.01
Delinquency index at round 1							
Unadjusted mean outcomes	1.58+	1.58*	1.32	1.21	1.26	1.06*	-0.26+	-0.26*
Adjusted outcomes after controls	1.48	1.54	1.32	1.20	1.27	1.13	-0.16	-0.22
How often respondent felt depressed in last month							
Unadjusted mean outcomes	1.51	1.47	1.44	1.40	1.36*	1.36+	-0.07	-0.03
Adjusted outcomes after controls	1.45	1.44	1.44	1.42	1.41	1.41	-0.01	0.00

Sources: ECLS-K (kindergarten outcomes) and NLSY97 (adolescent outcomes).

Note: Significance indicates difference between children born to mothers age 20–21 and all other groups.

a. Adjusted outcome models control for maternal and child factors listed in tables 5.1 and 5.2.

+ *p* < .10; * *p* < .05; ** *p* < .01; *** *p* < .001

Table 5.5. Family Environment Outcomes among Kindergartners and Adolescents by Maternal Age at First Birth, before and after Controls

	Age of Mother when Her First Child Was Born						Estimated Consequence of Teen Childbearing Relative to Delaying to Age 20–21	
	17 and under	18–19	20–21	22–24	25–29	30+	17 and under	18–19
Kindergarten Outcomes[a]								
Family environment index								
Unadjusted mean outcomes	3.23	3.05	3.15	3.25	3.47***	3.44***	−0.08	0.10
Adjusted outcomes after controls	3.51**	3.26	3.28	3.28	3.36	3.26	−0.23**	0.02
Adolescent Outcomes								
Physical environment risk								
Unadjusted mean outcomes	1.76*	1.55	1.38	1.03***	0.76***	0.78***	−0.38*	−0.17
Adjusted outcomes after controls	1.42	1.42	1.31	1.11+	1.04*	1.15	−0.11	−0.11

Enriching environment								
Unadjusted mean outcomes	1.49*	1.53*	1.69	1.83*	2.07***	2.14***	0.20* ·	0.16*
Adjusted outcomes after controls	1.70	1.64	1.73	1.79	1.89*	1.90*	0.03	0.09
Maternal monitoring and awareness								
Unadjusted mean outcomes	9.87*	9.85**	10.69	10.74	10.83	11.28*	0.82*	0.85**
Adjusted outcomes after controls	10.17	10.02+	10.66	10.63	10.55	10.89	0.49	0.64+
Family routines								
Unadjusted mean outcomes	16.09	15.66	15.75	15.60	15.43	14.89+	−0.34	0.09
Adjusted outcomes after controls	16.80	15.97	15.80	15.47	15.08+	14.45**	−1.00	−0.17

Sources: ECLS-K (kindergarten outcomes) and NLSY97 (adolescent outcomes).

Note: Significance indicates difference between children born to mothers age 20–21 and all other groups.

a. Adjusted outcome models control for maternal and child factors listed in tables 5.1 and 5.2.

+ $p < .10$; * $p < .05$; ** $p < .01$; *** $p < .001$

Table 5.6. Relationship Outcomes among Kindergartners and Adolescents by Maternal Age at First Birth, before and after Controls

	Age of Mother when Her First Child Was Born						Estimated Consequence of Teen Childbearing Relative to Delaying to Age 20–21	
	17 and under	18–19	20–21	22–24	25–29	30+	17 and under	18–19
Kindergarten Outcomes[a]								
Interpersonal skills								
Unadjusted mean outcomes	2.82**	2.85*	2.94	2.95	3.10***	3.04**	0.12**	0.09*
Adjusted outcomes after controls	2.92	2.92+	2.98	2.95	3.06*	2.99	0.06	0.06+
Adolescent Outcomes								
Positive peer environments								
Unadjusted mean outcomes	1.53	1.66	1.65	1.72	1.82*	1.94***	0.12	−0.01
Adjusted outcomes after controls	1.66	1.73	1.68	1.72	1.75	1.81	0.02	−0.05
Negative peer environments								
Unadjusted mean outcomes	3.30	3.12	3.06	3.01	2.84*	2.49***	−0.24	−0.06
Adjusted outcomes after controls	3.11	3.08	3.11	2.99	2.95+	2.76**	0.00	0.03

Mother-teen relationship								
Unadjusted mean outcomes	8.98	8.84	9.08	9.11	9.09	9.57*	0.10	0.24
Adjusted outcomes after controls	9.01	8.88	9.01	9.07	9.08	9.53*	0.00	0.13
Married or cohabited by age 20								
Unadjusted mean outcomes	0.35**	0.37***	0.23	0.20	0.14***	0.16**	−0.12**	−0.14***
Adjusted outcomes after controls	0.28+	0.32***	0.21	0.20	0.16*	0.18	−0.07+	−0.11***
Closeness to dating partner/spouse								
Unadjusted mean outcomes	8.92	9.05	9.02	8.88	8.82+	8.76+	0.10	−0.03
Adjusted outcomes after controls	8.91	9.01	8.99	8.85	8.77	8.74	0.08	−0.02
Caring behavior of dating partner/spouse								
Unadjusted mean outcomes	9.33	9.44	9.34	9.29	9.16+	9.20	0.01	−0.10
Adjusted outcomes after controls	9.27	9.42	9.32	9.30	9.15	9.21	0.05	−0.10
Amount of conflict with dating partner/spouse								
Unadjusted mean outcomes	3.93*	3.55	3.29	3.27	3.16	3.16	−0.64*	−0.26

Sources: ECLS-K (kindergarten outcomes) and NLSY97 (adolescent outcomes).

Note: Significance indicates difference between children born to mothers age 20–21 and all other groups.

a. Adjusted outcome models control for maternal and child factors listed in tables 5.1 and 5.2.

$^+ p < .10$; $^* p < .05$; $^{**} p < .01$; $^{***} p < .001$

Table 5.7. Health Outcomes among Kindergartners and Adolescents by Maternal Age at First Birth, before and after Controls

	Age of Mother when Her First Child Was Born						Estimated Consequence of Teen Childbearing Relative to Delaying to Age 20–21	
	17 and under	18–19	20–21	22–24	25–29	30+	17 and under	18–19
Kindergarten Outcomes[a]								
Low birth weight								
Unadjusted mean outcomes	0.10**	0.06	0.05	0.06	0.06	0.05	-0.05**	-0.02
Adjusted outcomes after controls	0.08*	0.06	0.05	0.06	0.06	0.06	-0.03*	-0.01
Disabilities								
Unadjusted mean outcomes	0.14	0.13	0.13	0.12	0.12	0.12	0.00	0.01
Adjusted outcomes after controls	0.13	0.13	0.13	0.12	0.12	0.12	0.00	0.01
Risk of obesity								
Unadjusted mean outcomes	0.26	0.27	0.29	0.31	0.25	0.25	0.03	0.02
Adjusted outcomes after controls	0.23	0.24	0.26	0.30	0.27	0.28	0.04	0.02

				Adolescent Outcomes				
Overall health assessment (parent report)								
Unadjusted mean outcomes	4.20	4.19*	4.28	4.34	4.44***	4.47***	0.08	0.10*
Adjusted outcomes after controls	4.33	4.27	4.32	4.34	4.39	4.40+	0.00	0.05
Risk of obesity (age 12–16)								
Unadjusted mean outcomes	0.10	0.11	0.12	0.11	0.10	0.09+	0.02	0.01
Adjusted outcomes after controls	0.09	0.11	0.13	0.12	0.13	0.11	0.04	0.02
Used birth control at first sex[b]								
Unadjusted mean outcomes	0.74	0.75	0.79	0.79	0.80	0.86*	0.05	0.04
Adjusted outcomes after controls	0.76	0.76	0.79	0.78	0.79	0.85+	0.03	0.03

Sources: ECLS-K (kindergarten outcomes) and NLSY97 (adolescent outcomes).

Note: Significance indicates difference between children born to mothers age 20–21 and all other groups.

a. Adjusted outcome models control for maternal and child factors listed in tables 5.1 and 5.2.

b. Adjusted model controls for age at first sex along with controls listed in table 5.2.

+ $p < .10$; * $p < .05$; ** $p < .01$; *** $p < .001$

at child's birth, and then presents outcomes after controlling for child, mother, and grandparent characteristics. The last two columns of each table present the estimated consequence of teen childbearing compared with delaying childbirth to at least age 20–21. Tables 5.3–5.7 reflect predicted probability estimates based on full multivariate models for each outcome; the full models are presented in appendix tables A.5.1–A.5.5.

Cognitive Development and Academic Achievement

Kindergarten Outcomes. Table 5.3 indicates that children of younger and older teen mothers have lower cognitive attainment and proficiency scores at kindergarten entry relative to children of mothers age 20–21, both before and after controlling for maternal and child characteristics. Specifically, bivariate analyses indicate lower performance among children born to mothers age 17 or younger and to mothers age 18–19 on all kindergarten outcomes except approaches to learning (a parent report on how often her child exhibits task persistence, eagerness to learn new things, and creativity). After controlling for mother and child background characteristics, the differences are smaller and less significant (demonstrated in the last two columns of the table), but children of teen mothers still score lower on multiple outcomes. For example, children of younger and older teen mothers score significantly lower than do children of mothers age 20–21 on reading and general knowledge tests. In addition, children whose mothers were 17 or younger score marginally lower on letter recognition and awareness of beginning sounds than do children born to mothers age 20–21 ($p = .083$ and $p = .088$, respectively).

We find a significant interaction between maternal age and gender on children's knowledge of beginning sounds (in analyses not shown here). This finding indicates significantly lower scores on knowledge of beginning sounds among daughters of mothers who were age 17 and younger at birth, relative to daughters of women age 20–21 at birth, after controlling for maternal and child outcomes. However, gender interactions suggest no significant effect for male children. Children of mothers who were age 18–19 also have lower math test scores than do children of mothers who were age 20–21, net of controls. Unexpectedly, after controlling for mother and child background characteristics, we find that children born to the youngest mothers performed significantly *better* on approaches to learning than did children born to mothers age 20–21; however, the difference was only .06 on a 5-point scale. Note also that children of mothers age 22 and older score higher than do children of mothers age 20–21 on all outcomes except approaches to learning, even net of controls.

Other factors associated with cognitive outcomes among kindergarten children are shown in appendix table A.5.1 and include age of child, educational attainment of both the mother and maternal grandmother, and mother's marital status at the birth of the focal child, all of which were associated with positive kindergarten outcomes. These analyses also showed that being male, a member of a minority group, part of a multiple birth, or from a non-English-speaking home were associated with lower cognitive development.

Adolescent Outcomes. Before controlling for mother and child background characteristics, adolescent children of teen mothers have significantly lower Peabody Individual Achievement Test (PIAT) math and Armed Services Vocational Aptitude Battery (ASVAB) test scores than do adolescent children of mothers age 20–21 at first birth. The PIAT math test is a widely used, age-appropriate mathematics assessment, and the ASVAB assessment evaluates respondents' knowledge in a series of topic areas.[7] Children of teen mothers are also less likely than children of 20- to 21-year-old mothers to receive a high school diploma by age 19. However, after controlling for maternal and child background characteristics, we find no significant differences between adolescent children of teen mothers and adolescent children of mothers who were 20–21 at birth on cognitive and academic outcomes. Interaction models by gender (not shown here) indicate that a lower percentage of daughters of mothers who were age 18–19 at birth earn a high school diploma (71 percent) than do daughters of mothers who were in their early 20s at birth (80 percent), net of controls.

We find no comparable effect for adolescent male children. However, children born to delayed childbearers have a relative advantage compared with children of mothers age 20–21. Children born to mothers age 22 and older have significantly higher ASVAB scores and educational attainment than children born to mothers age 20–21, net of controls.

Appendix table A.5.1 also shows that mothers' and grandmothers' higher levels of education, along with mother's marital status at birth, are associated with more positive cognitive and academic outcomes among adolescents, while having a grandmother who was a teen at the mother's birth is associated with more negative cognitive outcomes. In addition, black adolescents and Hispanic adolescents have lower test scores than do other teens, and male respondents have significantly lower odds of academic achievement than do female respondents. Other factors associated with at least one negative cognitive outcome among adolescents included being older and having a mother who grew up in a central city or suburb.

Behavior Outcomes

Kindergarten Outcomes. Table 5.4 shows that a mother's age at first birth is minimally associated with behavioral outcomes at kindergarten. Before controlling for background factors, children born to teen mothers have significantly higher internalizing problem behaviors and lower levels of self-control than children born to mothers age 20–21. After taking into consideration mothers' and children's background characteristics, however, we find that children born to mothers age 17 or younger reportedly behave no differently than children born to mothers age 20–21. However, children born to mothers age 18–19 continue to have lower levels of self-control and marginally worse internalizing problem behaviors ($p = .057$) than do children born to mothers age 20–21, net of controls. These differences, however, are small—.06 and .08, respectively, on a 5-point scale. Interactions by gender (analyses not shown here) also indicate marginally worse internalizing problem behaviors among male (but not female) children of mothers age 17 and younger at first birth, and significantly lower self-control among male (but not female) children of mothers who were age 18–19 at first birth compared with children of mothers who were age 20–21 at first birth, net of controls. Further, the pattern of results suggests no better behavioral outcomes for children born to older mothers.

Appendix table A.5.2 indicates that age and maternal marital status at birth are associated with fewer negative behavioral outcomes. Male children have fewer problem behaviors than do females, and black children have higher levels of externalizing problem behaviors and lower levels of self-control—and of internalizing problem behaviors—than do white children. Other factors associated with fewer behavioral problems include being part of a multiple birth, having a mother who speaks a language other than English at home, and having a mother with higher educational attainment.

Adolescent Outcomes. Teen motherhood also has only a small association with behavioral outcomes among adolescents. Bivariate analyses indicate that children of teen mothers are significantly more likely to have a teen birth themselves than children of older mothers. These analyses also indicate that children of mothers age 18–19 at their first birth have significantly higher average scores on measures of delinquency than do children of mothers age 20–21 at their first birth. After controlling for mother and child background characteristics, however, these differences either disappear or reduce in magnitude.

One notable difference remains: children of mothers age 17 or younger when they first gave birth have marginally higher odds—and children of mothers age 18–19 at first birth have significantly higher odds—of having a teen birth themselves than do children of mothers who were 20–21 when they first had a child, net of controls. An estimated 13 percent of children of mothers age 17 and younger and an estimated 15 percent of children of mothers age 18–19 have a birth by age 18, after controlling for maternal and child background characteristics. This compares with an estimated 9 percent of children of mothers age 20–21 who have a birth by age 19. Also, as we found for kindergartners, adolescent children of older mothers have relatively few advantages over children born to mothers age 20–21, but children born to older mothers are significantly less likely to be sexually experienced or to have a baby by age 18.

Appendix table A.5.2 indicates that an older age is associated with more problem behaviors among adolescents. Factors associated with fewer problem behaviors include having a mother who was married at birth of focal child; spoke a language other than English; lived with both biological parents until age 14; grew up in a town, rural area, reservation, or military base (compared with a central city or suburb); or had higher educational attainment, although specific predictors differ by outcome. Additionally, having a grandmother with less education or who was a teen mother is negatively associated with at least one adolescent behavior problem. Finally, males have more delinquent behavior than do females, but females are more likely than males to become a parent by age 18. Black adolescents are less likely to have used substances by Round 3 than are white adolescents, but they are more likely to have had or fathered a child by age 18.

Home and Family Environment Outcomes

Kindergarten Outcomes. The family environment index shown in table 5.5 measures the number of activities such as reading books, telling stories, singing songs, and playing games and sports in which the kindergartner and his or her family members participate at least three times a week. Bivariate analyses show no association between having a teen mother and family environment. Interestingly, however, children born to the youngest teen mothers are significantly *more* likely to participate regularly in activities with family members such as having books read to them or stories told to them, playing sports, or playing games than are children born to mothers age 20–21, once controls are added to the model. We find no such differences between children born to mothers age 18–19 and their peers born to mothers age 20–21. The advantages associated with having an older mother found in bivariate analyses all disappear when we included multivariate controls.

Other factors associated with the family environment index are shown in appendix table A.5.3. More family activities are associated with younger child age, being female, being white, speaking only English at home, and greater educational attainment achieved by the mother and maternal grandmother.

Adolescent Outcomes. Before controlling for mother and child background characteristics, children of teen mothers have lower average scores on enriching environment and maternal monitoring and awareness measures do than their counterparts with 20–21-year-old mothers. In addition, children of mothers age 17 and younger have higher average physical environment risk scores than did children of 20–21-year-old mothers. However, once we control for background characteristics, we find no significant disadvantages faced by children of teen mothers.

In analyses not shown here, we find one significant gender interaction in multivariate models of family environments. Specifically, we find that female (but not male) children of mothers age 18–19 at first birth experience significantly higher physical environment risks than do female children of mothers age 20–21 at first birth. (The physical risk index was created from a combination of interviewer and youth reports on such items as how well kept the respondent's home and neighborhood appeared, how safe the interviewer felt in the neighborhood, how often the respondent heard gunshots, and whether the respondent regularly had electricity and heat.) Except for family routines, children of older mothers show clear advantages over children of mothers who were age 20–21 at their first birth before controlling for background factors. However, once controls are added to the models, only the enriching environment variable remains.

Other notable findings reported in appendix table A.5.3 are that child age, having a mother who was not married at birth, and being a member of a racial or ethnic minority are associated with more negative family environment outcomes. Having a mother who was born in the United States, who speaks a language other than English at home, had fewer siblings, or had higher educational attainment is associated with at least one positive family environment outcome. Having a mother who grew up in a suburb is associated with a lower score on measures of physical risk and with fewer family routines. In addition, being male is associated with less maternal monitoring and awareness than is being female.

Relationship Quality Outcomes

Kindergarten Outcomes. Table 5.6 indicates that before controlling for background characteristics, teacher assessments of the interpersonal skills of children born to teen mothers are significantly lower than teacher assessments of the interpersonal skills of children born to mothers age 20–21. However, after controlling for mother and child background characteristics, we find no significant differences in interpersonal skills between children born to the youngest teen mothers and only marginally significant differences ($p = .093$) between children born to mothers age 18–19 and children born to mothers age 20–21; these differences are small (.06 on a 5-point scale). Children born to mothers age 25–29 retain a slight advantage, but this is not the case for children born to mothers age 30 and over.

Appendix table A.5.4 indicates that child age, being female, having a mother who was married at first birth, and having a mother with at least a high school degree or GED are all associated with kindergartners' greater interpersonal skills.

Adolescent Outcomes. Teen motherhood has no association with adolescent relationship quality for any outcomes examined here, with one notable exception. Children of teen mothers have significantly greater odds of marrying or cohabiting by age 20 than do children of mothers age 20–21, both before and after controls. Specifically, an estimated 28 percent of children born to mothers age 17 and younger and an estimated 32 percent of children born to mothers age 18–19 have married or cohabited by age 20, after controls, compared with an estimated 21 percent of children born to mothers age 20–21. In addition, in separate multivariate models (not shown here), we find a significant interaction between maternal age and gender for models assessing how caring the adolescent's dating partner/spouse is perceived to be. Specifically, we find that daughters of mothers who were age 18–19 at first birth report *higher* levels of caring in their relationships reported at Round 6 or 7 of the NLSY97 (when ages ranged from 18 to 24) than do daughters of mothers age 20–21 at first birth. In contrast, adolescent sons of mothers who were age 18–19 at first birth report marginally *lower* levels of caring in these relationships than do sons of mothers who were age 20–21 at first birth.

In addition, we find that children of older mothers have advantages over children of teen mothers on three variables. Children of the oldest mothers have, on average, fewer negative peers and a higher-quality average mother-teen relationship than do children who have been born to 20–21-year-old mothers, while children who have been born to 25–29-year-old mothers are less likely to have married or cohabited by age 20 than are children born to mothers age 20–21.

Appendix table A.5.4 shows what other factors are associated with relationship quality outcomes in adolescents. Older adolescents and black adolescents have poorer relationship-quality outcomes. Factors positively associated with at least one relationship-quality outcome include being of non-Hispanic mixed race and having a mother with higher educational attainment. Factors associated with at least one negative relationship quality outcome include having a mother who was born in the United States, who had more siblings, who grew up in a suburb, and who had married at the child's birth.[8] Additionally, we find that males have fewer negative peers than do females but also that males have a lower-quality mother-teen relationship than do females.

Physical Health and Well-Being Outcomes

Kindergarten Outcomes. Table 5.7 indicates that children born to teenagers age 17 or younger are at a statistically significant disadvantage on one of four kindergarten health outcomes—low birth weight—compared with children born to mothers age 20–21. Although the magnitude of the difference drops after controlling for mother and child background characteristics (from 5 to 3 percentage points), children of the youngest mothers continue to be at a disadvantage regarding low birth weight compared with children born to mothers age 20–21. Mothers who gave birth at age 18–19 give a lower assessment of their child's overall health status than do mothers who were age 20–21 when their child was born; however, after controlling for mother and child background characteristics, this difference disappears. Mothers over age 30 at first birth report somewhat better health status for their child, but we find no other advantages in multivariate models.

Other factors associated with kindergarten health and well-being are shown in appendix table A.5.5. Factors associated with better health outcomes include an older age of child, female gender, Hispanic or other race/ethnicity, and higher educational attainment by the mother and maternal grandmother. Black children have lower odds of having a disability but higher odds of being low birth weight and of having lower health assessment scores than do white children. Additionally, children who are part of a multiple birth have higher odds of being of low birth weight and having a disability, but lower odds of being obese, than do children who are not part of a multiple birth. Children whose mothers speak a language other than English at home have lower odds of having a disability but also have assessments of poorer health than do children of mothers who speak only English.

Adolescent Outcomes. In the areas of physical health and well-being, children of young mothers do not differ, on average, from children of mothers age 20–21 at their first birth. In addition, after controlling for background characteristics, children of the oldest mothers have no advantages over children of younger mothers when it comes to being obese. And, again after controlling for background characteristics, the adolescent children of mothers who gave birth when they were 30 and older are only marginally more likely to have used contraception the first time that they had sex than are the children of younger mothers.

Appendix table A.5.5 shows that male gender, black or Hispanic race/ethnicity, having a mother who was born in the United States, having a mother with lower educational achievement, and having a grandmother who had a teen birth are all associated with greater odds of obesity. Additionally, adolescents who are older when they first had sex are more likely to use contraception (Abma et al. 2004).

Discussion

Table 5.8 synthesizes the findings of the bivariate and multivariate analyses of children of younger and older teen mothers compared with children of mothers who were age 20–21 at birth. Here, we summarize outcomes among kindergarten children using the ECLS-K data and among adolescent children using the NLSY97, by discussing answers to each research question that we posed.

Table 5.8. Outcomes of Birth to a Mother Age 20–21 Relative to Birth to a Teen Mother

	ECLS-K				NLSY97			
	Bivariate		Multivariate		Bivariate		Multivariate	
	≤17	18–19	≤17	18–19	≤17	18–19	≤17	18–19
Cognitive development								
IRT reading score	√	√	√	√				
IRT math score	√	√	0	√				
IRT general knowledge score	√	√	√	√				
Approaches to learning	0	0	x	0				
Letter recognition	√	√	(√)	0				
Beginning sounds	√	√	(√), F	0				
Ending sounds	√	√	0	0				
PIAT math score					√	√	0	0
ASVAB score					√	√	0	0
High school diploma by age 19					√	√	0	0, F
Four-year college by age 19					0	0	0	0
Behavior								
Internalizing problem behaviors	√	0	0, (M)	(√)				
Externalizing problem behaviors	0	0	0	0				
Self-control	√	√	0	√, M				
Sexually experienced by age 18					0	0	0	0
Birth by age 18					√	√	(√)	√
Ever used alcohol					0	0	x	0
Ever smoked a cigarette					0	0	0	0
Ever used marijuana					0	√	0	0
Delinquency index					(√)	√	0	0
Frequency of depression					0	0	0	0

Outcome						
Home environment						
Family environment index	0	0	0	√	0	0, F
Physical environment risk		0	0	√	√	0
Enriching environment				√	√	(√)
Maternal monitoring and awareness	x	0	0	0	0	0
Family routines	0					
Relationships						
Interpersonal skills	√	√	(√)	0	0	0
Positive peer environments				0	0	0
Negative peer environments				0	0	0
Mother-teen relationship	√	√	0	√	√	√
Married or cohabited by age 20	0			0	0	0
Closeness to dating partner/spouse				0	0	0, (M), xF
Caring behavior of dating partner/spouse	0			√	0	0
Amount of conflict with dating partner/spouse				0	0	0
Health						
Low birth weight	√	0	0	√		0
Disabilities	0	0	0	0		0
Overall health assessment	0	√	0	0		
Risk of obesity	0	0	0	0	0	0
Used birth control at first sex	0		0	0	0	0

Key:

√: A relative advantage among children born to mothers age 20 to 21

(√): A marginal advantage among children born to mothers age 20 to 21

0: No significant association

x: A relative advantage among children born to mothers age 17 or younger, or age 18 to 19

M, F: An interaction with gender and a relative advantage for male or female children born to mothers age 20–21

xF: An interaction and a relative advantage among female children born to teen mothers

On Average, Do Children of Teen Mothers Differ from Those Whose Mothers First Gave Birth in Their Early Twenties?

Our findings indicated differences, though not for all outcomes. In bivariate analyses, kindergarten-age and adolescent children of teen mothers exhibit relative disadvantages on most cognitive and academic outcomes (with lower scores on six of seven kindergarten outcomes and on three of four adolescent outcomes), and on three of four adolescent home environment outcomes. Findings in other domains are more mixed. Analyses suggest children of teen mothers are relatively disadvantaged on some behavioral outcomes (including two of three kindergarten outcomes and two of seven adolescent outcomes) and on some relationship outcomes (including poorer interpersonal skills among kindergarten-age children and relationship conflict and early marriage/cohabitation among adolescents). Findings also show a relative disadvantage for children of teen mothers on two of four health outcomes, including lower reported birth weight among children of the youngest teen mothers and lower overall health assessment among children of older teen mothers; however, there were no bivariate associations for the two adolescent health measures.

Do Differences in Child Outcomes by Maternal Age Remain after Controlling for Family Background Characteristics?

After controlling for maternal and child background characteristics (multivariate analyses), associations between teen parenthood and child outcomes are concentrated in the cognitive and academic domains, especially among kindergarten children. Children of younger and older teen mothers have poorer scores on five of seven kindergarten outcomes (including one marginal association and one association that was significant for females only). The magnitude of the kindergarten effects, however, is fairly small, representing only about one-tenth of a standard deviation. While only one of the three adolescent educational outcomes remains significant, it is a critical outcome; daughters of 18- to 19-year-old mothers have lower odds of completing high school than do children of 20- to 21-year-old mothers. The associations between adolescent motherhood and more negative cognitive and educational outcomes concur with findings from other data files (Haveman et al. 1997; Levine et al. 2001; Moore et al. 1997; Moore and Snyder 1991).

Among kindergarten children, net of controls, having a young mother is associated with lower scores on four of nine noncognitive outcomes, including two behavioral outcomes (lower self-control among sons of 18- to 19-year-old mothers at birth and marginally higher internalizing problem behaviors), the measure of interpersonal skills (a marginal association), and one health outcome (low birth weight among babies of younger teen mothers). Among adolescent children of teen mothers, having a young mother is associated with only 5 of the 20 noncognitive outcomes, net of controls, including greater odds of having a baby before age 18, more physical environment risks (among daughters of 18- to 19-year-old mothers at birth), marginally reduced maternal monitoring and awareness (among 18- to 19-year-old teen mothers at birth), greater odds of marrying or cohabiting before age 20, a marginally lower reported level of caring within a relationship among sons, and a *higher* reported level of caring within a relationship among daughters of mothers who gave birth as 18- to 19-year-olds (see gender difference discussion below). The intergenerational trend in teen parenthood supports other research (Haveman et al. 1997; Kahn and Anderson 1992; Manlove 1997) as does the link to parenting (Moore et al. 1997).

Do the Negative Consequences of Being Born to a Teen Mother Vary by Maternal Age or across the Stages of the Child's Life Cycle?

Our findings suggest similarly problematic outcomes among children of younger and older teen mothers for many outcomes examined. This result contrasts with results of other research that finds especially negative outcomes among children of mothers age 17 and younger at birth (Maynard 1997). The fact that we do not find more negative outcomes among children of the youngest teen mothers may partly result from their living situations. Our sample characteristics (reported in tables 5.1 and 5.2) show that older teen mothers were much more likely to be married at the birth of their child than were mothers age 17 and younger at birth. High marital dissolution rates among teen mothers may lead to greater turbulence in family situations for children of these mothers, which may be associated with more negative outcomes (Abma et al. 2004; Furstenberg, Brooks-Gunn, and Morgan 1987). In contrast, children of the youngest teen mothers may be more likely to stay in their family home, which may be associated with improved child outcomes.

Our analyses indicate more significant findings among kindergarten children than among adolescent children of teen mothers. These findings may reflect, in part, the larger sample of children in the ECLS-K data—more than 6,000 respondents, compared with fewer than 3,000 in the NLSY97. We are particularly troubled by the amount of missing data for parents of adolescents in this survey, and our analyses indicate that we may have excluded some of the highest-risk parents from the NLSY97 sample. One direction for future research is to test the effects of teenage motherhood on outcomes across the life course of a cohort of children instead of comparing outcomes among different samples of children and adolescents.

Do the Associations between Maternal Age and Child or Adolescent Outcomes Differ by Child Gender?

We find limited interaction effects by child gender, indicating that most effects of maternal age on child outcomes are similar for males and females. Table 5.8 shows that several outcomes are significant for males or females only, including negative associations between teenage motherhood and young female children's abilities to match the beginning sounds of letters with the appropriate words, with female adolescents' success in earning a high school diploma, with physical home risks for females but not for males, and with a relative disadvantage for sons of teen mothers on internalizing problem behaviors and self-control. Interestingly, one interaction shows opposite associations between adolescent motherhood and reported caring by a relationship partner; it shows marginally *lower* reported caring for a relationship partner among sons and *higher* reported caring among daughters of mothers who gave birth when they were age 18–19. Additional analyses (not shown here) suggest that the higher reports of caring among these daughters partly results from the greater likelihood that they are in a marital or cohabiting relationship at an early age.

Is Delaying Childbearing Associated with Especially Positive Outcomes?

Child outcomes continue to improve with increasing maternal age, especially in the cognitive domain, even after controlling for maternal and child background characteristics. In particular, children of mothers age 22 and older at birth have more positive cognitive and academic outcomes than do children of mothers age 20–21 at birth in six of the seven kindergarten outcomes and in three of the four adolescent outcomes. The other outcome domains do not show a similar linear trend between maternal age and child outcomes.

These findings in the cognitive domain suggest that delaying childbearing until mothers are in their mid- to late 20s may be associated with even more positive child outcomes, especially if delaying childbearing is accompanied by mothers' improved educational attainment and a greater likelihood of having a child within a stable marriage. High rates of nonmarital childbearing in the early 20s, combined with poorer cognitive outcomes among children of these mothers relative to older mothers, suggest that mothers who give birth in their early 20s may be another target group for intervention. The high rates of nonmarital childbearing among teens and young adults is reflected in the sample characteristics among mothers of the kindergarten cohort from the late 1990s. For this cohort, women had to reach age 22 before the majority of them were married when they gave birth.

Limitations

Our analyses have some limitations, primarily due to data quality. As noted above, while we excluded almost no firstborn children of teen mothers in our kindergarten sample (less than 1 percent), our adolescent sample was missing much more data. Because of missing data on biological mothers, we removed one-quarter of the NLSY97 sample, including 10 percent of adolescents because they did not live with their biological mothers and 17 percent of adolescents because their mothers did not fill out the parent survey. Our analyses indicate that those excluded from the sample are more likely to be children of teen mothers and to have mothers with low education levels.

In addition, we were limited in the number and range of measurable controls for the kindergarten and adolescent surveys. In particular, neither survey included a measure of the mother's cognitive ability, which other studies have shown is strongly associated with both maternal age at first birth and child outcomes (Levine et al. 2001; Moore and Snyder 1991). However, we did have a strong set of maternal, child, and even grandparent controls for each survey. Finally, even net of a strong set of controls, the remaining associations between parental age and child outcomes may be endogenous. For example, unobserved factors may be associated with both teen parenthood and child well-being. Thus, future analyses should employ methods to help control for endogeneity. These limitations were offset by the strengths of using recently available, nationally representative data to assess the potential influence of maternal age on child outcomes in recent cohorts of children and adolescents.

Conclusion

These findings have several implications. One conclusion is that a young maternal age represents a clear marker for children who will experience challenges and disadvantages. Without controlling for confounding factors, the bivariate results clearly indicate that children born to teen mothers are a disadvantaged group and that delaying these pregnancies would foster child well-being. Another conclusion flows from the pattern of findings. When social, economic, and demographic factors are controlled, many findings diminish or go away, which suggests that improving mother's educational and social circumstances would contribute to better outcomes for children. In other words, delaying the first birth is part of the story but not the whole story.

Description of Dependent Variables

Table A.5.6 provides the mean, standard error, and range for all measures.

Early Child Longitudinal Study, Kindergarten Class of 1998–99

Cognition, Knowledge, and Academic Achievement

The assessments used to measure children's reading, math, and general knowledge skills were based on item response theory (IRT). IRT tests are designed to compare the scores of children receiving questions of varying levels of difficulty. In part 1, children answered general questions to determine the difficulty level of the second stage of questioning. Questions in part 2 focused on the topic area of interest (e.g., reading, math, and general knowledge). See Westat et al. (2001) for more information.

IRT reading test score (direct assessment) measures the child's reading knowledge at kindergarten entry.

IRT math test score (direct assessment) measures the child's math knowledge at kindergarten entry.

IRT general knowledge test score (direct assessment) measures the child's general knowledge of the social, physical, and natural world at kindergarten entry.

text continues on page 212

Table A.5.1. Odds Ratios and Coefficient Estimates for Cognitive and Academic Achievement Outcomes

	ECLS-K			
	IRT reading	IRT math	IRT general knowledge	Approaches to learning
Age of mother at focal child's birth[a]				
Under 17	−0.78*	−0.35	−0.89**	0.07*
18–19	−0.77*	−0.68*	−0.73**	0.02
22–24	1.17**	0.72*	0.75*	−0.02
25–29	2.36***	2.07***	2.05***	−0.05*
30+	3.51***	2.66***	3.25***	−0.03
Child characteristics				
Age	5.10***	5.35***	5.86***	0.05**
Male	−1.63***	−0.22	0.03	−0.10***
Race/ethnicity[b]				
Black	−0.16	−1.69***	−4.85***	0.00
Hispanic	−0.80*	−1.61***	−1.64***	−0.03
Non-Hispanic mixed (NLSY)/ other (ECLS-K)	0.86	−0.10	−2.79***	−0.02
Child part of multiple birth	−2.22***	−1.73***	−1.75*	−0.07
Mother characteristics				
Born in the United States	—	—	—	—
Speaks language other than English at home	−0.79+	−1.06***	−2.92***	−0.08***
Lived with both bio parents until age 14	—	—	—	—
Number of siblings	—	—	—	—
Grew up in a city, town, or rural area[c]				
Central city	—	—	—	—
Suburb	—	—	—	—
Married at birth of focal child	1.39***	0.86***	0.53*	0.04*
Highest grade completed (1–20 NLSY)[d]				
Less than high school	−2.35***	−2.03***	−2.17***	−0.09***
Vocational degree	1.16***	1.16***	1.17***	0.07***
College graduate	4.52***	3.49***	3.29***	0.09***

				NLSY97		
Letter recognition	Beginning sounds	Ending sounds	PIAT math	ASVAB	High school diploma by 19	Enrolled in 4-year college by 19
−0.04+	−0.03+	−0.01	−4.15	−2.19	0.78	1.13
−0.04	−0.02	−0.02	−4.21	−2.71	0.83	1.04
0.05*	0.07***	0.04**	2.61	5.68**	1.36+	1.83***
0.12***	0.11***	0.07***	5.15*	7.46***	1.88***	2.94***
0.14***	0.15***	0.11***	4.68	9.33***	1.95**	2.77***
0.15***	0.21***	0.17***	−4.74***	−0.04	0.98	0.96
−0.07***	−0.08***	−0.06***	2.93*	−0.54	0.67***	0.68***
0.01	−0.01	0.00	−16.40***	−17.97***	1.06	1.14
−0.06***	−0.02	−0.01	−9.46**	−12.04***	1.17	0.80
0.00	0.02	0.03	−2.62	3.20	1.13	1.01
−0.09**	−0.06+	−0.07**	—	—	—	—
—	—	—	−1.98	−2.20	0.64+	0.77
−0.08**	−0.03+	−0.01	0.13	0.73	0.87	1.02
—	—	—	−0.17	−0.26	1.05	0.99
—	—	—	−0.26	−0.20	0.98	0.99
—	—	—	−1.58	−2.38	0.71*	0.83
—	—	—	3.05	2.25	0.72*	1.06
0.06***	0.06***	0.04***	5.79**	4.76**	1.70***	1.59***
			2.66***	2.77***	1.18***	1.23***
−0.14***	−0.07***	−0.04***	—	—	—	—
0.07***	0.06***	0.04***	—	—	—	—
0.15***	0.21***	0.16***	—	—	—	—

(continued)

Table A.5.1. *(Continued)*

	ECLS-K			
	IRT reading	IRT math	IRT general knowledge	Approaches to learning
Grandparent characteristics				
Highest grade completed by maternal grandmother (1–7 NLSY, 1–22 ECLS-K)	0.11**	0.12***	0.17***	0.01***
Grandmother a teen at mom's birth	—	—	—	—
F/Wald chi square (degrees of freedom in parentheses)	95.28*** (17, 421)	86.69*** (17, 425)	182.44*** (17, 420)	16.74*** (17, 429)
Intercept	−9.56***	−13.97***	−13.61***	2.81***
R^2	0.22	0.29	0.36	0.05
N	5,707	5,985	5,688	6,227

$^+p < .10$; $^*p < .05$; $^{**}p < .01$; $^{***}p < .001$

a. Omitted mother's age category is 20–21.

b. Omitted race/ethnicity category is nonblack/non-Hispanic.

c. Omitted category for mother's environment growing up is town or other.

d. Omitted ECLS-K mother's education category is high school graduate/GED.

			NLSY97			
Letter recognition	Beginning sounds	Ending sounds	PIAT math	ASVAB	High school diploma by 19	Enrolled in 4-year college by 19
0.00	0.01***	0.00***	1.52*	1.49***	1.19***	1.13**
—	—	—	−5.52**	−5.45**	0.63**	0.95
63.98***	134.00***	75.68***	30.31***	55.55***	241.37***	285.11***
(17, 421)	(17, 421)	(17, 421)	(20, 187)	(20, 2315)	(20)	(20)
−0.26**	−1.03***	−0.88***	77.09***	13.61+	—	—
0.18	0.22	0.19	0.24	0.29	—	—
5,707	5,707	5,707	1,898	2,336	2,572	2,555

Table A.5.2. Odds Ratios and Coefficient Estimates for Behavior Outcomes

	ECLS-K		
	Internalizing problem behaviors	Externalizing problem behaviors	Self-control
Age of mother at focal child's birth[a]			
Under 17	0.03	0.01	−0.04
18–19	0.06[+]	0.02	−0.08*
22–24	0.04	−0.04	−0.02
25–29	0.01	−0.06*	0.04
30+	0.05*	0.01	−0.03
Child characteristics			
Age	−0.06**	−0.07**	0.14***
Male	0.04**	0.29***	−0.22***
Race/ethnicity[b]			
Black	−0.07**	0.10**	−0.10*
Hispanic	−0.02	0.00	−0.04
Non-Hispanic mixed (NLSY)/other (ECLS-K)	−0.03	0.01	−0.05
Child part of multiple birth	−0.07	−0.15*	0.14[+]
Mother characteristics			
Born in the United States	—	—	—
Speaks language other than English at home	−0.07**	−0.07*	0.03
Lived with both bio parents until age 14	—	—	—
Number of siblings	—	—	—
Grew up in a city, town, or rural area[c]			
Central city	—	—	—
Suburb	—	—	—
Married at birth of focal child	−0.06**	−0.10***	0.12***
Highest grade completed (1–20 NLSY)[d]			
Less than high school	0.09*	0.07[+]	−0.09*
Vocational degree	−0.02	0.01	0.01
College graduate	−0.05**	−0.02	0.01
Grandparent characteristics			
Highest grade completed by maternal grandmother (1–7 NLSY, 1–22 ECLS-K)	0.00	−0.01[+]	0.00
Grandmother a teen at mom's birth	—	—	—
F/Wald chi square (degrees of freedom in parentheses)	4.41*** (17, 415)	23.26*** (17, 415)	19.37*** (17, 414)
Intercept	1.88***	1.93***	2.38***
R^2	0.02	0.08	0.07
N	5,728	5,799	5,640

[+]$p < .10$; *$p < .05$; **$p < .01$; ***$p < .001$

a. Omitted mother's age category is 20–21.

b. Omitted race/ethnicity category is nonblack/non-Hispanic.

c. Omitted category for mother's environment growing up is town or other.

d. Omitted ECLS-K mother's education category is high school graduate/GED.

			NLSY97			
Sex by 18	Birth by 18	Ever drank by round 3	Ever smoked by round 3	Ever used marijuana by round 3	Delinquency at round 1	Depression at round 6
1.20	1.62+	0.66*	1.05	0.77	0.16	0.00
1.47	1.86*	0.92	1.11	0.96	0.22	0.00
0.84	0.67	0.96	0.93	0.92	−0.13	−0.02
0.66*	0.80	0.86	0.88	0.85	−0.05	−0.03
0.69+	0.63	0.97	0.97	1.01	−0.19	−0.03
1.01	1.04	1.55***	1.37***	1.38***	0.23***	0.00
0.98	0.35***	0.89	0.93	1.05	0.72***	−0.08**
1.31	1.52*	0.44***	0.47***	0.67**	−0.03	0.07
1.42+	1.08	1.48*	0.91	1.17	0.05	−0.07
1.71	4.14*	0.88	0.90	1.27	−0.11	0.18
—	—	—	—	—	—	—
1.30	1.54	1.12	1.06	1.14	−0.05	0.00
0.68+	1.23	0.60**	0.69*	0.68+	−0.31*	0.09
0.74*	1.03	0.94	1.03	0.75**	−0.08	0.02
1.03	1.01	1.00	1.01	0.99	0.01	0.01**
0.92	1.31	1.12	0.97	1.28*	0.10	0.07+
0.84	0.81	1.05	1.00	1.22+	0.19*	0.04
0.68**	0.50***	0.87	0.80*	0.69**	−0.17+	−0.07+
0.95+	0.89***	0.99	0.97	0.99	0.00	−0.01*
—	—	—	—	—	—	—
—	—	—	—	—	—	—
—	—	—	—	—	—	—
0.97	0.86*	1.05	1.00	1.07+	0.01	−0.01
1.05	1.37	1.06	1.27+	1.13	0.11	0.10*
108.42***	233.83***	210.71***	148.13***	144.43***	11.52***	3.54***
(20)	(20)	(20)	(20)	(20)	(20, 2874)	(20)
—	—	—	—	—	−2.18***	1.65***
—	—	—	—	—	0.10	0.03
2,757	2,894	2,895	2,896	2,895	2,895	2,580

Table A.5.3. Odds Ratios and Coefficient Estimates for Family Environment Outcomes

	ECLS-K	NLSY97			
	Family environment index	Physical risk	Enriching environment	Maternal monitoring/ awareness	Family routines
Age of mother at focal child's birth[a]					
Under 17	0.24**	0.11	-0.03	-0.49	1.00
18–19	-0.02	0.11	-0.09	-0.65+	0.17
22–24	0.01	-0.20+	0.06	-0.04	-0.34
25–29	0.09	-0.27*	0.16*	-0.12	-0.72+
30+	-0.01	-0.16	0.17*	0.22	-1.35**
Child characteristics					
Age	-0.12*	-0.03	-0.05*	-0.56***	-0.90***
Male	-0.08*	0.04	-0.06+	-0.60***	0.42
Race/ethnicity[b]					
Black	-0.35***	0.43***	-0.11*	-0.48+	-0.32
Hispanic	-0.20**	0.19	-0.17*	-0.34	-0.71
Non-Hispanic mixed (NLSY)/other (ECLS-K)	-0.30***	0.77**	-0.35	-0.26	0.15
Child part of multiple birth	0.10	—	—	—	—
Mother characteristics					
Born in the United States	-0.31***	0.25+	-0.05	0.10	1.24*
Speaks language other than English at home	—	0.12	-0.02	0.00	1.61**
Lived with both bio parents until age 14	—	-0.03	0.01	0.16	0.23
Number of siblings	—	0.03*	-0.01+	0.05	0.10+

	(1)	(2)	(3)	(4)	(5)
Grew up in a city, town, or rural area[c]					
Central city	—	-0.04	-0.01	0.30	-0.31
Suburb	—	-0.17*	0.07	0.20	-0.65*
Married at birth of focal child	0.03	-0.25**	0.19***	0.68**	1.28***
Highest grade completed (1–20 NLSY)[d]					
Less than high school	-0.26***	-0.09***	0.07***	0.05	0.09
Vocational degree	0.16***	—	—	—	—
College graduate	0.37***	—	—	—	—
Grandparent characteristics					
Highest grade completed by maternal grandmother (1–7 NLSY, 1–22 ECLS-K)	0.03***	0.00	0.03+	0.06	-0.18
Grandmother a teen at mom's birth	—	0.20+	-0.05	-0.01	-0.31
F/Wald chi square (degrees of freedom in parentheses)	22.74*** (17, 429)	13.03*** (20, 1598)	20.68*** (20, 1638)	5.18*** (20, 1625)	3.76*** (20, 1625)
Intercept	3.61***	2.65***	1.37***	16.74***	24.22***
R^2	0.07	0.16	0.20	0.07	0.05
N	6,227	1,619	1,638	1,646	1,646

+$p < .10$; *$p < .05$; **$p < .01$; ***$p < .001$

a. Omitted mother's age category is 20–21.

b. Omitted race/ethnicity category is nonblack/non-Hispanic.

c. Omitted category for mother's environment growing up is town or other.

d. Omitted ECLS-K mother's education category is high school graduate/GED.

Table A.5.4. Odds Ratios and Coefficient Estimates for Relationship Quality Outcomes

	ECLS-K		
	Interpersonal skills	Positive peer environments	Negative peer environments
Age of mother at focal child's birth[a]			
Under 17	−0.06	−0.02	0.01
18–19	−0.06+	0.05	−0.02
22–24	−0.03	0.05	−0.11
25–29	0.08*	0.08	−0.16+
30+	0.00	0.14	−0.35**
Child characteristics			
Age	0.12***	−0.13***	0.63***
Male	−0.24***	−0.06	−0.31***
Race/ethnicity[b]			
Black	−0.05	0.06	0.31**
Hispanic	−0.03	0.02	0.23+
Non-Hispanic mixed (NLSY)/other (ECLS-K)	−0.04	−0.30	0.10
Child part of multiple birth	0.12	—	—
Mother characteristics			
Born in the United States	—	−0.24*	0.15
Speaks language other than English at home	−0.01	−0.17	0.07
Lived with both bio parents until age 14	—	0.00	0.00
Number of siblings	—	−0.02*	0.00
Grew up in a city, town, or rural area[c]			
Central city	—	−0.01	0.09
Suburb	—	−0.03	0.08
Married at birth of focal child	0.09***	0.08	−0.11
Highest grade completed (1–20 NLSY)[d]		0.04***	−0.02
Less than high school	−0.08*	—	—
Vocational degree	0.04	—	—
College graduate	0.06+	—	—
Grandparent characteristics			
Highest grade completed by maternal grandmother (1–7 NLSY, 1–22 ECLS-K)	0.00	0.00	−0.01
Grandmother a teen at mom's birth	—	−0.20**	0.16+
F/Wald chi square (degrees of freedom in parentheses)	26.16*** (17, 414)	6.79*** (20, 2784)	53.91*** (20, 2763)
Intercept	2.32***	3.27***	−5.55***
R^2	0.07	0.05	0.30
N	5,622	2,805	2,784

+$p < .10$; *$p < .05$; **$p < .01$; ***$p < .001$

a. Omitted mother's age category is 20–21.

b. Omitted race/ethnicity category is nonblack/non-Hispanic.

c. Omitted category for mother's environment growing up is town or other.

d. Omitted ECLS-K mother's education category is high school graduate/GED.

	NLSY97			
Mother-teen relationship	Married or cohabited by 20	Closeness to partner/spouse	Caring behavior of partner/ spouse	Amount of conflict with partner/spouse
0.00	1.52+	−0.08	−0.04	0.49
−0.13	1.88***	0.02	0.10	0.25
0.06	0.92	−0.14	−0.02	0.02
0.07	0.69*	−0.22	−0.17	−0.03
0.52*	0.82	−0.25	−0.11	−0.05
−0.39***	1.12**	0.03	0.05+	0.04
−0.30*	0.37***	−0.12	−0.12+	−0.01
0.29	0.38***	−0.41**	−0.16	0.78***
−0.35	0.98	0.12	0.13	0.42
−0.74	1.45	0.63*	0.65***	0.79
—	—	—	—	—
−0.03	1.46	0.25+	0.17	−0.37
0.20	0.73	−0.10	−0.03	0.06
−0.08	0.90	0.01	0.02	0.02
0.00	1.04*	0.00	0.00	−0.01
−0.32	1.12	0.11	−0.10	−0.17
−0.21	0.77+	−0.10	0.00	0.39*
0.38+	0.75*	−0.05	−0.24**	−0.21
−0.03	0.91***	0.00	0.01	0.01
—	—	—	—	—
—	—	—	—	—
—	—	—	—	—
0.04	0.90*	−0.04	0.00	−0.01
−0.15	1.47**	−0.03	−0.04	0.25
2.50***	231.55***	1.86*	3.74***	2.00**
(20, 1624)	(20)	(20, 1805)	(20, 1806)	(20, 1806)
14.45***		8.54***	8.57***	2.87***
0.03		0.02	0.02	0.03
1,645	2,897	1,826	1,827	1,827

Table A.5.5. Odds Ratios and Coefficient Estimates for Health Outcomes

	ECLS-K				NLSY97	
	Low birth weight	Disabilities	Risk of obesity	Health assessment	Risk of obesity (1997)	Used birth control at first sex
Age of mother at focal child's birth[a]						
Under 17	1.81*	1.01	0.82	0.00	0.67	0.82
18–19	1.21	0.95	0.89	-0.05	0.82	0.82
22–24	1.18	0.88	1.19	0.02	0.95	0.96
25–29	1.33	0.86	1.03	0.06	1.06	1.00
30+	1.20	0.89	1.08	0.08+	0.90	1.50+
Child characteristics						
Age	1.70**	1.51**	1.06	0.00	0.98	1.03
Male	0.93	1.72***	1.08	-0.07***	1.99***	0.86
Race/ethnicity[b]						
Black	2.85***	0.56***	1.12	-0.11*	2.23***	1.33
Hispanic	1.70**	0.87	1.41**	-0.10**	1.85*	0.91
Non-Hispanic mixed (NLSY)/other (ECLS-K)	1.40	0.72*	1.14	-0.24***	1.94	0.70
Child part of a multiple birth	20.67***	1.91*	0.46**	-0.07	—	—
Mother characteristics						
Born in the United States	0.78	0.58**	0.95	-0.10*	2.60***	1.06
Speaks language other than English at home	—	—	—	—	1.06	0.82
Lived with both bio parents until age 14	—	—	—	—	1.12	1.06
Number of siblings	—	—	—	—	0.97	1.01

Grew up in a city, town, or rural area[c]						
Central city	—	—	—	—	1.11	0.80
Suburb	—	—	—	—	0.71+	0.85
Married at birth of focal child	1.02	0.84	0.87+	0.04	1.16	1.03
Highest grade completed (1–20 NLSY)[d]						
Less than high school	1.26	1.19	0.87	-0.18***	—	—
Vocational degree	1.05	1.05	0.96	0.06+	—	—
College graduate	0.83	1.05	0.81+	0.10**	—	—
Grandparent characteristics						
Highest grade completed by maternal grandmother (1–7 NLSY, 1–22 ECLS-K)	1.01	1.01	0.97**	0.01**	0.91	1.03
Grandmother a teen at mom's birth	—	—	—	—	1.56*	1.01
Age at first sex	—	—	—	—	—	1.08**
F/Wald chi square (degrees of freedom in parentheses)	12.32*** (17, 429)	5.89*** (17, 429)	3.36*** (17, 426)	16.27*** (17, 429)	97.02*** (20)	44.18** (21)
Intercept	—	—	—	4.20***	—	—
R²	—	—	—	0	—	—
N	6,215	6,228	6,049	6,227	2,796	2,411

+p < .10; *p < .05; **p < .01; ***p < .001

a. Omitted mother's age category is 20–21.

b. Omitted race/ethnicity category is nonblack/non-Hispanic.

c. Omitted category for mother's environment growing up is town or other.

d. Omitted ECLS-K mother's education category is high school graduate/GED.

Table A.5.6. Descriptive Statistics for Dependent Variables

	ECLS-K			NLSY97		
	Mean	Standard error	Range	Mean	Standard error	Range
Cognitive development						
IRT reading score	23.60	0.21	0–72			
IRT math score	19.85	0.16	0–64			
IRT general knowledge score	23.19	0.20	0–52			
Approaches to learning	3.15	0.01	1–4			
Letter recognition	0.72	0.01	0–1			
Beginning sounds	0.36	0.01	0–1			
Ending sounds	0.21	0.01	0–1			
PIAT math score				54.29	0.78	0–100
ASVAB score				55.04	0.60	0–100
High school diploma by age 19				0.79	0.01	0–1
Four-year college by age 19				0.33	0.01	0–1
Behavior						
Internalizing problem behaviors	1.54	0.01	1–4			
Externalizing problem behaviors	1.65	0.01	1–4			
Self-control	3.08	0.01	1–4			
Sexually experienced by age 18				0.78	0.01	0–1
Birth by age 18				0.08	0.00	0–1
Ever used alcohol				0.71	0.01	0–1
Ever smoked a cigarette				0.55	0.01	0–1
Ever used marijuana				0.37	0.01	0–1
Delinquency index				1.29	0.03	0–10
Frequency of depression				1.40	0.01	1–4
Home environment						
Family environment index	3.31	0.01	0–5			
Physical environment risk				1.07	0.03	0–7
Enriching environment risk				1.88	0.02	0–3
Maternal monitoring and awareness				10.69	0.08	0–16
Family routines				15.49	0.12	0–28

Table A.5.6. *(Continued)*

	ECLS-K			NLSY97		
	Mean	Standard error	Range	Mean	Standard error	Range
Relationships						
Interpersonal skills	2.98	0.01	1–4			
Positive peer environments				1.75	0.02	0–4
Negative peer environments				2.93	0.03	0–5
Mother-teen relationship				9.13	0.07	0–12
Married or cohabited by age 20				0.21	0.01	0–1
Closeness to dating partner/spouse				8.89	0.04	0–10
Caring behavior of dating partner/ spouse				9.27	0.03	0–10
Amount of conflict with dating partner/spouse				3.31	0.06	0–10
Health						
Low birth weight	0.06	0.00	0–1			
Disabilities	0.12	0.01	0–1			
Overall health assessment	4.35	0.01	1–5			
Risk of obesity	0.27	0.01	0–1	0.11	0.01	0–1
Used birth control at first sex				0.79	0.01	0–1

Approaches to learning (parent assessment). The Social Rating Scale (SRS) assesses kindergartners' approaches to learning, a concept that targets how ready children are to engage meaningfully in school.[9] The child's parent assesses how often their kindergartner exhibits the following behaviors (scaled from 1 "never" to 4 "very often"): task persistence, eagerness to learn new things, and creativity (Westat et al. 2001).

Letter recognition (direct assessment) measures whether the child is proficient for his or her age in recognizing upper- and lowercase letters.

Beginning sounds (direct assessment) measures whether the child is proficient for his or her age in identifying the corresponding letter to sounds at the beginning of words.

Ending sounds (direct assessment) measures whether the child is proficient for his or her age in identifying the corresponding letter to sounds at the end of words.

Behavior and Delinquency

All three measures included in the kindergarten outcome section of behavior and delinquency were created based on the Social Rating Scale, which is based on the teacher's assessment of how frequently the child exhibited each behavior and social skill.

Internalizing problem behaviors (teacher report) measures how often the child exhibits anxiety, loneliness, low self-esteem, and sadness (scaled from 1 "never" to 4 "very often").

Externalizing problem behaviors (teacher report) measures how often the child exhibits arguing, fighting, getting angry, acting impulsively, and disturbing ongoing activities (scaled from 1 "never" to 4 "very often").

Self-control (teacher report) measures how often the child exhibits self-control (scaled from 1 "never" to 4 "very often").

Home Environment and Family Integration

Family environment index (parent report) is a summative index measuring how many of the following five activities a family member and the child participate in at least three days a week: reading books to the child, telling stories to the child, singing songs with the child, playing sports with the child, and playing games with the child.

Relationship Outcomes

Interpersonal skills (teacher report) measures how frequently the child forms and maintains friendships; gets along with people who are different; comforts or helps other children; expresses feelings, ideas, and opinions in positive ways; and shows sensitivity to the feelings of others (scaled from 1 "never" to 4 "very often").

Physical Health and Well-Being

Low birth weight (parent report) measures whether the child weighed less than 5.5 lbs at birth.

Disabilities (parent report) measures whether the child has any disabilities (as diagnosed by a professional) including those relating to paying attention, activity level, use of limbs, or ability to communicate, hear, and see, or if the child has received therapy services or taken part in a program for children with disabilities.

Risk of obesity (direct assessment). Each child's height and weight is used to calculate body mass index (BMI), which is then compared with growth charts produced by the Centers for Disease Control to determine whether the child's weight for height percentage is greater than the 95th percentile for his or her age group.

Overall health assessment (parent report) measures the parent's report of the child's overall health (scaled from 1 "excellent" to 5 "poor").

National Longitudinal Survey of Youth–1997 Cohort

Cognition, Knowledge, and Academic Achievement

Peabody Individual Achievement Test math score (1997) is a standardized assessment that measures math proficiency at round 1.

Armed Services Vocational Aptitude Battery (1997–98) is a standardized test given between summer 1997 and spring 1998 that evaluates the respondent's knowledge in several topic areas including arithmetic reasoning, assembling objects, auto information, coding speed, electronics information, general science, mathematics knowledge, mechanical comprehension, numerical operations, paragraph comprehension, shop information, and word knowledge.

Received high school diploma by age 19 is based on the respondent's reports of his or her highest degree ever received at the round of the NLSY97 in which he or she was 19. Respondents who had not yet turned 19 by round 7 or who were not interviewed at age 19 were excluded from this measure.

Enrolled in a four-year college or higher at age 19 is based on the respondent's report of whether s/he graduated from, or is enrolled in, a four-year college or graduate program at the round in which s/he was 19. Respondents who had not turned 19 by round 7 or were not interviewed at age 19 were excluded from this measure.

Behavior and Delinquency

Sexually experienced by age 18 is based on the respondent's report of whether s/he has ever had sex, and at what age. We excluded from this measure respondents who did not have a valid age of first sex or who were not interviewed through age 18.

Teen birth by age 18 is based on the respondent's report of the date of birth of her first child. We excluded from this measure respondents who were not interviewed through age 18.

Ever used alcohol (1997–99) is based on the respondent's report of whether s/he has ever drunk a can or bottle of beer, a glass of wine, a mixed drink, or a shot of liquor in rounds 1, 2, or 3 (respondents were age 12–16 in round 1 to 14–20 in round 3).

Ever smoked a cigarette (1997–99) is based on the respondent's report of whether s/he has ever smoked a cigarette in rounds 1, 2, or 3 (respondents were age 12–16 in round 1 to 14–20 in round 3).

Ever used marijuana (1997–99) is based on the respondent's report of whether s/he has ever used marijuana in rounds 1, 2, or 3 (respondents were age 12–16 in round 1 to 14–20 in round 3).

Delinquency index (1997) is a summative index measuring how many of the following 10 delinquent acts the respondent has ever done by round

1: run away from home, carried a handgun, belonged to a gang, purposely damaged or destroyed property, stolen something worth less than $50, stolen something worth more than $50, committed other property crimes, attacked or assaulted someone with the intent to do serious harm, sold drugs, or been arrested for an illegal or delinquent offense.

Frequency of depression (2002) is based on the respondent's report of how often s/he felt depressed in the month before the round 6 interview (respondents were age 18–23 in this round) (scaled from 1 "none of the time" to 4 "all of the time").

Home Environment and Family Integration

Physical environment risk (1997) is based on the following five items: whether the respondent's home regularly has electricity and heat (youth report), how well kept the buildings on the street appear (interviewer report), how well kept the interior of the building in which the youth lives appears (interviewer report), whether the interviewer feels safe in the respondent's neighborhood (interviewer report), and how many days a week the youth can hear gunshots in his or her neighborhood (youth report) (Moore et al. 1999) (scaled from 0 "no/low risk" to 7 "high risk").

Enriching environment (1997) is based on youth reports of the following three items: whether their home usually had a computer, whether their home usually had a dictionary, and whether the child spent any time in the past month participating in such activities as music lessons, dance lessons, or foreign language classes (Moore et al. 1999).

Maternal monitoring and awareness (1997, alpha = .71) is based on the youth's responses to the following four questions in round 1: "How much does your mother know about close friends, that is, who they are?"; "How much does your mother know about close friends' parents, that is, who they are?"; "How much does your mother know about who you are with when not at home?"; and "How much does your mother know about your teachers and what you are doing at school?" (each item is scaled from 0 "knows nothing" to 4 "knows everything").

Family routines (1997) is based on the respondent's report in round 1 of how many days a week (from 0 to 7) s/he eats dinner with their family; housework is completed when it was supposed to be; s/he participates in some sort of family activity, such as playing a game or attending a sporting event; and s/he does something religious as a family, such as pray or attend church.

Relationship Outcomes

Positive peer environments (1997) is based on the respondent's report in round 1 about whether most of his or her peers attend church regularly, plan on attending college, belong to a club or sports team, and volunteer.

Negative peer environments (1997) is based on the respondent's report in round 1 about whether 25 percent or more of his or her peers smoke one or more times a month, drink alcohol one or more times a month, use illegal drugs, cut class regularly, and belong to a gang.

Mother-teen relationship (1997) is based on the respondent's rating of three items (scaled from 0 "strongly disagree" to 4 "strongly agree") in round 1: respondent thinks highly of mother, enjoys spending time with mother, and wants to be like mother.

Married or cohabiting by age 20 is based on the respondent's report of his/her marital/cohabitation status and his/her age at the first marriage or cohabitation. We excluded from this measure respondents who were not interviewed through age 20.

Closeness to dating partner or spouse (2002–03) is based on the respondent's report of how close s/he feels to his/her current dating partner or spouse (scaled from 0 "not close at all" to 10 "very close"). This measure is valid only for those respondents who report currently being in a relationship, being married, or having a cohabiting partner.

Caring behavior of dating partner or spouse (2002–03) is based on the respondent's report of how caring his/her current dating partner or spouse is (scaled from 0 "not caring at all" to 10 "very caring"). This measure is valid only for those respondents who report currently being in a relationship, being married, or having a cohabiting partner.

Amount of conflict with dating partner or spouse (2002–03) is based on the respondent's report of how much conflict there is in his/her relationship with his/her current dating partner or spouse (scaled from 0 "no conflict" to 10 "a lot of conflict"). This measure is valid only for those respondents who report currently being in a relationship, being married, or having a cohabiting partner.

Physical Health and Well-Being

Risk of obesity (1997). Each child's height and weight is used to calculate BMI, which is then compared with growth charts produced by the Centers for Disease Control and Prevention to determine if the child's weight for height percentage is greater than the 95th percentile for his or her age group.

Used birth control at first sex is based on the respondent's report of using birth control during his/her first sexual intercourse. Respondents who never had sexual were excluded from this measure.

NOTES

The research on which this chapter is based was supported by grant FPR006015-01 from the Office of Population Affairs of the U.S. Department of Health and Human Services. The conclusions and opinions expressed here are those of the authors and not necessarily those of the funding agency.

1. Data are from U.S. Census Bureau, "Table MS-2. Estimated Median Age at First Marriage, by Sex: 1890 to the Present," http://www.census.gov/population/socdemo/hh-fam/ms2.pdf, September 21, 2006.

2. Child Trends, "Child Trends Databank: Educational Attainment," http://www.childtrendsdatabank.org/indicators/6EducationalAttainment.cfm; and National Center for Education Statistics, "Digest of Education Statistics, 2004," http://nces.ed.gov/programs/digest/d04/intro.asp (retrieved April 24, 2006).

3. Of the 14,884 children who were excluded because they were not firstborns, 763 reported no older siblings, but their date of birth occurred more than one year after the mother's reported year of first birth. Given this uncertainty in the independent variables, we chose to exclude these cases.

4. The 287 firstborn respondents dropped from the sample because they were not first-time kindergarteners or did not live with their biological mothers differed from the 6,228 respondents that remained in the sample. They were, on average, older, more likely to be male, and had mothers with lower educational attainment than were respondents who remained in the sample. However, they were no more likely to be born to a teen mother than respondents in the final sample.

5. To discover how many adolescents were first born, we compared an adolescent's birth date with the date of the mother's first birth. If these two dates did not match ($n = 4,279$) or if a respondent was missing information on date of mother's first birth ($n = 732$), we assumed that the adolescent was not first born. Respondents who did not live with their biological mothers or did not have a biological mother complete the parent survey also were excluded because we controlled for several mother and maternal grandparent characteristics that could only be found in the parent survey.

6. The 1,076 firstborn respondents dropped from our sample because they did not live with their biological mothers or their biological mothers did not complete the parent survey differed from the 2,897 respondents that remained in the sample. Those removed from the sample were more likely to have been born to a teen mother (23 percent versus 18 percent) and to a mother with a lower level of education. They were also more likely to

be of mixed race, and marginally more likely to be male or of Hispanic ethnicity than were those included in the final sample. Those adolescents removed from the sample also were marginally older, on average, than were those who remained in the sample.

7. See appendix A.5 for a complete description of outcomes discussed above.

8. We find a counterintuitive negative association between mother's marital status at birth and adolescents' reports of caring from their current partner or spouse at round 6 (age 18–24). On average, children of married mothers report 9.22 out of 10 on partner caring, compared with 9.41 among children of unmarried mothers; this small difference remains in multivariate models. Analyses of gender differences indicate that this association is significant only for male children.

9. The SRS is composed from the Social Skills Rating Scale (Gresham and Elliott 1990), a copyright-protected instrument, and is not available for review.

REFERENCES

Abma, Joyce C., Gladys M. Martinez, William D. Mosher, and Brittany S. Dawson. 2004. "Teenagers in the United States: Sexual Activity, Contraceptive Use, and Childbearing, 2002." Vital and Health Statistics 23(24). Hyattsville, MD: National Center for Health Statistics.

Bureau of Labor Statistics. See U.S. Department of Labor. Bureau of Labor Statistics.

Campbell, Frances A., Craig T. Ramey, Elizabeth Pungello, Joseph Sparling, and Shari Miller-Johnson. 2002. "Early Childhood Education: Young Adult Outcomes from the Abecedarian Project." Applied Developmental Science 6(1): 42–57.

Furstenberg, Frank F., Jr., Jeanne Brooks-Gunn, and S. Phillip Morgan. 1987. Adolescent Mothers in Later Life. Cambridge: Cambridge University Press.

Furstenberg, Frank F., Jr., Judith A. Levine, and Jeanne Brooks-Gunn. 1990. "The Children of Teenage Mothers: Patterns of Early Childbearing in Two Generations." Family Planning Perspectives 22(2): 54–61.

Geronimus, Arline T., and Kristin A. Moore. 1992. "The Socioeconomic Consequences of Teen Childbearing Reconsidered." Quarterly Journal of Economics 107:1187–1214.

Geronimus, Arline T., Sanders Korenman, and Marianne Hillemeier. 1994. "Does Young Maternal Age Adversely Affect Child Development? Evidence from Cousin Comparisons in the United States." Population and Development Review 20(3): 585–609.

Goerge, Robert M., and Bong Joo Lee. 1997. "Abuse and Neglect of the Children." In Kids Having Kids: Economic Costs and Social Consequences of Teen Pregnancy, edited by Rebecca A. Maynard (205–30). Washington, DC: Urban Institute Press.

Gresham, Frank, and Stephen Elliott. 1990. Social Skills Rating System Manual. Circle Pines, MN: American Guidance Service.

Haveman, Robert, Barbara Wolfe, and Karen Pence. 2001. "Intergenerational Effects of Nonmarital and Early Childbearing." In Out of Wedlock: Causes and Consequences of Nonmarital Fertility, edited by Lawrence L. Wu and Barbara Wolfe (287–316). New York: Russell Sage Foundation.

Haveman, Robert H., Barbara Wolfe, and Elaine Peterson. 1997. "Children of Early Childbearers as Young Adults." In Kids Having Kids: Economic Costs and Social Con-

sequences of Teen Pregnancy, edited by Rebecca A. Maynard (257–84). Washington, DC: Urban Institute Press.

Hofferth, Sandra L., and Lori Reid. 2002. "Early Childbearing and Children's Achievement and Behavior over Time." *Perspectives on Sexual and Reproductive Health* 34(1): 41–49.

Hoffman, Saul D. 1998. "Teen Childbearing Isn't So Bad after All . . . or Is It? A Review of the New Literature." *Family Planning Perspectives* 30(5): 236–39, 243.

Kahn, Joan R., and Kay E. Anderson. 1992. "Intergenerational Patterns of Teenage Fertility." *Demography* 29(1): 39–57.

Levine, Judith A., Harold Pollack, and Maureen E. Comfort. 2001. "Academic and Behavioral Outcomes among the Children of Young Mothers." *Journal of Marriage and the Family* 63(2): 355–69.

Manlove, Jennifer. 1997. "Early Motherhood in an Intergenerational Perspective: The Experiences of a British Cohort." *Journal of Marriage and the Family* 59(2): 263–79.

Martin, Joyce A., Brady E. Hamilton, Paul D. Sutton, Stephanie J. Ventura, Fay Menacker, Sharon Kirmeyer, and Martha L. Munson. 2007. "Births: Final Data for 2005." National Vital Statistics Reports 56(6). Hyattsville, MD: National Center for Health Statistics.

Maynard, Rebecca A., ed. 1997. *Kids Having Kids: Economic Costs and Social Consequences of Teen Pregnancy.* Washington, DC: Urban Institute Press.

Moore, Kristin Anderson, and Nancy O. Snyder. 1991. "Cognitive Attainment among Firstborn Children of Adolescent Mothers." *American Sociological Review* 56(5): 612–24.

Moore, Kristin Anderson, Donna Ruane Morrison, and Angela Dungee Greene. 1997. "Effects on the Children Born to Adolescent Mothers." In *Kids Having Kids: Economic Costs and Social Consequences of Teen Pregnancy,* edited by Rebecca A. Maynard (145–80). Washington, DC: Urban Institute Press.

Moore, Kristin Anderson, Sharon M. McGroder, Elizabeth C. Hair, and Marjorie L. Gunnoe. 1999. *NLSY97 Codebook Supplement Main File Round 1. Appendix 9: Family Process and Adolescent Outcomes Measures.* Washington, DC: Bureau of Labor Statistics, U.S. Department of Labor.

Moore, Kristin Anderson, David E. Myers, Donna Ruane Morrison, Christine Winquist Nord, Brett Brown, and Barry Edmonston. 1993. "Age at First Birth and Later Poverty." *Journal of Research on Adolescence* 3(4): 393–422.

National Center for Health Statistics. 1984. *Vital Statistics of the United States, 1980, Public Health Service.* Vol. 1. DHHS Pub. (PHS) 85-1100. Washington, DC: U.S. Government Printing Office.

Pogarsky, Greg, Alan J. Lizotte, and Terence P. Thornberry. 2003. "The Delinquency of Children Born to Young Mothers: Results from the Rochester Youth Development Study." *Criminology* 41(4): 1249–86.

Pogarsky, Greg, Terence P. Thornberry, and Alan J. Lizotte. 2006. "Developmental Outcomes for Children of Young Mothers." *Journal of Marriage and the Family* 68(2): 332–44.

StataCorp. 2001. *Stata Statistical Software: Release 7.0.* Station, TX: Stata Corporation.

Terry-Humen, Elizabeth, Jennifer Manlove, and Kristin Anderson Moore. 2005. *Playing Catch-Up: How Children Born to Teen Mothers Fare.* Washington, DC: The National Campaign to Prevent Teen Pregnancy.

Turley, Ruth N. L. 2003. "Are Children of Young Mothers Disadvantaged Because of Their Mother's Age or Family Background?" *Child Development* 74(2): 465–74.

U.S. Department of Labor. Bureau of Labor Statistics. 2005. *NLSY97 User's Guide: A Guide to the Rounds 1–7 Data.* Columbus: Center for Human Resource Research, Ohio State University.

Ventura, Stephanie J., Joyce C. Abma, William D. Mosher, and Stanley Henshaw. 2004. "Estimated Pregnancy Rates for the United States, 1990–2000: An Update." National Vital Statistics Reports 52(23). Hyattsville, MD: National Center for Health Statistics.

———. 2006. "Recent Trends in Teenage Pregnancy in the United States, 1990–2002." Health E-stats. Hyattsville, MD: National Center for Health Statistics. http://www.cdc.gov/nchs/products/pubs/pubd/hestats/teenpreg1990–2002/teenpreg1990–2002.htm.

Westat, National Center for Education Statistics, Educational Testing Services, University of Michigan, Education Statistics Services Institute, and National Center for Education Statistics. 2001. *ECLS-K Base Year Public-Use Data Files and Electronic Codebook (User's Manual).* Washington, DC: U.S. Department of Education.

Wolfe, Barbara, and Maria Perozek. 1997. "Teen Children's Health and Health Care Use." In *Kids Having Kids: Economic Costs and Social Consequences of Teen Pregnancy,* edited by Rebecca A. Maynard (181–204). Washington, DC: Urban Institute Press.

6

Children's Health and Health Care

Barbara Wolfe and Emilie McHugh Rivers

In the press and in today's common wisdom, teen childbearing is associated with negative outcomes for the mothers: teen mothers are less likely to graduate from high school and more likely to live in poverty than are older mothers. They are also less likely to marry and remain in stable long-term relationships. However, little is known about the effect of teenage motherhood on the children born to teen mothers.[1]

This chapter explores some possible health and medical care consequences of having a teenage mother. For example, children of teen mothers may face an increased risk of medical problems. This increased risk may result from the relatively poor parenting skills of teen mothers, which may arise from their lower education levels. Poorer parenting and lower income among teen mothers may lead to poorer nutrition, later detection of health problems, and greater risk of accidents among their children. Or, teen childbearing may be associated with fewer medical problems during childbirth and a higher probability of giving birth to a healthy infant. These positive effects of teen childbearing might help offset the negative effects of poorer parenting skills and lower income levels.

Even if children of teens are more likely to be in poor health than are the children of older mothers, they will not necessarily incur higher medical costs or use more medical care. There are several possible explanations for this. First, people with lower incomes and those without insurance are less likely to take their children to medical care providers

(Wolfe 1994). Second, if these parents do take their children, they are more likely to use lower-cost providers such as subsidized clinics and primary care providers, rather than specialists (Mitchell 1991). Finally, since Medicaid and the State Children's Health Insurance Programs (SCHIP) generally reimburse providers at a lower level than private insurers do, reported expenditures are likely to be lower for children covered by Medicaid or SCHIP.

Teen mothers are more likely than others to have public insurance (Medicaid or SCHIP) or to have no insurance coverage. If the cost of their children's medical care is paid by Medicaid or SCHIP or is shifted to other payers, then other members of society are paying for these costs. Hence, the difference in the probability of having public health insurance coverage multiplied by how often children of teen mothers use public care provides an estimate of the additional cost to the public of teen parenting.

The teen birth rate continues to decline in most developed countries. In the United States, for example, the rate in 2004 was 22.1 per 1,000 for 15–17-year-olds, compared with 37.5 in 1990; the rates for 18–19-year-olds were 70.0 and 88.6, respectively, for those years. U.S. rates continue to be far higher than rates in other developed countries. United Nations data, averaged over 2000–05, suggest that the rate for 15–19-year-olds was 50 per 1,000 in the United States. Other English-speaking countries have much lower rates: the United Kingdom at 26, New Zealand at 24, Australia at 15, and Canada at 14 (in each case per 1,000). Other western European countries have rates of 5–13; Japan and China are even lower, at 4 and 5 per 1,000, respectively.[2]

Data and Descriptive Results

This chapter uses a nationally representative dataset, the 2002 Medical Expenditure Panel Survey (MEPS), to investigate the consequences of teen parenting for the health and medical care costs of the children. At the time of this analysis, the 2002 MEPS was the most recent source of detailed data on medical care use, health status, and insurance coverage for a national sample. We use these data to construct a sample of 4,249 children who were less than 15 years old at the time of the most recent interview and who had mothers at least 12 but less than 45 years old. Information is taken from three rounds of interviews over the year. We use the data as it was consolidated by MEPS for the year, except as described below. The unit of analysis is a child, and maternal characteristics are merged with the child's observation to complete the analysis file. The sample is restricted to children and mothers for whom complete information is available.

Unfortunately, the MEPS dataset is not ideally suited for studying the fertility decisions of the women in the sample. We know very little about their fertility histories. Instead, we infer the age at which women had their first child by subtracting the age of the mother's oldest child in the sample from the mother's age. Clearly, this approach has several problems. First, since the sampling unit is the household, we only observe the mother and the child if they are living in the same household at the time of the first interview. Therefore, if the mother's oldest child moved away from home some time before the initial interview, we would overestimate the age at which the mother had her first child. To address this problem, we restrict the sample of mothers to those who were less than 44 years old at the time of the last interview. This restriction minimizes the chances that one or more of the mother's children would no longer be living in the household.

A second problem results from restricting our sample to children whose mothers live in the same household; we thus omit children who live only with their fathers or other relatives. It seems reasonable to assume that children of teen mothers might disproportionately live with other family members. To the extent that this is true, we do not have a representative sample of children of teen mothers.

We use these data to compare the characteristics of children born to young teen mothers (< age 18), older teen mothers (18–19), and older mothers (20–21). (Table 6.1 presents the overall means and standard deviations of the variables used from these data.) We limit our analysis to women who first gave birth before age 22 since we believe these groups are the more relevant. Policy may attempt to influence postponement of first births from the teen years to older teen years or possibly ages 20–21, but further postponement is unlikely, and there is no clear evidence that it has advantages for women at risk of giving birth as a teen.[3] In particular, for these three groups, we study differences in health status, medical care use and expenditures, insurance coverage, and public cost of medical care for their children.

To make these comparisons, we present the results from a descriptive analysis and then from multivariate regression analysis. First, we present average (mean) use and medical expenditure figures for the following

Table 6.1. Definitions, Means, and Standard Deviations of Variables Used in Tobit Estimates on Sample of All Children of Women Age 12–44 as of 2002

	Full Sample		First Births Only	
	Mean	Standard deviation	Mean	Standard deviation
Dependent variables				
Total number of medical care visits	2.38	4.40	2.56	5.06
Total medical care expenditures	$683.61	$2,282.10	$719.71	$2,454.54
Total paid by society	$398.00	$1,741.40	$417.73	$2,013.03
Independent variables				
Age of child	6.80	4.22	7.28	4.25
Race of child is white	0.30	0.46	0.32	0.46
Race of child is black	0.22	0.41	0.21	0.41
Race of child is Hispanic	0.43	0.49	0.42	0.49
Race of child is other	0.05	0.22	0.05	0.23
Sex of child is male	0.50	0.50	0.48	0.50
Child has excellent health	0.41	0.49	0.43	0.49
Child has fair/poor health	0.02	0.15	0.02	0.14
Child has a chronic condition	0.20	0.49	0.22	0.51
Child has an acute condition	1.44	1.65	1.51	1.65
Mother first gave birth when 17 or younger	0.30	0.46	0.27	0.45
Mother first gave birth when 18–19	0.36	0.48	0.37	0.48
Mother first gave birth when 20–21	0.34	0.47	0.35	0.48
Child born when mother was 17 or younger	0.11	0.31	0.27	0.45
Child born when mother was 18–19	0.19	0.39	0.37	0.48
Child born when mother was 20–21	0.23	0.42	0.35	0.48
Other variables				
Mother a high school graduate upon entry to MEPS	0.51	0.50	0.52	0.50
Mother's age in 2002	29.55	5.64	26.32	4.58
Mother's number of children in 2002	2.94	1.37	2.13	1.06
Sample size	4,249		1,540	

Source: Medical Expenditure Panel Survey (MEPS).

three groups of children: (1) children born to mothers who first gave birth as young teens (less than 18; *young teen mother*), (2) children born to mothers who first gave birth as older teens (age 18–19; *older teen mother*), and (3) children born to mothers who never gave birth as a teen but did so between the ages of 20 and 21 (*older, or nonteen, mother*). Further, we present these means for children stratified by the following six age groups: 0–1 year, 2–3 years, 4–5 years, 6–7 years, 8–10 years, and 11–14 years. The first group (0–1 year) comprises children who are most likely to receive well-baby care. The second group (2–3 years) is at the age when vaccinations are usually given. Four- to 5-year-olds are at nursery school age, 6- to 7-year-olds are in their first years of elementary school, 8- to 10-year-olds have completed most of elementary school, and 11- to 14-year-olds are entering their early adolescent years. In each case, when we compute weighted averages we weight the data so each age has an equal weight, removing any differences in the age profile of children from the analysis.

Although the descriptive analysis provides insight into the consequences of teen childbearing, it does not control for many important variables. Hence, we also conduct multivariate regression analysis on medical care use, total medical expenditures, and total social expenditures. Since the dependent variable is censored at zero for a substantial fraction of the observations, we use tobit analysis.

Health Status

We use four measures of health status. The first two are based on parents' self-assessments and are perhaps the most widely used of all health status measures.[4] The first measure is a dummy variable for whether the child is reported to be in excellent health (excellent), and the second measure is a dummy variable for whether the child is reported to be in poor or fair health (poor-fair). Both variables are based on questions asked of parents. We also use two other indicators of health problems, one that indicates the number of acute health conditions (acute) and a second that indicates the number of chronic health conditions (chronic) reported during the year. The categories of acute and chronic conditions are built up from individually reported conditions and grouped via ACG/ADG software that maps International Classification of Diseases (ICD-9) codes into groupings based on need for specialty care, severity, and chronicity.[5] (See the glossary in appendix A.6 and the ICD-9 codes in appendix B.6 for more detail.) Weighted means for the prevalence of each health status measure for our three groups are presented in table 6.2.

Table 6.2. Children's Health Status, by Mother's Age at Birth of First Child (weighted means)

	Excellent health	Fair or poor health	Health Condition		N
			Acute	Chronic	
Young teen mother					
Age of child (years)					
0 to 1	0.46	0.02	1.75	0.16	169
2 to 3	0.37	0.03	1.68	0.25	194
4 to 5	0.40	0.02	1.31	0.19	168
6 to 7	0.44	0.02	1.17	0.17	181
8 to 10	0.42	0.00	1.02	0.20	257
11 to 14	0.37	0.03	1.03	0.26	301
All	0.41	0.02	1.27	0.21	1,270
Older teen mother					
Age of child (years)					
0 to 1	0.39	0.03	1.73	0.15	200
2 to 3	0.41	0.02	1.75	0.19	221
4 to 5	0.45	0.02	1.28	0.12	231
6 to 7	0.40	0.02	1.49	0.20	209
8 to 10	0.43	0.03	1.22	0.19	308
11 to 14	0.45	0.02	1.25	0.26	367
All	0.43	0.02	1.41	0.20	1,536
Nonteen mother					
Age of child (years)					
0 to 1	0.47	0.02	1.91	0.13	187
2 to 3	0.44	0.02	1.99	0.17	199
4 to 5	0.39	0.03	1.76	0.22	192
6 to 7	0.41	0.03	1.68	0.19	206
8 to 10	0.43	0.02	1.38	0.18	286
11 to 14	0.36	0.02	1.33	0.24	373
All	0.41	0.02	1.61	0.19	1,443

Source: Authors' calculations based on 2002 MEPS.

The overall proportion of children in excellent health does not differ significantly by the age of the mother, though on average it appears that children born to older teen mothers are slightly more likely to be in excellent health than those born to young teen or nonteen mothers. The biggest difference is the higher probability that children age 11–14 born to older teen mothers are in excellent health relative to other children age 11–14.

We also find few differences in the proportion of children whose health status is reported to be poor or fair; around 2 percent of children in all three groups are reported to have poor or fair health on the five-point scale (table 6.2). The only exception is the zero percentage of children age 8–10 in poor or fair health and born to young teen mothers.

The pattern for acute and chronic conditions is rather different. Children born to young teen mothers, especially younger children, are less likely to be reported as having acute conditions than children born to older mothers but somewhat more likely to be reported with chronic conditions. The differences are, however, small; they may reflect real health differences or simply greater use of medical care and the diagnosis rendered at the site of care. Chronic conditions may be the most likely to be diagnosed and hence the most accurately reported of the health indicators.

Use

We use five measures of medical care use: outpatient visits to medical providers, outpatient visits to hospital clinics, visits to an emergency room, number of inpatient or hospital stays, and total number of visits. Much of the literature suggests that emergency room visits represent inappropriate use of medical care: in many cases, such visits take place when access to providers is restricted and care is postponed until it is an emergency. Further, some inpatient stays result from postponed medical care and may represent a *lack* of access—rather than access—to medical care. Finally, in some areas of the country, outpatient visits to hospitals may indicate both a lack of access to private providers and absence of a regular provider.

Table 6.3 presents the average pattern of use of medical providers. As in table 6.2, the reported values are weighted means. The results suggest that children born to mothers who never gave birth as a young teen visited medical care providers more frequently than children born to mothers in the youngest group. There is only one exception: children age 11–14 born to young teen mothers are more likely to visit medical providers than those age 11–14 born to older teen mothers. The differences between children born to mothers in the youngest group and those born to mothers in the other two groups are particularly large for infants and 1-year-olds. The overall differences are also sizeable: 2.11 and 2.12 for children of older and older teen mothers versus 1.74 for children born to young teen mothers.

Table 6.3. Health Care Use, by Mother's Age at Birth of First Child (weighted means)

	Medical provider visits	Hospital outpatient visits	Emergency room visits	Inpatient stays	All medical visits	N
Young teen mother						
Age of child (years)						
0 to 1	3.16	0.11	0.37	0.14	3.78	169
2 to 3	2.15	0.08	0.35	0.04	2.62	194
4 to 5	1.36	0.04	0.22	0.02	1.64	168
6 to 7	1.14	0.04	0.18	0.02	1.39	181
8 to 10	1.26	0.04	0.18	0.02	1.50	257
11 to 14	1.68	0.07	0.14	0.04	1.93	301
All	1.74	0.06	0.22	0.04	2.07	1,270
Older teen mother						
Age of child (years)						
0 to 1	3.67	0.38	0.36	0.15	4.55	200
2 to 3	2.32	0.13	0.31	0.04	2.80	221
4 to 5	2.04	0.03	0.17	0.01	2.26	231
6 to 7	2.01	0.15	0.18	0.02	2.36	209
8 to 10	1.74	0.05	0.13	0.01	1.93	308
11 to 14	1.60	0.23	0.20	0.01	2.05	367
All	2.12	0.16	0.21	0.03	2.53	1,536
Nonteen mother						
Age of child (years)						
0 to 1	3.79	0.06	0.35	0.11	4.32	187
2 to 3	2.42	0.09	0.35	0.03	2.87	199
4 to 5	2.22	0.23	0.26	0.02	2.73	192
6 to 7	1.68	0.10	0.17	0.04	1.99	206
8 to 10	1.37	0.08	0.12	0.02	1.59	286
11 to 14	1.81	0.25	0.12	0.02	2.20	373
All	2.11	0.15	0.21	0.03	2.49	1,443

Source: Authors' calculations based on 2002 MEPS.

In most tabulations, the same pattern exists: children of young teen mothers have the lowest use, whereas children born to later-fertility mothers have higher use. Children born to older mothers are far more likely to make hospital outpatient visits than young teen mothers' children. Emergency room visits may be an exception, and inpatient stays are so infrequent in this age group that the pattern is unclear. Finally, since total medical care visits are dominated by visits to a medical provider, the pattern of total visits is essentially identical to that for use of medical providers.

Table 6.4 provides information on the proportion of medical expenditures paid by three sources: self-payment (payment by the parents),

Table 6.4. Proportion of Medical Expenses Paid by Source, by Mother's Age at Birth of First Child (weighted means)

	Self-paid	Paid by private insurance	Paid by others in society	N
Young teen mother				
Age of child (years)				
0 to 1	0.06	0.24	0.70	169
2 to 3	0.03	0.20	0.77	194
4 to 5	0.11	0.12	0.77	168
6 to 7	0.13	0.31	0.56	181
8 to 10	0.08	0.44	0.48	257
11 to 14	0.19	0.37	0.44	301
All	0.11	0.29	0.60	1,270
Older teen mother				
Age of child (years)				
0 to 1	0.04	0.12	0.84	200
2 to 3	0.08	0.32	0.61	221
4 to 5	0.11	0.25	0.65	231
6 to 7	0.06	0.32	0.62	209
8 to 10	0.18	0.32	0.50	308
11 to 14	0.17	0.40	0.43	367
All	0.10	0.27	0.63	1,536
Nonteen mother				
Age of child (years)				
0 to 1	0.06	0.39	0.55	187
2 to 3	0.10	0.27	0.63	199
4 to 5	0.11	0.24	0.65	192
6 to 7	0.12	0.30	0.58	206
8 to 10	0.18	0.35	0.47	286
11 to 14	0.19	0.49	0.32	373
All	0.13	0.37	0.50	1,443

Source: Authors' calculations based on 2002 MEPS.

private insurance, and public payments. Public payments include payments made by Medicaid, SCHIP, the Civilian Health and Medical Program for the Uniformed Services (CHAMPUS), and Medicare (for a small
number of disabled children). (See the glossary in appendix A.6 for a
description of expenditure source types). The pattern here is clear: children born to nonteen mothers are more likely to have their care paid for
directly by their parents—13 percent of the cost in the weighted sample,
compared with 10 percent for children of older teen mothers and 11 percent for children born to young teen mothers.

The proportion covered by private insurance differs more dramatically
by mother's age at first birth. On average, 37 percent of the medical costs
of children born to nonteen mothers are paid by private insurance, compared with 29 and 27 percent, respectively, for children of young teen
mothers and older teen mothers. The high proportion (24 percent) of
expenditures covered by private insurance for infants of young teens is
consistent with a higher probability that young teen mothers will live with
parents before giving birth and after their children are born and will not
be eligible for public coverage.

The proportion paid by others in society is again consistent with expectations: a greater proportion of children born to teenage mothers has
publicly provided insurance. Public insurance paid 50 percent of the
medical care costs of children born to older-fertility mothers, 60 percent
of the costs for children born to young teen mothers, and 63 percent of
the costs for children born to older teen mothers. In all cases the proportion paid by others in society is highest for children less than 8 years old;
this is consistent with eligibility for these public programs, especially
Medicaid. Notable is the very large proportion of expenditures paid by
society for infants (0–1) born to older teen mothers.

Expenditures

Table 6.5 lists the total annual medical expenditures for all children in the
sample age 0–14, again weighted by children's ages for a uniform distribution across all three groups of children. As the use patterns suggest,
expenditures are greater for children born to older teen or nonteen mothers than for children born to young teen mothers: $703 and $682, respectively, for the first two groups versus $669 for children born to mothers
who first gave birth as young teens. The pattern is not consistent across
age groups. For infants (0–1), the highest average expenditures are among

Table 6.5. Average Total Annual Expenditures, by Mother's Age at Birth of First Child (2002 dollars)

	Young Teen Mother		Older Teen Mother		Nonteen Mother	
Age of child	$	N	$	N	$	N
0 to 1	1,112.27	169	1,548.12	200	890.64	187
2 to 3	865.85	194	657.99	221	597.50	199
4 to 5	479.31	168	444.62	231	805.70	192
6 to 7	375.29	181	893.39	209	675.09	206
8 to 10	469.91	257	367.04	308	426.88	286
11 to 14	740.92	301	589.05	367	754.59	373
All	669.26	1,270	703.04	1,536	682.46	1,443

Source: Authors' calculations based on 2002 MEPS.

children born to older teen mothers, the lowest among those born to non-teen mothers. These are the largest outlays and the largest differences across mothers' age at birth groups.

The final table of means, table 6.6, displays the average amount paid by public insurance per year. In this case, the amount paid is greatest for children born to teen mothers ($401 and $444 for young and older teens, respectively, compared with $342 for children born to nonteens). This amounts to about $100 less, on average, for those born to nonteen mothers. What may at first seem somewhat surprising is that the public medical expenditures of children born to older teen mothers are higher than those of children born to younger teen mothers. But this is consistent with the results of table 6.4, where we noted that this result is largely due to differential coverage of infants.

Acute and chronic health problems may explain differential medical expenditures (table 6.6). Children with chronic conditions only have far higher expenditures than children with acute conditions, no doubt because of the continuing nature of their illness.[6] In this case, children born to older teens impose the highest social cost (about $2,100) on average, whereas those born to young teen and nonteen mothers have far lower costs (about $850 and $450, respectively). Finally, for children with both chronic and acute conditions (this category includes the majority of children with chronic conditions), children born to young teen mothers impose the highest social cost, slightly more than $1,300 on average,

Table 6.6. Average Total Expenditures and Amount Paid by Others in Society, by Mother's Age at Birth of First Child and Child's Health (2002 dollars)

	Dollars paid by others	Total expenditures
Young teen mother		
Child's health conditions		
None	86.16	149.30
Acute only	309.44	493.24
Chronic only	848.47	1,908.54
Acute and chronic	1,319.37	2,103.34
All	400.53	669.26
Older teen mother		
Child's health conditions		
None	156.88	206.02
Acute only	392.66	684.86
Chronic only	2,099.39	2,339.27
Acute and chronic	1,062.92	1,640.81
All	443.52	703.04
Nonteen mother		
Child's health conditions		
None	55.38	137.54
Acute only	262.47	597.79
Chronic only	446.84	829.53
Acute and chronic	1,288.25	2,174.59
All	342.15	682.46

Source: Authors' calculations based on 2002 MEPS.

though this is only about $30 more than children of nonteen mothers with both types of conditions. In contrast, children of older teen mothers with both types of conditions cost society about $1,060 on average.

Multivariate Analysis

The means above display differences in health status, medical care use, and expenditures by whether a child was born to a young teen mother (younger than age 18), an older teen mother (age 18–19), or a mother who started childbearing after her teen years (20–21). Since the distribution of children's characteristics is not constant across these groups, we use multivariate analysis to better isolate the effect on children's medical care use of having a mother who first gave birth as a teen. We look at three measures of medical care use: total number of visits, total expenditures, and societal expenditures (expenditures paid by others). For all three dependent variables, a number of children have zero values; hence we used tobit analysis.

Five models are estimated for each dependent variable. Model 1, the simple, or limited, model, includes only the child's age at the time he or she is observed in 2002; dummy variables indicate that the child's mother first gave birth before age 18, at age 18–19, or at age 20–21 (the last category is omitted). Model 2 adds the child's race and sex to the equation. We have four categories for race: white non-Hispanic (*white*), black non-Hispanic (*black*), Hispanic, and other, which is the excluded category. We include these variables because race and sex are associated with some illnesses and may be associated with barriers to medical care. We also add region of the country and metropolitan residence; both indicators are associated with access to medical care. Model 3 adds two measures of a child's health to the estimates: a dummy variable for poor-fair health and a dummy variable for excellent health. The former is expected to lead to greater use of care, the latter to less use. Model 4 uses our alternative indicators of health: the number, if any, of a child's chronic conditions and the number, if any, of acute conditions. We expect both these numbers to be associated with greater use of medical care. Model 5 includes all four indicators of health. Other variables normally included in usage estimates, such as insurance coverage and income, are not included for several reasons: (1) both variables are likely endogenous to the mother's fertility decisions, (2) reported income may belong to the mother's parents as the mother may not have her own household, and (3) there are documented problems with the income imputations at the tails of the distribution.

The tobit estimates appear in tables 6.7–6.9, which present the estimated coefficients and t-statistics for each of the three dependent variables described above. Table 6.7 presents the estimates for the determinants of total medical care visits. The results are consistent with the means presented earlier: older children have fewer visits; children with mothers who first gave birth as older teens use more care, particularly compared with children born to mothers who first gave birth before age 18. Children's

234   Kids Having Kids

Table 6.7. Determinants of Total Medical Care Visits: Tobit Estimates ($n = 4{,}249$)

	Model 1		Model 2		Model 3		Model 4		Model 5	
Mother first gave birth when										
17 or younger	-0.90	(3.86)	-0.69	(2.98)	-0.67	(2.98)	-0.36	(1.80)	-0.36	(1.80)
18 to 19	-0.01	(0.06)	0.08	(0.36)	0.08	(0.39)	0.32	(1.74)	0.32	(1.73)
Child's age	-0.27	(12.16)	-0.27	(12.25)	-0.27	(12.56)	-0.21	(11.49)	-0.21	(11.47)
Child's sex = male			0.03	(0.15)	-0.04	(0.24)	-0.07	(0.48)	-0.08	(0.51)
Child's race										
White			0.98	(2.23)	1.08	(2.51)	0.20	(0.54)	0.22	(0.58)
Black			-0.61	(1.34)	-0.57	(1.27)	-0.07	(0.18)	-0.10	(0.26)
Hispanic			-0.29	(0.66)	-0.39	(0.92)	-0.18	(0.48)	-0.21	(0.58)
Child lives in										
Northeast			0.93	(3.02)	0.90	(3.01)	0.95	(3.64)	0.93	(3.59)
Midwest			0.37	(1.37)	0.36	(1.37)	0.12	(0.54)	0.13	(0.56)
West			-0.15	(0.64)	-0.23	(1.01)	0.05	(0.27)	0.02	(0.08)
Child lives in an MSA			-1.07	(4.65)	-0.98	(4.39)	-0.53	(2.72)	-0.52	(2.70)
Child's health										
Excellent					-1.26	(6.82)			-0.14	(0.89)
Fair to poor					6.44	(11.09)			2.79	(5.45)
Chronic health condition							3.16	(20.34)	2.96	(18.60)
Acute health condition							1.40	(29.13)	1.37	(28.31)
Constant	3.08	(14.27)	3.65	(7.28)	4.04	(8.20)	0.17	(0.38)	0.28	(0.64)
Log likelihood	-10,118.00		-10,067.00		-9,973.00		-9,398.00		-9,382.00	

Source: Authors' calculations based on 2002 MEPS.

Notes: Mean of the dependent variable = 2.38; standard deviation = 4.40. T-statistics are in parentheses.

health status plays the expected role, and both sets of measures are very significant when included separately. Self-reported fair-poor health and numbers of acute and chronic conditions are statistically significant and have the expected positive sign when all four are included. There is a suggestion that white non-Hispanic children made relatively more medical visits than children of other races or ethnicities, but this finding is no longer significant once the child's health conditions are controlled. This difference suggests that race or ethnicity and the presence of health conditions are correlated. Geographic location also appears to influence medical use; children living in the northeast and outside metropolitan areas use the greatest amount of care.

In table 6.8, we investigate the determinants of medical care expenditures. Results are similar to those for visits, with the following exception: even after a child's health is taken into account, the age of the mother at her first birth does not appear related to significant differences in the determinants of medical expenditures. This result contrasts with the lower level of care received by children born to mothers who gave birth as young teens. The major determinant of the pattern of expenditures is a child's health, followed by age and by whether a child lives in a metropolitan (urban) area, both tied to lower expenditures.

Finally, in table 6.9, we explore the determinants of medical care costs borne by other members of society. The public costs of care are significantly greater for children of mothers who first gave birth when younger than 20, compared with children of mothers who did not give birth until 20 or 21. Costs for children born to mothers under 18 are greater than those for children born to older teen mothers. But by far the most important determinant of public medical costs is the child's health status; this is especially the case when a child's overall general health is defined as fair or poor. Metropolitan residence and midwest residence are associated with lower societal costs, but residence in the northeast appears tied to higher societal costs. Race or ethnicity affects societal costs and use differently. Use suggests higher rates among white non-Hispanic children than among children of other races and ethnicities, but societal costs are higher for non-Hispanic black children.

As argued above, the health status of the child may vary systematically with the mother's age at birth. Indeed, the descriptive statistics in table 6.2 suggest that children of teenage mothers are less likely to report acute health problems than children of older mothers. However, the descriptive statistics do not allow us to control for such demographic variables as sex

Table 6.8. Determinants of Total Medical Expenditures: Tobit Estimates (n = 4,249)

	Model 1		Model 2		Model 3		Model 4		Model 5	
Mother first gave birth when										
17 or younger	−173.07	(1.63)	−107.54	(1.01)	−100.83	(0.97)	−47.74	(0.48)	−45.48	(0.46)
18 to 19	−14.84	(0.15)	9.39	(0.09)	11.78	(0.12)	71.02	(0.76)	68.58	(0.74)
Child's age	−55.82	(5.59)	−56.94	(5.71)	−56.32	(5.79)	−49.64	(5.32)	−48.52	(5.25)
Child's sex = male			83.71	(1.00)	58.78	(0.72)	2.10	(0.03)	2.61	(0.03)
Child's race										
White			547.89	(2.67)	566.81	(2.83)	322.25	(1.69)	317.33	(1.68)
Black			45.39	(0.21)	50.89	(0.25)	220.60	(1.12)	192.90	(0.99)
Hispanic			−5.25	(0.03)	−44.59	(0.23)	75.61	(0.40)	56.50	(0.30)
Child lives in										
Northeast			141.35	(0.99)	123.42	(0.89)	117.18	(0.89)	103.74	(0.79)
Midwest			−1.09	(0.01)	−3.51	(0.03)	−56.75	(0.49)	−56.38	(0.49)
West			−124.27	(1.15)	−161.36	(1.53)	−43.84	(0.44)	−67.90	(0.69)
Child lives in an MSA			−386.87	(3.66)	−354.51	(3.43)	−231.18	(2.36)	−228.56	(2.36)
Child's health										
Excellent					−390.10	(4.58)			10.47	(0.13)
Fair to poor					3,352.12	(12.35)			1,920.40	(7.38)
Chronic health condition							1,620.08	(20.56)	1,499.38	(18.62)
Acute health condition							385.34	(15.90)	367.56	(15.13)
Constant	$677.17	(6.80)	$763.87	(3.29)	$859.79	(3.75)	−$319.56	(1.44)	−$297.48	(−1.33)
Log likelihood	−31,628.00		−31,595.00		−31,501.00		−31,214.00		−31,187.00	

Source: Authors' calculations based on 2002 MEPS.

Notes: Mean of the dependent variable = $683.61; standard deviation = $2,282.10. *T*-statistics are in parentheses.

Table 6.9. Determinants of Medical Expenditures Paid by Society: Tobit Estimates ($n = 4,249$)

	Model 1		Model 2		Model 3		Model 4		Model 5	
Mother first gave birth when										
17 or younger	282.32	(2.47)	270.42	(2.34)	272.80	(2.42)	324.58	(2.98)	324.36	(3.00)
18 to 19	240.32	(2.19)	219.01	(1.99)	219.97	(2.05)	293.11	(2.83)	288.68	(2.81)
Child's age	−123.35	(11.30)	−126.59	(11.59)	−125.66	(11.78)	−118.38	(11.40)	−117.63	(11.42)
Child's sex = male			26.12	(0.29)	1.70	(0.02)	−35.24	(0.41)	−38.84	(0.46)
Child's race										
White			361.13	(1.62)	405.68	(1.86)	162.66	(0.77)	187.36	(0.90)
Black			647.17	(2.82)	665.82	(2.97)	784.52	(3.63)	771.84	(3.60)
Hispanic			203.94	(0.93)	162.48	(0.76)	266.70	(1.29)	238.49	(1.17)
Child lives in										
Northeast			293.65	(1.91)	274.72	(1.83)	248.95	(1.72)	240.71	(1.68)
Midwest			−185.73	(1.36)	−184.56	(1.38)	−226.03	(1.76)	−224.84	(1.77)
West			108.47	(0.93)	72.85	(0.64)	179.05	(1.63)	152.81	(1.40)
Child lives in an MSA			−683.02	(6.04)	−641.90	(5.81)	−532.16	(5.00)	−524.03	(4.97)
Child's health										
Excellent					−551.33	(5.92)			−199.74	(2.21)
Fair to poor					2,781.23	(10.03)			1,606.56	(5.96)
Chronic health condition							1,354.30	(16.2)	1,219.26	(14.28)
Acute health condition							339.73	(13.13)	316.59	(12.21)
Constant	−$171.35	(1.59)	$6.99	(0.03)	$173.41	(0.70)	−$939.70	(3.86)	−815.23	(−3.33)
Log likelihood	−20,975.00		−20,946.00		−20,872.00		−20,697.00		−20,675.00	

Source: Authors' calculations based on 2002 MEPS.

Notes: Mean of the dependent variable = $398.00: standard deviation = $1,741.41. *T*-statistics are in parentheses.

and race. Thus, we use probit and tobit models to examine the effect of teen motherhood on health status; the dependent variables are acute conditions, chronic conditions (tobit estimates), and self-reported poor-fair and excellent health (probit models).

Tables 6.10 and 6.11 report the coefficient estimates for these models. According to the results, the children of young teen mothers are less likely to have acute health conditions and more likely to have chronic conditions (though the latter is only marginally significant).

Simulations

This section uses the 2002 MEPS data to simulate changes to child health, medical use, and medical expenditures if teen mothers delay their childbearing. It also considers our analysis in the context of children who are the first born to each mother in our sample.

Table 6.10. Determinants of Child's Health Conditions ($n = 4,249$)

	Conditions: Tobit Results	
	Acute	Chronic
Mother first gave birth when		
17 or younger	−0.339**	0.163+
18 to 19	−0.182**	0.026
Child's age	−0.067**	0.034**
Child's sex = male	−0.155**	0.408**
Child's race		
White	0.643**	0.117
Black	−0.495**	−0.179
Hispanic	−0.008	−0.393**
Child lives in		
Northeast	−0.197+	0.202+
Midwest	0.221**	−0.098
West	−0.118	−0.204*
Child lives in an MSA	−0.377**	−0.1
Constant	1.87**	−2.006**

Source: Authors' calculations based on 2002 MEPS.
+significant at the .15 level; *significant at the .10 level; **significant at the .05 level

Table 6.11. Determinants of Child's General Health ($n = 4,249$)

| | Self-Reported Health: Probit Results | |
	Fair/Poor	Excellent
Mother first gave birth when		
17 or younger	−0.021	0.014
18 to 19	−0.001	0.025
Child's age	−0.007	−0.007+
Child's sex = male	0.066	−0.08**
Child's race		
White	0.1	0.322**
Black	0.122	0.25**
Hispanic	0.073	−0.109
Child lives in		
Northeast	0.128	0.054
Midwest	−0.011	0.004
West	0.163+	−0.034
Child lives in an MSA	−0.1	0.086*
Constant	−2.072**	−0.315**

Source: Authors' calculations based on 2002 MEPS.

+significant at the .15 level; *significant at the .10 level; **significant at the .05 level

All Children

The estimates in tables 6.10 and 6.11 can be used to simulate the expected number of chronic and acute conditions and the probability of reporting poor-fair health or excellent health if we allow the mother's age to increase. First, based on the tobit (probit) estimates, we calculate the expected value of the dependent variable for all children in the sample. Second, we "increase" the age of the mother at first birth from 17 or younger to 18–19 and then to 20–21, and recalculate the expected value of the dependent variable. The results, shown in table 6.12, suggest that were the mother's age at first birth to increase from 17 or younger to 20–21, the expected number of chronic health conditions for the child would decrease from 0.2 to 0.17, whereas the expected number of acute conditions would increase from 1.3 to 1.5. We also would expect the number of acute conditions to increase if women who gave birth at 18–19 were to wait until 20–21. We would expect little change in self-

Table 6.12. Expected Health of Child, Given Delay in Childbearing

| | | If Mother Delayed until Age | | |
	Baseline value	18 to 19	20 to 21	N
Chronic conditions				
Age of mother at birth of first child				
17 or younger	0.198	0.174	0.170	1,270
18 to 19	0.180		0.175	1,536
20 to 21	0.178			1,443
Acute conditions				
Age of mother at birth of first child				
17 or younger	1.292	1.391	1.511	1,270
18 to 19	1.427		1.549	1,536
20 to 21	1.591			1,443
Fair/poor health				
Age of mother at birth of first child				
17 or younger	2.1%	2.2%	2.2%	1,270
18 to 19	2.2%		2.2%	1,536
20 to 21	2.3%			1,443
Excellent health				
Age of mother at birth of first child				
17 or younger	40.6%	41.0%	40.0%	1,270
18 to 19	42.5%		41.5%	1,536
20 to 21	40.9%			1,443

Source: Authors' calculations based on 2002 MEPS.

Notes: Condition variables represent number of health conditions, therefore expected health results represent frequency of conditions. Self-reported health variables are indicators, therefore expected health results represent probability of health status.

reported health as we increase the mother's age when she first began childbearing.

The estimates in tables 6.7–6.9 and in table 6.10 can be used to simulate the expected effect of changes in the mother's age at birth on the children's medical expenses, use of care, and amount paid by others. The simulations are conducted like those for health status, above. First, based on the estimates, we calculate the expected value of the dependent variable for all children in the sample. Second, we increase the age of the mother at first birth and recalculate the expected value of the dependent variable. In all cases these simulations use model 5 from each table.[7]

The results of our simulations provide a range of expected effects. The first or upper bound of this range is calculated assuming that all covariates in the analysis are held constant except the age of the mother at first birth. But one might argue that this assumption is not very reasonable, because our simulations suggest that the health status of the child is also affected by a change in the mother's age at first birth. In particular, raising the age of the mother should result in improved health status (fewer chronic conditions) for the child. Hence, we also calculate a lower bound that incorporates the expected change in health status when the mother's age is changed. In table 6.13, the figures given in each cell that do not include the change in health status represent the upper bound, or simulated values holding all characteristics of mother and child constant except an increase in the mother's age at first birth. Table 6.13 also presents the lower bound, estimates that include a simulation of change in the probability of an acute or chronic health condition for a child based on the simulated increase in the mother's age at first birth.

The first set of rows in table 6.13 shows how average total medical visits would be expected to vary if the mother were older when she had her first child. As a baseline case, column 2 presents the average "expected" value (which uses the actual values for all variables) for different groups of children in the sample. The first row suggests that if a woman who first gave birth before age 18 postponed childbirth until she was 18–19 or 20–21 years old, expected medical visits for one of her children would increase from 2.41 to 2.78 and 2.60, respectively. Thus, a shift to a first birth as an older teen would increase medical visits by about 0.4 of a visit; a shift to a first birth at age 20–21 results in a small subsequent decline in expected medical visits.

The second set of rows in table 6.13 shows that as a woman's age at first birth is increased, the expected medical expenses of her children also increase—by about 5 percent as she moves from younger than 18 to age 18–19 at first birth and by about 2 percent as she moves to age 20–21. Increasing the age of a mother at first birth from 18–19 to 20–21 is simulated to lead to a slight decrease in expected medical expenditures of about $35.

The last set of rows in table 6.13 simulates the effects of an increase in a woman's age at first birth on the medical care costs borne by society. The cost to society decreases in every case, but the big decrease occurs

Table 6.13. Total Expected Medical Use and Expenditures

| | Baseline Value | | If Mother Delayed until Age | | | | |
| | | | 18 to 19 | | 20 to 21 | | |
	No change in child's health	Change in child's health	No change in child's health	Change in child's health	No change in child's health	Change in child's health	N
Total medical visits							
Age of mother at birth of first child							
17 or younger	2.41	2.15	2.78	2.57	2.60	2.47	1,270
18 to 19	2.91	2.64			2.73	2.54	1,536
20 to 21	2.93	2.59					1,443
Total medical expenditures							
Age of mother at birth of first child							
17 or younger	$1,100.75	$1,017.15	$1,159.51	$1,076.93	$1,123.94	$1,060.80	1,270
18 to 19	$1,187.63	$1,101.46			$1,151.54	$1,085.31	1,536
20 to 21	$1,201.01	$1,096.86					1,443
Expenditures paid by others							
Age of mother at birth of first child							
17 or younger	$720.36	$658.94	$706.81	$646.53	$603.89	$555.90	1,270
18 to 19	$714.06	$649.97			$610.42	$559.05	1,536
20 to 21	$630.93	$551.16					1,443

Source: Authors' calculations based on 2002 MEPS.

Notes: The figures in "no change" columns denote simulated expenses and number of medical visits assuming that the child's health does not change. The figures in the "change in child's health conditions" columns denote simulated expenses and number of medical visits assuming that the child's chronic and acute health conditions change as predicted by the tobit estimates in table 6.10. Expenditure figures are in 2002 dollars.

when a woman who gave birth when younger than 18 instead does not give birth until 20 or 21; the expected savings to society is $116 per child a year, or about 16 percent. The result is nearly as significant if age at first birth is raised from 18–19 to 20–21—potential savings of about $103 per child a year, or nearly 15 percent.

As noted above, some estimates in table 6.13 do not incorporate the potential improvement in the child's health status as the mother's age increases. When the expected change in health conditions is included in the simulations, the baseline for expected visits is reduced but the qualitative effect is similar as a women goes from giving birth as a young teen to an older teen and finally to age 20–21. For example, including changes in a child's health status, annual medical expenses borne by society would decrease by more than $100 or 16 percent if a mother who was under 18 at the time of her first birth were to postpone childbearing until she was 20–21 years old.[8]

The results from these simulations carry important implications for society: if a mother who was younger than 18 at her first birth were to postpone childbearing until after age 19, public medical expenses for one of her children would decrease by about 16 percent; in 2006 dollars, this is about $115 per birth a year. Thus, if a woman who first gave birth as a young teen were to wait until at least age 20 to first give birth, society would save $115 on average annually for each of her children. As noted above, the total medical expenses for each member of this group is expected to increase by about 4 percent, which implies that as the age of the mother increases, others in society pay an unambiguously lower percentage of the health expenses of her children.

Although the results of these simulations provide a measure of the effects of teen childbearing on the health status and health expenses of children, it is important to highlight the limitations of our simulations. The estimates on which the simulations are based are reduced-form regressions. Because we do not have a structural model of the process in which teen childbearing plays a major part, we cannot make policy predictions based on our simulations. For example, several important factors that may be correlated with both health care use and teen motherhood are necessarily omitted from our analysis. These include educational attainment, earnings opportunities, and mothers' incomes—all likely to be correlated with teen motherhood and health care use. Insurance status is another important omitted variable that is likely to be correlated with both medical use and teen motherhood. Hence, although our results usefully describe the differences in medical care use and expenses between children born to teenage mothers and other children, we are unable to predict behavioral responses to alternative policies.

Firstborn Children

We also consider our analysis in the context of children who are the first born to each mother in our sample. We expect that the negative consequences of being born to a teen mother at her youngest childbearing age are stronger than the consequences of merely being born to a woman who started her parental role as a teen.

The descriptive statistics for this smaller group of children are included in table 6.1 in the second set of columns. As would be expected, a far higher proportion of first births were to young teen mothers (27 percent of first births versus 11 percent of all births) and to mothers who were 18–19 (37 percent of first births versus 19 percent of all births). In every category of medical care, these firstborn children made higher use, on average— more visits, greater expenditures, and higher costs paid by society— although the differences are not large. The descriptive statistics for health suggest a mixed picture: a slightly higher number of conditions (both acute and chronic) is reported for the firstborn, but also a higher proportion is reported to be in excellent health.

For these 1,540 firstborn children, we conduct a similar analysis as for the larger group of 4,249 children born to the three groups of mothers (the tables are available upon request). Here we focus only on the results of the simulations in which we increase the age of the teenage mothers and examine the expected change in the number of visits, medical expenditures, and the amount paid by society. These results are presented in table 6.14.

The entries in table 6.14 that do not take changes in a child's health into account show that the number of visits would be higher for the first-born of teenage mothers than if the mother postponed giving birth until age 20–21. But that difference is rather small (.08 of a visit, on average). The highest number of visits is expected if the young teen mother postpones giving birth until age 18 or 19, but again the difference is very small (.06 of a visit). In all cases the number of visits is higher, on average, than it is for the entire set of children born to these mothers.[9] Expenditures would be less by about 6 percent for the firstborn child if the young teen (or older teen) postponed childbearing until age 20–21. This pattern is

Table 6.14. Total Expected Medical Use and Expenditures, First Births Only

| | Baseline Value | | If Mother Delayed until Age | | | | |
| | | | 18 to 19 | | 20 to 21 | | |
	No change in child's health	Change in child's health	No change in child's health	Change in child's health	No change in child's health	Change in child's health	N
Total medical visits							
Age of mother at birth of first child							
17 or younger	2.94	2.65	3.00	2.85	2.86	2.83	1,270
18 to 19	3.20	2.95			3.05	2.92	1,536
20 to 21	3.32	2.95					1,443
Total medical expenditures							
Age of mother at birth of first child							
17 or younger	$1,232.41	$1,177.11	$1,240.44	$1,216.11	$1,160.40	$1,164.23	1,270
18 to 19	$1,303.19	$1,257.54			$1,220.71	$1,205.14	1,536
20 to 21	$1,293.18	$1,223.02					1,443
Expenditures paid by others							
Age of mother at birth of first child							
17 or younger	$873.78	$819.63	$805.21	$773.38	$682.17	$668.74	1,270
18 to 19	$831.33	$789.52			$704.56	$683.50	1,536
20 to 21	$742.29	$675.66					1,443

Source: Authors' calculations based on 2002 MEPS.

Notes: The figures in "no change" columns denote simulated expenses and number of medical visits assuming that the child's health does not change. The figures in the "change in child's health conditions" columns denote simulated expenses and number of medical visits assuming that the child's chronic and acute health conditions change as predicted by the tobit estimates. Expenditure figures are in 2002 dollars.

similar to that for older teen mothers in the sample of all children but not younger teen mothers. For children born to younger teens, expenditures for all children are expected to increase by about 2 percent if the mother postponed her initial childbearing until age 20–21 in contrast to the expected decrease among firstborn children.

Our primary interest is in public expenditures. These expenditures on behalf of firstborn children are expected to decrease if the mother postpones her first birth to age 18–19 or 20–21 (for young teens) and age 20–21 (for older teens). The decrease is expected to be nearly 22 percent for young teens who postpone first births to age 20–21 and 15 percent for older teens who postpone first births to age 20–21. The savings are greater than those for subsequent children born to these mothers, though the pattern is consistent.

Table 6.14 also shows simulations that include changes in the child's health and medical care use as the mother's age at first birth increases. The health variables included are the number of acute and chronic conditions. Total expenditures are expected to decrease if a teen mother postpones childbearing to age 20–21; however, once health is taken into account, visits are expected to increase if a young teen postpones childbearing. Children of older teen mothers consistently have the greatest number of visits. Societal costs for medical care show a similar pattern of decrease as the mother postpones her childbearing. If a young teen mother were to postpone her first birth to age 20–21, the expected savings are more than 18 percent; for an older teen mother, expected savings are more than 13 percent.

Thus, as with all children born to teen mothers, the medical costs borne by society would be significantly reduced if teen mothers were to postpone their first births until age 20–21. And as expected, the potential savings are greater for firstborn children than for subsequent children. This finding is consistent with the hypothesis that the greatest negative effect on children of being born to a teen mother occurs when the mother is youngest.

Conclusion

Children of young teen mothers tend to have more chronic health problems than the children of older mothers. In addition, although the children of young teen mothers visit medical providers less frequently and have lower *total* medical expenses, a larger percentage of the expenses they incur is paid by others in society than is the case among children of older mothers. Hence, a greater proportion of medical expenses for children of teenage mothers is borne by other members of society.

The medical expenses paid by society would be reduced substantially—by about 16 percent—if teenage mothers were to wait until they were older (age 20–21) to have their first children. However, the simulations are based on the assumption that current teenage mothers will act like older mothers, not only in terms of their fertility behavior but also in their educational attainment, earnings, and insurance. If these assumptions do not hold, then our results may well overstate the savings to society from postponing the childbearing of current teenage mothers.

Glossary of Variables

Demographic Variables

Age	Child's age at last interview.
Mom age	Mother's age at last interview.
Young teen mom	1 if mother ever had a child when less than 18 years old; 0 otherwise.
Older teen mom	1 if mother had her first child when 18 or 19 years old; 0 otherwise.
Nonteen mom	1 if mother had her first child when 20 or 21; 0 otherwise.
White	1 if child is white, non-Hispanic; 0 otherwise.
Black	1 if child is black, non-Hispanic; 0 otherwise.
Hispanic	1 if child is Hispanic; 0 otherwise.
Male	1 if child is male; 0 otherwise.

Geographic Variables

Northeast	1 if child lives in northeast region of the United States; 0 otherwise.
Midwest	1 if child lives in midwest region of the United States; 0 otherwise.

West	1 if child lives in western region of the United States; 0 otherwise.
South	1 if child lives in southern region of the United States; 0 otherwise.
MSA	1 if child lives in a metropolitan statistical area; 0 otherwise.

Health Variables

Acute

This variable is intended to capture acute health problems. All medical conditions reported during the panel were categorized using ACG/ADG software based on International Classification of Diseases ICD-9 codes. The acute indicator is set to 1 if any condition reported for the child is categorized as one of the following:

- Time Limited: Minor
- Time Limited: Minor–Primary Infections
- Time Limited: Major
- Time Limited: Major–Primary Infections
- Likely to Recur: Discrete
- Likely to Recur: Discrete–Infections
- Dermatologic
- Injuries/Adverse Effects: Minor
- Injuries/Adverse Effects: Major
- Psychosocial: Time Limited, Minor
- Signs/Symptoms: Minor
- Signs/Symptoms: Uncertain
- Signs/Symptoms: Major

Chronic

This variable is intended to capture chronic health problems. All medical conditions reported during the panel were categorized using ACG/ADG software based on ICD-9 codes. The chronic indicator is set to 1 if any condition reported for the child is categorized as one of the following:
- Asthma
- Likely to Recur: Progressive

- Chronic Medical: Stable
- Chronic Medical: Unstable
- Chronic Specialty: Stable–Ortho
- Chronic Specialty: Stable–ENT
- Chronic Specialty: Stable–Eye
- Chronic Specialty: Unstable–Ortho
- Chronic Specialty: Unstable–Eye
- Psychosocial: Recur or Persist: Stable
- Psychosocial: Recur or Persist: Unstable
- Discretionary
- See and Reassure

Excellent 1 if self-reported health status (reported by primary respondent for the children) is excellent; 0 otherwise.

Fair-poor 1 if self-reported health status (reported by primary respondent for the children) is fair or poor; 0 otherwise.

Use

ER visits Total number of emergency room visits, measured over all rounds.

Hospital inpatient stays Total number of inpatient hospital stays, measured over all rounds.

Hospital outpatient visits Total number of hospital outpatient visits, measured over all rounds.

Medical provider visits Total number of visits to medical providers, measured over all rounds.

All medical visits Total of all reported visits to medical providers, hospital outpatient departments, emergency rooms, and inpatient hospital stays.

Expenditures

Self-paid Total out-of-pocket payments for medical care by the patient in 2002.

Paid by private insurance Total payments for medical care in 2002 made by private insurers on behalf of the patient.

Paid by others in society   Total payments for medical care in 2002 made by public sources on behalf of the patient. Here, public sources may include Medicare, Medicaid, the Veterans Administration, TRICARE, other federal, state, and local sources, and workers' compensation.

Total expenditures   Total payments for medical care in 2002 from all sources.

Condition Codes

Table B.6.1. ICD9 Condition Codes for Children Included in Our Sample (sorted by frequency in sample, including only those reported by 10+ children)

ICD9 code value	Frequency in sample	ICD9 code description
460	753	Acute nasopharyngitis
382	464	Otitis media, suppurative/NOS*
8	391	Intestinal infection NEC*
493	289	Asthma*
477	205	Allergic rhinitis*
780	193	General symptoms*
487	186	Influenza*
786	163	Respiratory system/other chest symptoms*
34	150	Strep throat/scarlet fever*
79	143	Viral infection classified elsewhere/NOS*
782	118	Skin/other integument symptoms*
490	106	Bronchitis NOS
478	93	Other upper respiratory disease*
314	83	Hyperkinetic syndrome*
536	83	Stomach function disorder*
462	82	Acute pharyngitis

(continued)

ICD9 code value	Frequency in sample	ICD9 code description
784	81	Symptoms involving head/neck*
787	77	Gastrointestinal system symptoms*
873	70	Other open wound of head*
959	63	Injury NEC/NOS*
486	62	Pneumonia, organism NOS
692	58	Contact dermatitis*
473	57	Chronic sinusitis*
V70	54	General medical exam*
372	53	Disorders of conjunctiva*
465	52	Acute upper respiratory infections multiple sites/NOS*
110	38	Dermatophytosis*
388	35	Disorders of ear NEC*
112	34	Candidiasis*
519	30	Other respiratory system diseases*
599	30	Other urinary tract disorders*
V20	30	Health supervision child*
V72	28	Special examinations*
463	26	Acute tonsillitis
785	26	Cardiovascular system symptoms*
V30	26	Single liveborn*
360	23	Disorders of the globe*
530	22	Diseases of esophagus*
564	22	Functional digestive disorders NEC*
78	21	Other viral disease*
276	20	Fluid/electrolyte disorder*
522	19	Pulp & periapical disease*
719	19	Joint disorder NEC & NOS*
311	18	Depressive disorder NEC
535	18	Gastritis and duodenitis*
729	18	Other soft tissue disorder*
136	17	Infections/parasite disease NEC/NOS*
525	17	Other dental disorder*
285	16	Anemia NEC/NOS*
346	16	Migraine*
464	16	AC laryngitis/tracheitis*
514	16	Pulmonary congestion/hypostasis
995	16	Certain adverse effects NEC*

(continued)

ICD9 code value	Frequency in sample	ICD9 code description
367	15	Disorders of refraction*
474	14	Chronic tonsil and adenoid disease*
783	14	Nutrition/metabolism/development symptoms*
789	14	Other abdomen/pelvis symptoms*
989	14	Toxic effects other nonmedicinal substances*
706	13	Sebaceous gland disease*
41	12	Bacterial infection classified elsewhere/NOS*
686	12	Other local skin infection*
814	12	Carpal fracture*
818	12	Fracture arm, multiple sites/NOS*
V40	12	Mental/behavioral problems*
52	11	Chickenpox*
315	11	Specific developmental delays*
521	11	Hard tissue disease of teeth*
523	11	Gingival/periodontal disease*
691	11	Atopic dermatitis*
709	11	Other skin disorders*
799	11	Other ill-defined morbidity/mortality*
V68	11	Administrative encounter*
74	10	Coxsackie viral disease*
345	10	Epilepsy*
520	10	Tooth develop/erupt*

NEC = not elsewhere classified; NOS = unspecified, or of unspecified site

NOTES

1. Exceptions include Wolfe and Perozek (1997), who explored a question like that addressed here using an earlier dataset with a smaller number of observations and less detailed health information; Levine, Pollack, and Comfort (2001), who primarily explore educational outcomes; and Lawler and Shaw (2002), who explore this issue for the United Kingdom, concentrating on adverse pregnancy outcomes.

2. For details on other countries, see http://www.unfpa.org/swp/2005/images/e_indicator1.pdf.

3. We conducted a similar analysis for the first child born to these women. The means and standard deviations are presented in the last columns of table 6.1. There are 1,540 children in this first-child-only sample. If the oldest child had left the household, we incorrectly labeled a subsequent child as the first child. Our age cut-off for mothers was designed to minimize such errors.

4. The validity of this measure has been tested for older population age groups. See, for example, Maddox and Douglass (1973) and Fylkesnes and Forde (1991).

5. We thank Nilay Shah and David Vanness for suggesting and implementing this approach.

6. Since there are just 160 children with chronic conditions only, expenditure estimates for this group should be viewed with some caution. In contrast, there are 554 children with both acute and chronic conditions and 2,261 children with acute conditions only.

7. Because all four health measures are significant in the model 5 tobit estimates, we use the result of this model as the basis for our simulations. However, since there was very little change simulated in self-reported health, we concentrate on the change in chronic and acute conditions in our expenditure simulations that allow for health to respond to the increase in mother's age at the birth of the child. Simulations using all four children's health measures with model 5 are nearly identical to those simulated by increasing the age of the mother and adding the child's health conditions only.

8. As noted above, simulations using all four children's health measures with model 5 differ only slightly from those presented in table 6.13. Expenditures paid by others decline by 1.8 percent as the mother is aged from a young teen to an older teen and by 15.6 percent as she is aged from a young teen to 20–21 at first birth. The expected reduction in these expenditures from increasing a mother's age at first birth from older teen to 20–21 and adding children's health measures is 14 percent.

9. In our analyses for all children, the greatest number of medical visits, on average, was made by children born to older teen mothers; this pattern is also consistent for the firstborn children.

REFERENCES

Fylkesnes, Knut, and Olav Forde. 1991. "The Tromso Study: Predictors of Self-Evaluated Health: Has Society Adopted the Expanded Health Concept?" *Social Science and Medicine* 32:141–46.

Lawler, Debbie A. and Mary Shaw. 2002. "Too Much Too Young? Teenage Pregnancy Is Not a Public Health Problem." *International Journal of Epidemiology* 31:552–53.

Levine, Judith A., Harold Pollack, and Maureen E. Comfort. 2001. "Academic and Behavioral Outcomes among the Children of Young Mothers." *Journal of Marriage and the Family* 63(2): 355–69.

Maddox, George L., and Elizabeth B. Douglass. 1973. "Self-Assessment of Health: A Longitudinal Study of Elderly Subjects." *Journal of Health and Social Behavior* 14(1): 87–93.

Mitchell, Janet B. 1991. "Physician Participation in Medicaid Revisited." *Medical Care* 29(7): 645–53.

Wolfe, Barbara L. 1994. "Reform of Health Care for the Nonelderly Poor." In *Confronting Poverty: Prescriptions for Change,* edited by Sheldon H. Danziger, Gary D. Sandefur, and Daniel H. Weinberg. Cambridge, MA: Harvard University Press.

Wolfe, Barbara, and Maria Perozek. 1997. "Teen Children's Health and Health Care Use." In *Kids Having Kids: Economic Costs and Social Consequences of Teen Pregnancy,* edited by Rebecca A. Maynard (181–203). Washington, DC: Urban Institute Press.

7

Consequences of Teen Childbearing for Child Abuse, Neglect, and Foster Care Placement

Robert M. Goerge, Allen Harden, and Bong Joo Lee

EDITORS' NOTE

In the first edition of Kids Having Kids, *we found a significant relationship between maternal age and the likelihood of substantiated child maltreatment and foster care placement (Goerge and Lee 1997). Since the mid-1990s, the child welfare system has undergone significant changes, and more is known about the long-term effects of foster care. For that reason, it is important to update the previous chapter.*

This chapter describes the current context of the child welfare system, in terms of practice and changes in the policy environment, and reviews the literature on parenting differences between adolescents and older mothers. It also discusses recent research on the effects of the child welfare system on children and youth. The chapter concludes with a discussion of data issues and the findings of the research. Statistical methods are discussed in an appendix.

In federal fiscal year 2004, an estimated 3 million children were reported to state child welfare agencies as abused or neglected; 872,000 of these reports were confirmed, with clear evidence of maltreatment under state law or reason to believe that maltreatment occurred (U.S. Department of Health and Human Services [HHS] 2006). Infants and toddlers (up to age 3) had the highest rate of victimization, at 16.1 per 1,000 children. Infants under age 1 accounted for 10 percent of victims of all age groups. Of the more than 500,000 children in the U.S. foster care system in 2003, 30 percent were under age 5.[1]

Federal policy largely governs the process and parameters under which states can remove children from a parent's home, while state policy is more influential in reporting and investigating child maltreatment. Families suspected of abusing or neglecting their children are typically reported to a centralized abuse and neglect hotline by a concerned party. These reports are most often investigated by public agency investigators or law enforcement personnel, who determine whether credible evidence of abuse or neglect exists. This decisionmaking process can vary by individual worker and region. These investigators decide whether the danger warrants taking custody of the child immediately or, if the danger is not imminent, whether the case should be referred to another professional who guides future decisions in the case. Some cases that are substantiated receive no service at all if the situation that led to abuse or neglect has been addressed without formal intervention. Once a child is removed from the home, a judicial determination is made quickly confirming the investigator's decision to remove the child.

Because of concerns that this investigatory response might create more harm in less serious cases, several states have implemented an alternative, family support–oriented approach that triages reported cases into appropriate response systems (Shusterman et al. 2005). Although serious cases of abuse still go through the evidentiary and judicial process, less severe cases receive a service response, which is unlikely to result in immediate removal of the child from the parent's home.

Policy Changes

The Adoption and Safe Families Act of 1997 (ASFA) led to rules promulgated by the U.S. Department of Health and Human Services to assess state outcomes in safety, permanency, and child well-being. The Child and Family Service Review (CSFR) is the vehicle by which the federal government and each state determines whether federal regulations are being followed, how children and families in the system are faring, and what steps should be taken for a state to be in compliance with required benchmarks. Many researchers have criticized this process because of a lack of reliable data and the potential misalignment of goals and strategies (Courtney, Needell, and Wulczyn 2004).

In addition to increasing the focus on outcomes, ASFA shortened timelines for deciding about placing children in permanent homes. States must now move toward terminating parents' rights if a child has been in foster care for 15 of the previous 22 months, unless there are extenuating circumstances. Previously, a child might languish in care for years before there was any action to facilitate permanency. Incentives to place children into adoptive homes now exist, and states are moving toward subsidized guardianship (permanence without formal adoption) as an alternative to a child living in long-term foster care.

ASFA codified in federal policy what was already happening in Illinois in the early to mid-1990s. The increase in adoption and subsidized guardianship has sharply reduced the number of children in foster care in Illinois, but it has also increased the number of children in adoptive and subsidized arrangements. Although the administrative responsibility for these cases is minimal, the payments to adoptive parents or guardians equal those made to foster parents. In addition, these payments continue until the child's 18th birthday, while payments to foster parents obviously end when children are reunified with their biological parents or age out of care, typically at age 18.

Literature Review

This section reviews recent literature on four topics: adolescent childbearing and child maltreatment, child maltreatment reporting and investigation, the effects of foster care on development and adult outcomes, and the educational experiences of foster children and abused and neglected children.

Adolescent Childbearing and Child Maltreatment

Several studies have shown that adolescent mothers are more likely than older mothers to be more stressed by parenting (Ketterlinus, Lamb, and Nitz 1991). Adolescent mothers are also more likely to engage in dysfunctional parenting that may lead to child maltreatment (Brooks-Gunn and Chase-Lansdale 1995; Flanagan et al. 1995; Stevens-Simon, Nelligan, and Kelly 2001).

Child Maltreatment Reporting and Investigation

It remains an open question whether the higher rates of abuse and neglect among adolescent parents result from a higher tendency to abuse or neglect, or whether the rates result from reporting bias. The child protective system depends greatly on mandated reporters (police, teachers, physicians, nurses, social workers). If these reporters are biased toward or against reporting certain parents, the families that come to the attention of the system may not reflect who is actually maltreating their children. A 1996 study of the national incidence of child abuse and neglect found that relatively few children (either 28 percent or 33 percent, depending on the criteria) who were abused or neglected received child protective service attention in response to their maltreatment (Sedlak and Broadhurst 1996). This, in addition to the fact that most reports are unsubstantiated, suggests that who comes to the attention of the child welfare system is not necessarily a function of how children have been treated.

Much recent research finds that race and ethnicity is also a frequent factor in who enters the child protective system. Fluke and colleagues (2003) find in a study of five large states that African American children are more likely to be reported, although not more likely to be substantiated once reported. Ards and colleagues (2003) caution that these effects may stem from aggregation bias and that the race effect is not as large when disaggregated. In Illinois, African American children are more likely to be placed in foster care, even when controlling for many potentially confounding factors (Goerge and Lee 2005). African American children also spend more time in foster care, again controlling for many other factors.

Less attention is paid to other characteristics of parents or parents-to-be that might lead to reports of abuse or neglect and subsequent removal from the home. The importance of adolescent parenthood on maltreatment has not been recognized by the child welfare research field (Flanagan et al. 1995). The National Survey of Child and Adolescent Well-Being (NSCAW) failed to collect basic demographic data on the biological parents of children who were reported for abuse or neglect or of children who had entered foster care.[2] Therefore, the largest study of child welfare ever completed in the United States fails to consider the age of the mother, either at her first birth or at the time of the abuse or neglect report.

The Effects of Foster Care on Development and Adult Outcomes

Child welfare professionals and researchers recognize the important developmental ramifications of child abuse or neglect (Wulczyn et al. 2005). As codified in ASFA, the government is paying more attention to mental health, cognitive, and social outcomes. In addition, child welfare practitioners are paying special attention to negative conditions at birth, such as substance exposure, and conditions that might require early intervention. Federal regulations require state child welfare agencies to screen children under age 3 to determine whether referral to the agency for early intervention is necessary.[3]

What research to date has not explored rigorously is whether the poorer outcomes of foster children stem from their pre-foster care experiences of maltreatment, poverty, and the poor human and social capital of their biological families or from their experiences in foster care. A recent study of foster children in Illinois employed an instrumental variable approach to estimating the causal effect of foster care.[4] It shows foster children are marginally more likely to experience teen childbearing, delinquency, and unemployment than maltreated children who are not placed in foster care.

A recent study of former and current 19-year-old foster care youth in Illinois, Wisconsin, and Iowa finds that their outcomes are significantly worse than a general population of youth examined in the nationally representative Adolescent Health Survey (Courtney et al. 2005). Foster youth are more than twice as likely as youth in the Adolescent Health Survey (AHS) to be disconnected from work and education. More than one-third have neither a high school diploma nor a general equivalency degree, compared with 10 percent in the general population. Of the national sample who are in school, nearly 66 percent are in a four-year college, while only 18 percent of the current and former foster youth are so enrolled.

Further, employment is sporadic; 40 percent of the foster youth are employed, compared with nearly 60 percent in the AHS sample. Of those working, foster youth are significantly less likely to earn more than $10,000 a year. They are more likely than other youth to experience financial hardships, such as difficulty paying their rent or utility bills.

Health outcomes for foster youth are also disappointing. Foster youth are more likely to report that their health conditions limit their abilities to engage in moderate activity, and they report more emergency room and other hospital visits. The hospitalizations are more likely to be for drug use or emotional problems. One-third of former foster youth suffer from serious mental illness. Nearly 50 percent of foster youth have been pregnant, compared with 20 percent of the AHS youth, and foster youth are twice as likely to have at least one child. They are also significantly less like to be married or cohabiting.

Educational Experiences of Foster Children and Abused and Neglected Children

Recent research in Chicago confirms previous statewide research that children in foster care are significantly more likely than children in the general population to be classified with an emotional or behavioral disturbance and placed in special education (Goerge et al. 1992; Smithgall et al. 2004). According to Smithgall and colleagues (2005), foster children are more than 10 times as likely to be classified as emotionally or behaviorally disturbed. More than half of those with emotional or behavioral disorders, regardless of their foster care status, are involved in disciplinary incidents in schools. Also, fewer than 20 percent of these children graduate by their 19th birthday. A striking finding of this study is that children who are victims of abuse or neglect and remain at home do not experience significantly better outcomes than children placed into foster care.

Other research on the well-being of children involved with the child welfare system finds they have more emotional and behavior problems than their peers (Kortenkamp and Ehrle 2002). Studies have also found that children in foster care are significantly more likely than their peers to have school behavior problems and that they have high rates of suspensions and expulsions from school (Barber and Delfabbro 2003; Dubowitz and Sawyer 1994; McMillen et al. 2003; Zima et al. 2000).

Data and Methods

This chapter uses data from the Integrated Database of Child and Family Programs in Illinois (IDB), specifically data from the Illinois Department of Children and Family Services, and Illinois aggregate birth certificate data. The IDB uses the computerized administrative data that contain demographic, family composition, case status, service status, outcomes, and cost information for the entire population of abuse and neglect cases and children in foster homes between 1982 and 2005. These data provide longitudinal information on case openings and subsequent experiences of all families and children receiving child protective services during the study period. In addition to child welfare data, the IDB has data on cash assistance, Medicaid, food stamps, juvenile and criminal justice, WIC, child care, regular and special education, and employment dating back to at least 1990.

The Illinois child protective and child welfare administrative data continue to be one of very few available data sources, even at the state level, that provide detailed family information, including mother's age and sibling information. The overall demographic characteristics of the Illinois child population are very comparable to those of the population in the nation, which makes Illinois data suitable for approximating national figures. Unfortunately, we were unable to find national or other state data to supplement our findings from Illinois. Other states included in the Center for State Foster Care and Adoption Data[5] and Adoption and Foster Care Reporting System (AFCARS) have no maternal age data, nor does the NSCAW, as mentioned above. Also unfortunate is that the many challenges present in the first analysis still exist, and new national data collection efforts have done little to address these challenges.[6]

Calculating Abuse and Neglect Incidence Rates

This study uses Illinois population-level data to investigate incidence rates of child abuse and neglect and foster care placement in the state. The population at risk in this study was defined in two ways: (1) at the individual level, all children born between 1982 and 1998; and (2) at the family level, all new families formed during the same period. A new family is defined as a family, either single-parent or two-parent, with its first child.

Because our administrative data contain information on all children and families who come to the attention of the child welfare system in Illinois, we can estimate population incidence rates of a particular birth cohort or new family cohort by using total live births or total first live births as the denominator. Further, we classify the birth certificate data by birth order, maternal age, race and ethnicity, sex, and region to estimate the population incidence rates for each stratum of a particular birth cohort.

Multivariate Analysis: Testing the Effect of Various Factors on a Child's Abuse and Neglect and Foster Care Experiences

Using the first base population, we use multivariate analysis to examine the effect of mother's age at birth on an individual child's probability of becoming an indicated victim of child abuse or neglect or of being placed in foster care before age 5 (see appendix A.7 for details of the multivariate analysis). The base population at the family level allows us to follow entire cohorts of new families and examine how a mother's age at first birth affects the family having a child abuse or neglect case or having a child placed in foster care. We used Illinois birth certificate data to calculate these two base population sizes.

The second stage of the analysis addresses whether children of teen mothers use more foster care once they are placed in that system. Specifically, we use proportional hazards models to examine the effect of teenage parenthood on the duration of the foster care spell. The study population again is all children placed in foster care from 1982 through 2005.

We controlled for the effects of minimal confounding demographic factors: the child's birth order, race or ethnicity, sex, and region. Ideally, one would include additional background factors such as poverty or education of mothers; however, because our analysis employs aggregate-level birth certificate data as at-risk population estimates, we were unable to disaggregate the birth certificate data from the other factors. Instead, rather than using poverty data directly, we employed race or ethnicity and region (Chicago versus the rest of the state) as proxies for the socioeconomic status of a child. Therefore, the results of our multivariate analyses should be interpreted as adjusted population incidence rate differences between teen mothers and nonteen mothers after controlling for basic demographic factors. Of course, we are not implying any causal inferences but rather presenting demographically adjusted incidence rates.[7]

We would prefer to link individual birth certificates to any child welfare system outcomes. Unfortunately, we have been unable to secure birth certificates in Illinois, in part because of statutory limitations, but also because of class-action lawsuit consent decrees that prevent the identification of mothers. Linking birth certificate and child welfare data has been possible, on a small scale, in other states, but not to identify the mother's characteristics.

Descriptive Findings

This section looks at the changes over time in birth rates, abuse and neglect rates, foster care incidence rates, and foster care duration, and at the variation of these indicators by simple sociodemographic predictor variables. The fact that these predictors are highly interrelated is one main reason for continuing with multivariate approaches in the following section.

Changes in Birth Rates

The number of live births in Illinois rose to 192,281 in 1990 before falling back to pre-1988 levels by 1995 (table 7.1). From 1982 to 1998, births to women under age 22 decreased from 46,077 to 38,441, while births to women older than 22 mirrored the trends in all live births in the state, ending with a general upward trend. Between 1982 and 1998, 40 percent of all newborns each year were born to first-time mothers. The percentage of births to teen mothers fell from 14.0 to 12.4 percent of all births and from 25.9 to 24.3 percent of first births. Although the teen birth rate increased in the latter half of the 1980s, it decreased 21.1 percent from 1991 to 1999 (Ventura, Mathews, and Hamilton 2001).

There are also major changes in the racial and ethnic distribution of births. The number of white, non-Hispanic births per year has declined 16 percent, the number of Hispanic births has increased more than 100 percent, and the number of black births has held fairly constant. The proportion of births that occurred to Chicago residents remained fairly stable.

Abuse and Neglect Rates

The incidence of a substantiated abuse or neglect report before a child's 5th birthday peaked in 1992 and 1993, registering a 75 percent increase over 1982 rates. By the later 1990s, the incidence had returned to rates in the early 1980s. Across the entire period (1982–98), the incidence rate was 53.4 per 1,000 live births in Illinois (table 7.2).

Although the pattern for teens during this period is similar, the incidence rate during the late 1990s dropped lower than the rates in the 1980s, while the incidence of substantiated abuse or neglect for older mothers (age 20+) increased from 1982 to 1998. Nevertheless, the incidence is still correlated with age, in that younger mothers have a higher incidence.

text continues on page 270

Table 7.1. Selected Charateristics of Illinois Live Births, Annual Birth Cohorts 1982–98

Birth year	Total births	First births (%)	Mother's Age at Birth (%)					Race/Ethnicity (%)				Chicago (%)	Female (%)
			Under 16	16–17	18–19	20–21	22+	White	Black	Hispanic	Other		
All births													
1982	181,856	40.9	1.0	4.4	8.6	11.4	74.7	67.4	21.2	9.1	2.2	30.2	48.7
1983	176,875	40.5	1.0	4.2	8.4	10.8	75.5	67.7	21.2	8.9	2.1	30.2	48.8
1984	177,932	39.9	1.0	4.0	8.0	10.4	76.6	67.7	21.2	9.0	2.0	30.1	48.7
1985	180,346	39.8	1.0	3.9	7.6	10.0	77.5	67.7	21.2	9.3	1.8	30.0	48.7
1986	176,103	39.8	1.1	3.9	7.6	9.6	77.9	66.7	21.7	9.9	1.8	30.5	48.8
1987	179,843	39.5	1.1	4.1	7.3	9.4	78.2	65.2	22.2	9.9	2.6	30.6	48.8
1988	184,194	39.5	1.1	4.1	7.4	8.9	78.5	64.4	22.5	10.3	2.8	30.6	48.7
1989	186,089	40.1	1.1	4.2	8.0	9.1	77.7	63.4	22.4	11.4	2.8	30.2	49.0
1990	192,281	40.0	1.0	4.0	8.2	9.3	77.6	62.3	22.5	12.4	2.9	30.6	48.8
1991	190,327	39.8	1.1	4.0	8.1	9.7	77.2	60.8	22.9	13.3	3.0	31.2	49.0
1992	189,689	39.3	1.2	4.0	7.8	9.7	77.3	59.4	23.1	14.3	3.2	31.1	48.7
1993	190,223	39.2	1.1	4.2	7.5	9.3	77.9	58.5	23.3	15.0	3.2	30.9	48.8
1994	188,798	39.7	1.2	4.3	7.6	8.8	78.1	58.0	22.4	16.0	3.5	30.3	48.8
1995	185,395	40.0	1.1	4.1	7.7	8.6	78.5	58.0	20.9	17.3	3.8	29.3	48.8
1996	182,716	39.9	1.0	4.1	7.6	8.7	78.6	57.6	20.6	17.9	3.8	28.8	49.0
1997	180,302	39.6	0.9	4.1	7.5	8.6	78.8	57.0	20.6	18.4	4.1	28.3	48.9
1998	182,076	39.1	0.9	3.9	7.6	8.7	78.9	56.3	20.5	19.1	4.1	28.2	48.9
Total period	3,125,045	39.8	1.1	4.1	7.8	9.5	77.6	62.2	21.8	13.1	2.9	30.1	48.8

First births

Year	First births												
1982	74,427	100.0	2.4	9.0	14.5	14.8	59.3	70.9	19.1	7.8	2.2	29.2	—
1983	71,590	100.0	2.4	8.8	14.5	13.9	60.4	70.8	19.7	7.3	2.2	29.4	—
1984	70,943	100.0	2.3	8.3	13.8	14.0	61.7	70.6	19.7	7.5	2.2	29.3	—
1985	71,816	100.0	2.4	8.1	13.1	13.3	62.9	70.5	19.8	7.7	2.0	29.3	—
1986	70,176	100.0	2.6	8.1	13.0	12.7	63.6	69.4	20.2	8.5	1.9	29.9	—
1987	71,099	100.0	2.6	8.5	12.5	12.2	64.1	67.7	20.7	8.6	3.0	29.7	—
1988	72,780	100.0	2.6	8.6	12.6	11.6	64.7	66.6	20.9	9.2	3.2	30.1	—
1989	74,661	100.0	2.6	8.6	13.5	11.7	63.6	65.5	20.8	10.5	3.2	29.7	—
1990	76,960	100.0	2.4	8.0	13.7	12.2	63.7	64.4	20.6	11.7	3.3	29.7	—
1991	75,676	100.0	2.5	8.1	13.5	12.5	63.4	63.0	20.4	13.0	3.6	30.2	—
1992	74,510	100.0	2.7	8.2	12.8	12.4	63.9	61.7	20.4	14.2	3.8	29.9	—
1993	74,495	100.0	2.6	8.6	12.8	11.6	64.3	60.8	20.5	14.9	3.8	29.5	—
1994	74,974	100.0	2.7	8.8	13.0	11.6	63.9	60.1	20.0	15.9	4.1	29.2	—
1995	74,203	100.0	2.7	8.6	13.1	11.4	64.2	59.7	18.9	17.0	4.4	28.3	—
1996	72,885	100.0	2.5	8.7	13.2	11.5	64.2	59.5	18.5	17.5	4.5	28.0	—
1997	71,447	100.0	2.3	8.7	13.2	11.3	64.5	58.8	18.7	17.6	4.9	27.8	—
1998	71,128	100.0	2.2	8.5	13.6	11.5	64.2	57.9	18.9	18.3	4.9	28.2	—
Total period	1,243,770	100.0	2.5	8.5	13.3	12.4	63.3	64.6	19.9	12.2	3.4	29.3	—

Source: Chapin Hall analysis of data provided by the Illinois Department of Public Health.

Table 7.2. Incidence Rates (per 1,000) of Indicated Child Abuse/Neglect and Foster Care Placement within Five Years

Cohort year	All children	Individual Child Birth Cohorts Mother's Age at Birth				All new families	New Family Cohorts Mother's Age at First Birth			
		Under 18	18–19	20–21	22+		Under 18	18–19	20–21	22+
Abuse/neglect										
1982	37.8	104.1	75.4	60.2	25.2	35.0	95.8	59.3	39.0	16.5
1983	42.0	113.2	85.0	68.7	28.4	37.1	103.6	62.3	44.7	16.9
1984	44.8	123.8	93.2	76.2	30.4	39.1	117.0	71.4	43.3	17.5
1985	46.1	116.2	96.5	80.6	32.2	40.6	110.2	74.1	50.6	19.8
1986	47.9	124.0	98.8	84.7	33.7	41.2	114.9	75.8	49.4	20.1
1987	52.4	121.5	107.5	93.3	37.8	43.9	120.1	81.0	54.8	21.4
1988	55.2	125.0	105.2	96.4	41.2	43.9	115.3	80.7	52.9	22.8
1989	58.9	123.0	105.6	98.4	45.2	45.9	114.4	79.9	56.5	24.6
1990	60.4	125.8	106.9	95.8	47.0	44.2	112.1	77.6	53.5	24.1
1991	64.5	121.2	108.3	101.0	51.6	45.8	107.9	76.4	56.0	26.8
1992	65.8	113.0	104.1	95.2	55.2	45.5	105.3	75.6	53.5	27.7
1993	65.0	114.8	99.2	95.0	54.8	44.6	102.6	73.8	51.9	27.3
1994	61.6	111.2	87.2	84.8	53.0	42.5	103.2	65.1	47.2	26.2
1995	55.7	90.5	83.2	77.8	48.2	37.9	85.8	62.3	45.2	23.2
1996	51.9	90.1	74.2	69.7	45.3	39.0	82.4	56.9	47.3	26.4
1997	48.7	94.4	76.5	71.1	40.6	37.7	90.2	62.9	45.0	22.3
1998	46.2	86.9	77.1	70.1	38.1	35.7	81.4	60.9	45.9	20.8
Total period	53.4	111.7	93.2	83.4	41.9	41.2	103.6	70.2	49.1	22.7

Foster care placement

1982	10.7	31.2	21.0	16.5	7.1	11.1	27.0	16.4	12.3	6.4
1983	12.4	32.0	25.7	18.5	8.7	11.6	26.0	18.9	13.1	6.9
1984	13.3	40.9	28.2	22.5	8.6	11.3	33.9	18.9	10.5	5.9
1985	15.0	40.8	32.5	26.8	10.1	13.6	33.2	22.3	16.3	8.0
1986	16.3	43.6	36.5	28.4	11.1	13.3	33.2	23.2	14.1	7.7
1987	19.0	43.8	39.2	35.9	13.5	14.9	36.5	23.7	18.7	8.6
1988	20.7	48.0	38.8	37.2	15.3	14.8	35.9	21.9	17.8	9.2
1989	22.9	50.3	38.4	38.7	17.6	15.8	37.1	23.8	17.4	10.0
1990	24.7	51.0	43.5	37.6	19.5	13.6	34.8	22.0	14.7	8.2
1991	26.3	51.9	40.4	38.6	21.6	14.6	37.7	19.7	14.8	9.6
1992	26.6	45.7	37.1	37.3	22.9	13.3	32.5	19.0	13.9	8.8
1993	26.6	45.0	34.3	36.1	23.5	13.4	32.9	19.5	16.1	8.3
1994	25.0	38.2	28.8	30.6	23.0	12.2	29.5	15.9	11.2	8.5
1995	22.6	32.4	26.3	26.2	21.2	10.6	24.5	15.3	10.4	7.3
1996	21.0	34.3	23.9	22.6	19.6	10.5	27.1	14.7	10.5	6.8
1997	18.7	34.2	23.6	21.9	16.9	10.0	28.8	15.5	9.3	5.8
1998	17.5	30.8	23.6	20.5	15.8	10.5	26.4	16.1	12.1	6.3
Total period	20.1	40.9	31.9	29.1	16.4	12.7	31.6	19.2	13.7	7.8

Source: Chapin Hall analysis of data provided by the Illinois Department of Children and Family Services and the Illinois Department of Public Health.

During the entire period, the incidence rate of a substantiated abuse or neglect report among women under age 18 was 111.7 per 1,000, or nearly three times the rate of older mothers.

For new families (i.e., first births), the trends are similar, although the increase in abuse or neglect cases over time for mothers who had their first child after age 20 is smaller. Among all mothers, young and older, the increase during the 1980s was as high as 30 percent. For the entire period, the incidence rate among new families was 41.2 per 1,000.

The rates of maltreatment for women with their first child by age are lower than those for all births, although the rates for women who give birth under the age of 18 are more similar. There is a wider difference by age for first births than all births when we analyze the age at first birth. Women who have had their first birth after age 22 have a rate of only 22.7 per 1,000 births—the least likely to have a substantiated abuse or neglect report within five years after the birth of their first child.

Foster Care Incidence Rates

Fewer than a third of children who are reported for abuse or neglect enter foster care, and the foster care incidence rates reflect this (HHS 2004). Between 1982 and 1998, for every 1,000 births in Illinois, 20.1 of the children entered foster care before age 5, with a maximum of nearly 27 per 1,000 in 1992 and 1993 (table 7.2). The rate is nearly twice as high for children of mothers under age 18 and 50 percent higher for children of mothers under age 22 than for mothers age 22 and older. For those under age 22, the trend has been consistently downward since 1991. For women over age 22, the decline came later, not until 1995.

For the new family cohorts, the general trend is similar, although the magnitudes are smaller. The overall rate is 12.7 per 1,000, and the rate for women under 18 is 31.6 per 1,000.

Of the 118,206 children who entered foster care during the period, about 62 percent were born to mothers younger than age 20 at the time of first birth. The data in table 7.3 also show that about 63 percent placed were African American, 52 percent were living in Chicago, and 24 percent were infants at the time of placement. About 39 percent of children placed during the period had an abuse allegation. Those children who were not indicated cases of maltreatment (25.8 percent) are those who have one or more siblings who were also victims of abuse or neglect.

Table 7.3. Selected Charateristics of Illinois Children Placed in Foster Care, 1982–2003 (118,206 first placements)

Characteristic	Percentage of total	Characteristic	Percentage of total
Mother's age at first birth		Child's age at placement	
15 and under	13.5	Less than 1	24.0
16–17	24.9	1–2	17.1
18–19	23.1	3–5	18.5
20–21	13.9	6–8	13.7
22 and over	24.6	9–11	10.6
		12–14	10.0
Race/ethnicity		15–17	6.1
White	28.6		
Black	63.4	Gender of child	
Hispanic	6.0	Male	50.2
Other	1.9	Female	49.9
Region		Birth order	
Rest of state	47.6	First birth	34.4
Chicago	52.4	Second or higher birth	65.6
Indicated harms before		Years of placement	
placement		1982–85	11.5
Abuse	12.20	1986–89	17.4
Neglect	35.30	1990–94	32.5
Abuse and neglect	26.60	1995–99	26.9
Not identified	25.80	2000–03	11.9

Source: Chapin Hall analysis of data provided by the Illinois Department of Children and Family Services.

Foster Care Duration

Table 7.4 presents summary statistics on the duration of the first foster care placement, reported by the median time in care.[8] The amount of time differs significantly between children of teen mothers and those of older mothers. The median duration of the first spell in substitute care of children born to mothers who were 16 or 17 at first birth was nearly 1,000 days, whereas the median first spell in substitute care of children born to mothers age 20–21 was around 700 days. Our results also indicate

Table 7.4. Duration of First Substitute Care Placement Spell, Illinois 1982–2003

	Median duration (days)	95% Confidence Bounds	
		Lower	Higher
Total state	801	791	812
Mother's age at first birth			
15 and under	1,086	1,053	1,119
16–17	962	944	983
18–19	745	726	768
20–21	668	645	695
22 and over	638	617	653
Type of indicated harm			
Abuse	687	657	714
Neglect	947	930	964
Abuse and neglect	885	868	904
Not identified	449	396	602
Child's age at placement			
Less than 1	994	980	1,007
1–2	805	780	834
3–5	778	751	806
6–8	769	736	810
9–11	735	697	772
12–14	598	567	631
15–17	397	372	424
Region			
Rest of state	380	370	390
Chicago	1,266	1,254	1,277
Race/ethnicity			
White	296	288	305
Black	1,149	1,136	1,162
Hispanic	610	576	652
Other	478	421	550
Gender of child			
Male	822	807	837
Female	780	764	796

Table 7.4. *(Continued)*

	Median duration (days)	95% Confidence Bounds	
		Lower	Higher
Birth order			
First birth	521	505	536
Second or higher birth	945	932	957
Years of placement			
1982–84	196	182	206
1985–89	263	250	276
1990–94	1,340	1,318	1,359
1995–99	1,004	995	1,015
2000–03	749	730	766

Source: Chapin Hall analysis of data provided by the Illinois Department of Children and Family Services.

that children with neglect allegations, children first placed as infants, children from the Chicago area, African American children, and second or higher birth-order children tended to stay longer in foster care.

Our descriptive findings for this period agree largely with the findings from our earlier work. For the most part, the magnitude statistics have increased: there is a higher overall rate of abuse and neglect incidence, foster care placement, and foster care duration.

Multivariate Analysis Findings

Maternal age-specific incidence rates or duration measures do not necessarily reflect the independent effect of maternal age on maltreatment and foster care placement rates or duration of foster care. Duration of foster care varies considerably by factors other than maternal age. To calculate the independent effect of maternal age on child abuse or neglect and foster care, we controlled for the other factors in our multivariate methods.

Indicated Abuse and Neglect Reports

We present four models, where each adds additional variables to the previous one (table 7.5). The estimated effects for all models are expressed as

Table 7.5. Relationship between Mother's Age at Birth and an Indicated Child Abuse/Neglect Report, Illinois Birth Cohorts 1989–98

	Model 1	Model 2	Model 3	Model 4
Mother's age at birth				
15 and under	1.69	1.53	2.43	1.75
16–17	1.30	1.24	1.70	1.41
18–19	1.13	1.11	1.29	1.18
20–21	1.00	1.00	1.00	1.00
22 and over	0.48	0.50	0.43	0.51
Birth year				
1982		1.00	1.00	1.00
1983		1.13	1.13	1.13
1984		1.22	1.22	1.21
1985		1.27	1.27	1.26
1986		1.32	1.32	1.31
1987		1.45	1.45	1.43
1988		1.54	1.54	1.50
1989		1.64	1.64	1.62
1990		1.68	1.68	1.66
1991		1.80	1.79	1.77
1992		1.84	1.83	1.80
1993		1.83	1.81	1.78
1994		1.73	1.73	1.72
1995		1.56	1.57	1.59
1996		1.46	1.46	1.48
1997		1.37	1.37	1.39
1998		1.30	1.30	1.31
Region				
Chicago		1.64	1.55	1.03
Rest of state		1.00	1.00	1.00
Gender of child				
Male			1.00	1.00
Female			0.98	0.97
Birth order				
First birth			0.41	0.46
Second or higher birth			1.00	1.00

Table 7.5. *(Continued)*

	Model 1	Model 2	Model 3	Model 4
Race/ethnicity				
White				1.00
Black				3.18
Hispanic				0.70
Other				1.68

Source: Chapin Hall analysis of data provided by the Illinois Department of Children and Family Services and the Illinois Department of Public Health.

Note: All estimates are significant at the 0.05 level.

changes in the expected incidence rate of being an indicated victim of child abuse or neglect, relative to a baseline group. For example, model 1, which includes only mother's age at the birth of the child, shows the relative odds of having an indicated abuse/neglect report for the mother's age group. In this case, for mothers age 15 or younger the relative odds are 1.69; in other words, children born to mothers age 15 and younger are two-thirds more likely to become an indicated case of child abuse or neglect before age 5 than are children born to mothers age 20–21 (the baseline category). Mothers who have a child while under the age of 20 are also more likely to experience an indicated case of abuse or neglect.

Because model 1 includes no other demographic factors, it should be interpreted as "unadjusted" differences in the incidence rate of child abuse or neglect across the mothers' age groups.

Model 2 adds the child's birth year and region to the model. After controlling for the birth cohort and region effects, we still find significant differences in odds ratios between teen and nonteen mothers. As with the descriptive analysis, the results of model 2 show that incidence rates of indicated child abuse or neglect increased during the early 1990s and decreased after 1993. For instance, an infant in the 1992 birth cohort was 1.84 times as likely to suffer abuse or neglect as a child in the birth cohort of 1982. In model 2, region is a significant factor predicting the incidence rate of child abuse and neglect, with children in Chicago 1.64 times as likely to suffer abuse or neglect as children in the balance of the state.

Model 3 adds two more factors: sex and birth order of the child. First-born children are approximately half (0.41) as likely to become indicated cases of abuse and neglect as subsequent children. After controlling for birth order of the child, the effect of young motherhood on the rate of child abuse or neglect increases significantly, to 1.7 for 16–17-year-old mothers. As mentioned earlier, this is likely because the child protection system responds less forcefully to reports involving first children and young mothers with only one child, perhaps because it is assumed they have more support from their families.

From the results in model 3, we can conclude that once we take into account the fact that most births to teens are first births, the relative effect of having a child as a teen is greater. This makes sense since teens are more likely to have first births than subsequent births.

Model 4 adds race and ethnicity. African American children are more than three times as likely to suffer child abuse or neglect as non-Hispanic white children, and Hispanic children are less likely than white children to have an indicated case of maltreatment. Because the composition of cases reported to child protective services differs from the composition of teen parents, race and ethnicity account for the maternal age differences that we saw in model 3. We also find that the effect of living in Cook County almost disappears once we control for race and ethnicity. This is a result of the high concentration of African American children in the group of indicated children in the Chicago area.

After controlling for all the other demographic factors, we still find that children born to teen mothers are significantly more likely to have an indicated report of child abuse or neglect during their early childhood than are those born to nonteen mothers. Our results also suggest that children born to younger teen mothers are at greater risk of abuse or neglect than are children born to older teen mothers. For example, children born to mothers age 15 or younger are nearly two times (1.75) as likely as children born to mothers age 20–21 to have an indicated child abuse or neglect report, and children born to mothers age 16–17 are 1.41 times as likely to become victims of child abuse or neglect, even after controlling for the other demographic factors.

When focusing on the new family cohort, we find that families with mothers whose first birth was during their teen years are much more likely to be reported for child abuse or neglect than are families with nonteen mothers (table 7.6). We employ a similar strategy to control for other demographic characteristics, and the effect of having a first child as a teen persists as the mother ages. Delaying birth to after age 21 decreases by half the likelihood of an indicated case of abuse or neglect, compared with first-time mothers age 20 or 21. Controlling for year of birth, region of the state, and race/ethnicity has a weaker effect in this analysis than in the previous

Table 7.6. Relationship between Mother's Age at First Birth and an Indicated Child Abuse or Neglect Report, Illinois New Families, 1989–98

Characteristic	Model 1	Model 2	Model 3
Mother's age at first birth			
15 and under	2.92	2.85	2.32
16–17	2.05	2.02	1.81
18–19	1.46	1.46	1.39
20–21	1.00	1.00	1.00
22 and over	0.45	0.45	0.46
First birth year			
1982		1.00	1.00
1983		1.07[a]	1.06[a]
1984		1.15	1.15
1985		1.22	1.21
1986		1.24	1.23
1987		1.33	1.31
1988		1.33	1.31
1989		1.38	1.37
1990		1.34	1.33
1991		1.38	1.39
1992		1.38	1.39
1993		1.35	1.37
1994		1.27	1.30
1995		1.13	1.17
1996		1.17	1.22
1997		1.13	1.17
1998		1.07[a]	1.10[a]
Region			
Chicago		1.08	0.93
Rest of state		1.00	1.00
Race/ethnicity			
White			1.00
Black			1.76
Hispanic			0.55
Other			1.89

Source: Chapin Hall analysis of data provided by the Illinois Department of Children and Family Services and the Illinois Department of Public Health.

a. These estimates are not significant at the 0.05 level.

one, meaning that the effect of having a first birth during one's teen years is a robust one—other characteristics of the teen explain a small amount of the fact that she is more likely to maltreat her child.

Entry into Foster Care

Given the tight relationship between having an indicated case of abuse or neglect and entry into foster care, we would expect that the multivariate models of the two would be similar. In fact, they are, although the effects are not as strong as with abuse and neglect report (table 7.7). Again, we see a declining likelihood of foster care entry as the age of the mother increases. A 16- or 17-year-old is 28 percent more likely to have a child placed in foster care than is a 20- or 21-year-old (model 1).

As controls for birth year and region are added, we again see trends similar to those in the descriptive analysis, with the likelihood of placement increasing through 1993 and then decreasing, but still remaining higher in the late 1990s than in the early 1980s.

Controlling for birth order increases the magnitude of the teen parenthood effect, as we saw in the abuse and neglect model. The fact that second or later births are more likely to bring children in that family into foster care increases the effect of early childbearing. The fact that a woman's first births happen at younger ages than subsequent births explains this shift in the effect sizes from model 2 to model 3.

In the fourth model, we see the large effect of being African American. This, again, reduces the effect of maternal age, given the fact that a teen birth is more likely to occur among African American women than white women.

The magnitude of the coefficients for the new family cohort analysis (table 7.8), and therefore the differences between the maternal age groups, are larger than for all births. Having one's first child as a teen seems to have a strong and permanent effect on the placement of all a mother's children.

Duration of Foster Care

We pursue a similar strategy in analyzing foster care duration. Model 1 (table 7.9) simply includes age of the mother at her first birth. The effect of having a child under the age of 20 is clear. For example, mothers who had their first child at 16 or 17 years old had children who stayed in care

Table 7.7. Relationship between Mother's Age at Birth and Placement in Substitute Care, Illinois Birth Cohorts 1989–98

Characteristic	Model 1	Model 2	Model 3	Model 4
Mother's age at first birth				
15 and under	1.99	1.65	2.34	1.51
16–17	1.28	1.16	1.47	1.13
18–19	1.10	1.06[a]	1.18	1.04[a]
20–21	1.00	1.00	1.00	1.00
22 and over	0.56	0.62	0.55	0.76
Birth year				
1982		1.00	1.00	1.00
1983		1.17	1.17	1.17
1984		1.26	1.26	1.25
1985		1.44	1.44	1.43
1986		1.56	1.56	1.54
1987		1.83	1.82	1.78
1988		2.00	1.99	1.94
1989		2.21	2.21	2.16
1990		2.39	2.39	2.34
1991		2.52	2.51	2.46
1992		2.56	2.54	2.47
1993		2.57	2.55	2.47
1994		2.42	2.42	2.38
1995		2.22	2.22	2.25
1996		2.07	2.07	2.10
1997		1.86	1.86	1.88
1998		1.74	1.74	1.76
Region				
Chicago		2.67	2.56	1.30
Rest of state		1.00	1.00	1.00
Gender of child				
Male			1.00	1.00
Female			0.99[a]	0.98[a]
Birth order				
First birth			0.51	0.63
Second or higher birth			1.00	1.00

(continued)

Table 7.7. *(Continued)*

Characteristic	Model 1	Model 2	Model 3	Model 4
Race/ethnicity				
White				1.00
Black				6.12
Hispanic				0.82
Other				1.53

Source: Chapin Hall analysis of data provided by the Illinois Department of Children and Family Services and the Illinois Department of Public Health.

a. These estimates are not significant at the 0.05 level.

20 percent longer than those who had a first child at age 20 or 21 (1.00 − .83/.83). The effect of age of mother at first birth remains the same in model 2 when the maltreatment type variables are added. The maternal age effect weakens when region of the state is entered, suggesting that the age effect is partly because young mothers are more likely to live in Chicago. When child's age at first placement is added, we no longer see a statistically significant difference between young first-time mothers (age 18–19) and those who have their first birth at older ages. In the final model (5), which adds birth order, gender, and race, being a first-time mother at age 18 or younger is associated with only a 5–10 percent longer stay in care, albeit still a statistically significant difference, than those who had their first child at older ages.

The importance of adding additional variables to control for confounding factors is twofold. First, we do not want to overstate the effect, given that other factors may be explaining the longer duration we see for children of younger first-time mothers. Adolescent parenthood in Chicago among African American women is more prevalent than in other parts of the state, and African Americans are more likely to be reported, substantiated, placed, and to have longer durations in foster care. It is difficult, at best, to untangle these factors. Second, adding variables one or two at a time better clarifies where we might intervene to better address disparities or reduce overall duration of foster care. These more targeted interventions could have more pronounced effects on social and psychological outcomes, as well as fiscal burdens. The family and neighborhood context for children of African American teen parents in Chicago may be an important place for policymakers and practitioners to intervene to improve child well-being.

Table 7.8. Relationship between Mother's Age at First Birth and Placement in Substitute Care, Illinois New Families 1989–98

Characteristic	Model 1	Model 2	Model 3
Mother's age at first birth			
15 and under	3.52	3.28	2.22
16–17	2.00	1.90	1.53
18–19	1.41	1.38	1.25
20–21	1.00	1.00	1.00
22 and over	0.57	0.58	0.68
First birth year			
1982		1.00	1.00
1983		1.06[a]	1.04[a]
1984		1.04[a]	1.02[a]
1985		1.27	1.25
1986		1.23	1.21
1987		1.38	1.34
1988		1.38	1.32
1989		1.46	1.42
1990		1.27	1.24
1991		1.36	1.33
1992		1.24	1.21
1993		1.25	1.22
1994		1.22	1.11
1995		0.99[a]	0.99[a]
1996		0.98[a]	0.99[a]
1997		0.94[a]	0.94[a]
1998		0.98[a]	0.98[a]
Region			
Chicago		1.41	0.94
Rest of state		1.00	1.00
Race/ethnicity			
White			1.00
Black			3.28
Hispanic			0.71
Other			1.62

Source: Chapin Hall analysis of data provided by the Illinois Department of Children and Family Services and the Illinois Department of Public Health.

a. These estimates are not significant at the 0.05 level.

Table 7.9. Duration of First Placement Spells, Illinois 1982–2003

Characteristic	Risk Ratios				
	Model 1	Model 2	Model 3	Model 4	Model 5
Mother's age at first birth					
15 and under	0.78	0.78	0.83	0.84	0.91
16–17	0.83	0.84	0.89	0.89	0.95
18–19	0.95	0.95	0.96	0.97	0.99[a]
20–21	1.00	1.00	1.00	1.00	1.00
22 and over	1.03	1.02	0.99[a]	0.99[a]	0.97
Indicated allegation type					
Abuse		1.00	1.00	1.00	1.00
Neglect		0.94	1.00[a]	0.99[a]	1.03
Not identified		1.54	1.55	1.53	1.57
Year of placement					
1982–83			1.00	1.00	1.00
1984–85			0.97	0.97[a]	0.97[a]
1986–87			1.02	1.01[a]	1.04
1988–89			0.89	0.89	0.93
1990–91			0.76	0.76	0.81
1992–93			0.73	0.73	0.79
1994–95			0.83	0.83	0.89
1996–97			0.97	0.98[a]	1.05
1998–99			1.03	1.04	1.10
2000–01			1.04	1.05	1.10
2002–03			1.08	1.09	1.12
Region of Illinois					
Chicago			0.59	0.59	0.67
Rest of state			1.00	1.00	1.00
Child's age at first placement					
Less than 1				1.00	1.00
1–2				0.98	0.96
3–5				0.95	0.92
6–8				0.88	0.85
9–11				0.87	0.82
12–14				0.97	0.89
15–17				1.35	1.19
Birth order					
First birth					1.11
Second or higher birth					1.00

Table 7.9. *(Continued)*

Characteristic	Model 1	Model 2	Model 3	Model 4	Model 5
			Risk Ratios		
Gender of child					
Male					1.00
Female					1.03
Race/ethnicity					
White					1.00
Black					0.69
Hispanic					0.95
Other					0.94

Source: Chapin Hall analysis of data provided by the Illinois Department of Children and Family Services and the Illinois Department of Public Health.

a. These estimates are not significant at the 0.05 level.

Summary

There is some reason to believe that early childbearing results in a child being reported and substantiated by the child welfare system, being placed into foster care, and remaining in foster care for a period longer than women who have their first child over the age of 20. Without more rigorously designed research focused on identifying the causes of teens' children's poorer outcomes, we cannot be certain that delaying parenthood would reduce the burden on the child welfare system—in part because we do not know whether the delay would improve parenting. However, an intervention that would delay childbearing might also allow teen mothers to complete some of the developmental tasks that they are not because of the birth of their child. Further, if mandated reporters are focusing more on women who had their first child as an adolescent for whatever reason, as these women get older and escape that surveillance, their likelihood of receiving child welfare system attention might be reduced simply because of their age. One can imagine that a teacher would have a different response to a 21-year-old mother with three children than a 28-year-old mother in the same circumstance. Finally, one cannot discount the support of the family of the adolescent mother. If a delay in childbearing would at all extend or bolster the connection of an adolescent with her parents, the added social capital of the family might also prevent the events that would lead to the child welfare system.

Multivariate Analysis

W e use logistic regression to examine the independent effect of maternal age on child abuse or neglect and foster care incidence rates. We then use a proportional hazards model to estimate the independent effect of mother's age at first birth on the foster care duration.

For the study of first contact with service systems, we use logistic regression analysis to approximate the log-linear Poisson regression. This method allows us to investigate the effects of early childbearing on the probability of having a substantiated abuse or neglect report and being placed in foster care. Poisson regression is a statistical method of analyzing the relationship between an observed count with a Poisson distribution and a set of explanatory variables (Koch, Atkinson, and Stokes 1986). This method has been widely used in the studies of infant morbidity, mortality, and cancer incidence with aggregate data that are cross-classified according to demographic and other factors (Breslow and Day 1975; Frome 1983; James and Segal 1982). The general form of a log-linear Poisson regression model is given by:

$$\mu(x) = [N(x)][\exp(x'\beta)]$$

where $\mu(x)$ is the expected value of the number of events $n(x)$ from the subpopulation corresponding to known vector x of explanatory variables, $N(x)$ is the known (estimated) total exposure to risk of the subpopulation, where the events occur, and ß is the vector of unknown regression parameters.

In the model, $N(x)$ is regarded as fixed numbers sufficiently large and events $n(x)$ sufficiently rare that the data are well represented by the Poisson distribution.

Given that we have base population estimates and the number of children experiencing their first indicated abuse/neglect report or foster care placement with corresponding demographic factors, we can fit the logistic Poisson regression to estimate the unknown vector β.

To determine the effect of teen parenthood on the duration of foster care, we employed a particular type of event-history model, a proportional hazards model (Kalbfleisch and Prentice 1980). This regression-like model allows us to determine the effects of covariates on the risk of exiting foster care. We can estimate the coefficients using censored data, which is necessary in this case because many children in our population were still in foster care as of June 30, 1994 (when our observation of foster care spells ended in the data). The proportional hazards model is nonparametric in the specification of the variation of the hazard rate with time, given that it uses an unspecified distributional form for the baseline hazard function. The equation of the proportional hazard function that must be estimated is

$$\lambda_z = \lambda_0 \beta_x^t$$

where z is a vector of covariates, β is the coefficient vector, and t is the associated failure time.

NOTES

1. Data are from U.S. Department of Health and Human Services, Administration for Children and Families, "The AFCARS Report," http://www.acf.hhs.gov/programs/cb/stats_research/afcars/tar/report10.htm.

2. See the National Survey of Child and Adolescent Well-Being, 1997–2007, at http://www.acf.hhs.gov/programs/opre/abuse_neglect/nscaw/index.html.

3. Available online at http://www.acf.hhs.gov/j2ee/programs/cb/laws_policies/laws/cwpm/policy_dsp.jsp?citID=354.

4. The instrumental variable was removal tendency of child maltreatment investigators. This combined with a rotational system of assigning investigators to cases is proposed as essentially random assignment of cases to investigators. Doyle cautions against using point estimates for quantifying these effects (James Doyle, "Child Protection and Child Outcomes: Measuring the Effects of Foster Care," unpublished manuscript, Massachusetts Institute of Technology, 2005).

5. The Center for State Foster Care and Adoption Data, a partnership of the American Public Human Services Association (APHSA) and Chapin Hall Center for Children at the University of Chicago, was established to bring member child welfare agencies cutting-edge information technology for performance measurement. Developed at Chapin Hall, the Center's pioneering information management tools provide agencies with an evidence base to assess their program initiatives and monitor the impact of innovation.

6. Weaknesses in the current data include not having income and richer demographic variables in the birth and child welfare data. In many cases, having individual-level birth certificate data would allow other administrative data to be linked with the mother and child data.

7. Given our previous experience with these demographic variables, poverty may account for additional variance but would not greatly change the effects of teen parenthood on child protective and child welfare service experiences.

8. To account for the effect of the many incomplete cases (right censoring of the data), the median was calculated using the Kaplan-Meier method.

REFERENCES

Ards, Sheila D., Samuel L. Myers, Allan Malkis Erin, and Li Zhou. 2003. "Racial Disproportionality in Reported and Substantiated Child Abuse and Neglect: An Examination of Systemic Bias." *Children and Youth Services Review* 25(5/6): 375–92.

Barber, James G., and Paul H. Delfabbro. 2003. "The First Four Months in a New Foster Placement: Psychosocial Adjustment, Parental Contact, and Placement Disruption." *Journal of Sociology and Social Welfare* 30(2): 69–85.

Breslow, N. E., and N. E. Day. 1975. "Indirect Standardization and Multiplicative Models for Rates, with Reference to the Age Adjustment of Cancer Incidence and Relative Frequency Data." *Journal of Chronic Disease* 28:289–303.

Brooks-Gunn, Jeanne, and P. Lindsay Chase-Lansdale. 1995. "Adolescent Parenthood and Parenting: Development in Context." In *Handbook of Parenting: Vol. 3. Status and Social Conditions of Parenting,* edited by Marc H. Bornstein (113–49). Hillsdale, NJ: Lawrence Erlbaum Associates.

Courtney, Mark E., Barbara Needell, and Fred Wulczyn. 2004. "Unintended Consequences of the Push for Accountability: The Case of National Child Welfare Performance Standards." *Children and Youth Services Review* 26(12): 1141–54.

Courtney, Mark E., Amy Dworsky, Gretchen Ruth, Thomas Keller, Judy Havlicek, and Noel Bost. 2005. *Midwest Evaluation of the Adult Functioning of Former Foster Youth: Outcomes at Age 19.* Chicago, IL: Chapin Hall Center for Children at the University of Chicago.

Dubowitz, Howard, and Richard J. Sawyer. 1994. "School Behavior of Children in Kinship Care." *Child Abuse and Neglect* 18(11): 899–911.

Flanagan, P., C. T. García Coll, L. Andreozzi, and S. Riggs. 1995. "Predicting Child Maltreatment among Children of Teenage Mothers." *Archives of Pediatrics and Adolescent Medicine* 144(4): 451–55.

Fluke, John D., Ying-Ying T. Yuan, John Hedderson, and Patrick A. Curtis. 2003. "Disproportionate Representation of Race and Ethnicity in Child Maltreatment: Investigation and Victimization." *Children and Youth Services Review* 25(5/6): 359–73.

Frome, E. L. 1983. "The Analysis of Rates Using Poisson Regression Models." *Biometrics* 39(3): 665–74.

Goerge, Robert M., and Bong Joo Lee. 1997. "Abuse and Neglect of the Children." In *Kids Having Kids: Economic Costs and Social Consequences of Teen Pregnancy,* edited by Rebecca A. Maynard (206–30). Washington DC: Urban Institute Press.

———. 2005. "The Entry of Children from the Welfare System into Foster Care: Differences by Race." In *Race Matters in Child Welfare: The Overrepresentation of African American Children in the System,* edited by Dennette M. Derezotes, John Poertner, and Mark F. Testa (173–86). Washington, DC: CWLA Press.

Goerge, Robert M., John Van Voorhis, Stephen Grant, Katherine Casey, and Major Robinson. 1992. "Special-Education Experiences of Foster Children: An Empirical Study." *Child Welfare* 71(5): 419–37.

James, I. R., and M. R. Segal 1982. "On a Method of Mortality Analysis Incorporating Age-Year Interaction, with Application to Prostate Cancer Mortality." *Biometrics* 38(2): 433–43.

Kalbfleisch, J., and R. Prentice. 1980. *The Statistical Analysis of Failure Time Data.* New York: John Wiley & Sons.

Ketterlinus, Robert D., Michael E. Lamb, and Katherine Nitz. 1991. "Developmental and Ecological Sources of Stress among Adolescent Parents." *Family Relations* 40(4): 435–41.

Koch, G. G., S. S. Atkinson, and M. E. Stokes. 1986. "Poisson Regression." In *Encyclopedia of Statistical Sciences,* vol. 7, edited by Samuel Kotz, Norman Lloyd Johnson, and Campbell B. Read. New York: John Wiley & Sons.

Kortenkamp, Katherine, and Jennifer Ehrle. 2002. "The Well-Being of Children Involved with the Child Welfare System." *Assessing the New Federalism* Brief B-43. Washington, DC: The Urban Institute. http://www.urban.org/url.cfm?ID=310413.

McMillen, Curtis, Wendy Auslander, Dian Elze, Tony White, and Ronald Thompson. 2003. "Educational Experiences and Aspirations of Older Youth in Foster Care." *Child Welfare* 82(4): 475–95.

Sedlak, Andrea J., and Diane D. Broadhurst. 1996. *Executive Summary of the Third National Incidence Study of Child Abuse and Neglect.* Washington, DC: U.S. Department of Health and Human Services, Administration for Children and Families, Administration on Children, Youth and Families, National Center on Child Abuse and Neglect.

Shusterman, Gila R., Dana Hollinshead, John D. Fluke, and Ying-Ying T. Yuan. 2005. *Alternative Responses to Child Maltreatment: Findings from NCANDS.* Washington DC: U.S. Department of Health and Human Services, Office of the Assistant Secretary for Planning and Evaluation.

Smithgall, Cheryl, Robert Matthew Gladden, Duck Hye Yang, and Robert M. Goerge. 2005. *Behavior Problems and Educational Disruptions among Children in Out-of-Home Care in Chicago.* Chicago, IL: Chapin Hall Center for Children at the University of Chicago.

Smithgall, Cheryl, Robert Matthew Gladden, Eboni Howard, Robert M. Goerge, and Mark E. Courtney. 2004. *Educational Experiences of Children in Out-of-Home Care.* Chicago, IL: Chapin Hall Center for Children at the University of Chicago.

Stevens-Simon, Catherine, Donna Nelligan, and Lisa Kelly. 2001. "Adolescents at Risk for Mistreating Their Children. Part I: Prenatal Identification." *Child Abuse and Neglect* 25(6): 737–51.

U.S. Department of Health and Human Services. Administration on Children, Youth and Families. 2006. *Child Maltreatment 2004.* Washington, DC: U.S. Government Printing Office.

Ventura, Stephanie J., T. J. Mathews, and Brady E. Hamilton. 2001. "Births to Teenagers in the United States, 1940–2000." National Vital Statistics Reports 49(10). Hyattsville, MD: National Center for Health Statistics.

Wulczyn, Fred, Richard P. Barth, Ying-Ying T. Yuan, Brenda Jones Harden, and John Landsverk. 2005. *Beyond Common Sense: Child Welfare, Child Well-Being, and the Evidence for Policy Reform.* New Brunswick, NJ: Aldine Transaction.

Zima, Bonnie T., Regina Bussing, Stephanny Freeman, Xiaowei Yang, Thomas R. Belin, and Steven R. Forness. 2000. "Behavior Problems, Academic Skill Delays, and School Failure among School-Aged Children in Foster Care: Their Relationship to Placement Characteristics." *Journal of Child and Family Studies* 9(1): 87–103.

Consequences of Teen Childbearing for Incarceration among Adult Children

"Incarceration-Related Costs of Early Childbearing" by Jeffrey Grogger explored the relationship between early fertility and rates of male imprisonment and estimated the costs of this phenomenon to society. Grogger used data from the National Longitudinal Survey of Youth to examine this issue by following a cohort of young males age 14 to 21 as of 1979 until they were age 26 to 33 in 1991. Using various empirical techniques, he estimated the causal impact of a teen birth. Based on Grogger's most rigorous and conservative technique, he estimated that if mothers delayed their first birth from age 16 to 20.5, it would reduce the probability of incarceration of the sons by 11.8 percent. This change, in turn, would reduce the overall incarceration rate by 3.5 percent.

Grogger's 1997 chapter is included here in its entirety. The included materials describe the context, data, and especially the innovative methodology used in the analysis. Following the original chapter is a short update and extension of Grogger's analysis by Lauren Sue Scher and Saul Hoffman. Scher and Hoffman use the same dataset as Grogger to follow the men through 2002, when they were in their late 30s and early 40s. This extension more completely depicts each respondent's criminal history and allows the authors to analyze the impact of a teen birth on total prison time as well as on the probability of ever being in prison. Scher and Hoffman's results are generally consistent with, but slightly stronger than, those of Grogger and confirm that a teen birth has an effect, net of other risk factors, on the probability of incarceration of sons.

Approach and Estimates through 1991

Jeffrey Grogger

Two of the most troubling trends facing society are an increase in early fertility and a concomitant rise in reported crime. Between 1950 and 1975, the proportion of births to teenage mothers rose from 12 to 19 percent of all births (National Center for Health Statistics various years). Since 1965, when children born in 1950 would have reached their crime-prone teenage years, the reported crime rate has risen from about 2.5 crimes per 1,000 residents to nearly 6 per 1,000 (Freeman 1991).

A natural question to ask is whether these trends are linked—that is, whether early fertility on the part of the mother actually leads to increased crime on the part of her children. Equivalently, one could ask whether the amount of crime committed by an adolescent would have been less if that adolescent's mother had delayed her childbearing. It is hard to imagine otherwise. Teen childbearing has been shown to reduce the mother's educational attainment, her employment, her earnings, and her likelihood of marriage (Geronimus and Korenman 1992; Grogger and Bronars 1993). Single parents with lower human capital and lower income may transmit to their children the economic and social disadvantages that give rise to adolescent crime. Further, a young mother simply may lack the maturity required to be a good parent. As a result, her children may act out; as adolescents, they may commit crime.

In this chapter, I focus on one of the most socially costly aspects of the crime problem: imprisonment. I first ask whether a mother's early fertility leads to a greater likelihood that her son will be incarcerated at some point during his teens or 20s. I then estimate the incarceration-related costs that early childbearing imposes on the economy.

Unfortunately, the importance of these questions is nearly matched by the difficulty of obtaining valid answers. Studying the intergenerational link between early childbearing and crime imposes stringent data demands; the analyst requires data linking the fertility history of mothers to the criminal careers of their children. Indeed, valid measures of crime are themselves hard to come by. The subjective self-reports of criminals are tainted by obvious incentive problems, whereas police records and the like capture only a fraction of all crime. No ideal solution exists to this measurement problem: ultimately, criminal justice researchers must choose between objectivity and completeness.

Finally, there arises the methodological problem posed by confounding factors. The question of whether delayed fertility on the part of the mother would reduce the amount of crime committed by her children necessarily involves an unobserved counterfactual. Measuring the causal effect of early fertility requires an estimate of how many children born to a young mother would have committed less crime if that same mother had delayed her childbearing. Simply comparing the children of two mothers, one who started her family early and one who waited, is not the same. The same factors that lead different mothers to initiate their childbearing at different ages may also influence the subsequent behavior of their children. Failing to control for such influences would lead to overstating the effect of early fertility on crime, for one would also attribute the effects of the confounding factors to early childbearing.

A strategy for estimating the intergenerational effect of early fertility on crime must confront all these potential problems. For the requisite intergenerational data, I use the National Longitudinal Survey of Youth (NLSY79), an annual panel study. This survey provides fertility histories for the mothers of most of its respondents. It also includes an objective if incomplete measure of respondents' criminal behavior from 1979 to 1991.

The NLSY also provides some background information on the mothers of the survey respondents, which allows me to use multivariate statistical methods to control for some factors that confound the relationship between maternal age and final crime. Because the NLSY focuses on youths, however, the information on their mothers is rather limited. As a result, many confounding factors are not observed. To deal with this problem, I propose a simple statistical approach designed to hold constant the effect of unobservables as well.

Data

The National Longitudinal Survey of Youth began in 1979 as a survey of 12,686 youth age 14 to 21. It is stratified, providing an oversampling of minorities and disadvantaged whites. When properly weighted, however, it yields estimates that are representative of the entire population of its age cohort. Survey respondents have been reinterviewed annually. This study uses data through 1991, the most recent data available when this study was begun.

One source of crime data in the NLSY is its 1980 crime module, which queried respondents about the crimes they had committed over the previous year. A major problem with these data, however, as with almost all self-reported offending (SRO) data, concerns their validity. Criminologists have noted that SRO data differ in several ways from police records. Most notably, in SRO surveys, blacks and whites appear to participate in crime in roughly the same proportion, a feature that stands in sharp contrast to estimates based on police records (Blumstein et al. 1986). While in principle several explanations could reconcile this discrepancy, an extensive cross-checking study of self-reports and police records concluded that it was due largely to underreporting by young black men (Hindelang, Hirschi, and Weis 1981).

Because of the questionable validity of the NLSY self-report data, I do not use them for the main component of the analysis. Rater, I use a different, albeit more limited, source of information to measure crime among the survey respondents. At each annual interview between 1979 and 1991, survey interviewers recorded the type of residence—including jails and prisons—in which the respondent was housed. By 1991, members of the sample ranged from 27 to 34 years old. Since crime is disproportionately the pursuit of men in their late teens and early 20s, the jail interview data provide a measure that spans most of the criminal careers of most sample criminals.

The jail interview data also have the benefit of objectivity, although this benefit comes with a cost. First, the data limit the scope of the analysis to incarceration rather than to more general aspects of crime. Further, they provide no information about the offense that led to the observed jail spell. Finally, using these data I can observe only jail spells that are ongoing at the time of the annual interview; I may miss many short stays in jail. Although this is clearly a limitation of the data, I am able to provide some evidence below on how it affects my cost estimates.

The NLSY provides better measures of maternal childbearing. Indeed, two different measures can be constructed: the mother's age at the respondent's birth and her age at her first birth. Both these measures require data on the mother's age. Also, the former requires the age of the respondent, and the latter requires the age of the oldest sibling in the family.

For respondents who lived with their parents in 1979, the mother's age, generally reported by the mother herself, is available from the household enumeration conducted that year. The 1987 and 1988 questionnaires included further questions about the mother's age, to which the respondent provided answers. When the 1979 data were available, I used them in the analysis.

Not all respondents were certain about their mother's age, however, as was revealed by analysis of the responses of siblings in the survey. Sibling data are available because the NLSY was initially a household survey and included all youths in the target age group in all the households it sampled. When siblings disagreed about their mother's age, choosing any one sibling's report was difficult to rationalize. The approach I took was to use the average among all siblings for whom data were available. The average of the mother's age across siblings was then assigned to each sibling within the family.

Siblings likewise disagreed about the age of their oldest sibling. I averaged these responses as well and assigned the average to each child in the family. For each respondent, the mother's age at her first birth is simply the mother's (average) age in 1979 less the (average) age of the oldest sibling in 1979. The mother's age at the respondent's birth was constructed similarly.

Descriptive Statistics

Incarceration rates and birth rates to teen mothers among all males in the NLSY, weighted to provide estimates representative of the entire population of males who were 14 to 21 years old in 1979, are shown in table 8.1. Throughout the study, I restrict the analysis to males, because males account for over 90 percent of the jail and prison population in the United States.

Over the 13 years from 1979 to 1991, nearly 5 percent of all men in the NLSY age cohort were interviewed in jail at least once. Given that the incarceration measure misses many short spells, this 5 percent *observed* incarceration rate may imply a very high rate of *actual* incarceration. Since respondents are interviewed annually, spells that last one year or more are observed with certainty. Data from various sources, however, suggest that the average incarceration spell, among the roughly 10 million spells completed annually, lasts only 46 days.[1] Since the probability of observing a

Table 8.1. Incarceration and Young Teen Birth Rates, Young Male Population

Sample	Total number	% of total sample	% white	% black	% Hispanic
Full sample					
Ever interviewed in jail	6,403	4.82	2.99	14.23	6.85
Analysis sample					
Born to young teen mother (17 or younger)	5,204	12.06	9.07	27.89	15.89
Ever interviewed in jail	5,204	4.58	2.82	14.18	6.29
Born to young teen mother (17 or younger)	851	10.32	6.97	17.71	6.76
Born to older mother	4,353	3.80	2.41	12.82	6.20
Differential		6.52	4.56	4.89	0.56

Source: Based on data from the NLSY, 1979–91, weighted to provide estimates representative of the population of males age 14 to 21 in 1979.

46-day spell by sampling on any randomly chosen day over a one-year period is only 12.6 percent (46 ÷ 365), the 5 percent observed incarceration rate in the NLSY reflects what must be a substantially larger underlying rate of actual incarceration. The observed incarceration rate varies substantially by race, a pattern consistent with data from police records.

Data from the sample to be analyzed include only those respondents for whom the mother's age at first birth could be calculated. The overall incarceration rate in the analysis sample is 4.58 percent, only slightly lower than the full sample. Variation by race is similar to that from the full sample as well.

The fraction of males of this age group born to young teen mothers, whom I define as women 17 years old or younger at the age of their *first* birth, is shown in row 4 of table 8.1. Roughly one-eighth of the children in this cohort were born to young teens. Early teen births vary substantially by race, which is consistent with data from *Vital Statistics of the United States* (National Center for Health Statistics) and various fertility surveys.

Overall, the incarceration rate for children of young teen mothers was 10.32 percent, which is 6.52 percentage points, or 2.7 times, higher than the 3.8 percent incarceration rate among the children of older mothers.

This differential varies substantially by race. Whereas among whites the children of young teens are nearly three times more likely to be observed in jail than their counterparts, among blacks the differential is only 38 percent. Among Hispanics, the association between maternal age and filial incarceration is negligible.

Thus the raw data show a clear intergenerational association between maternal age and the likelihood of incarceration, at least among whites and blacks. It would be improper to attribute this correlation entirely to the mother's early fertility, however, because of the possibility that the same factors that contributed to the mother's early childbearing also influenced her children's proneness to delinquency.

Multivariate Analyses

In this section, I provide estimates of the effect of early fertility that attempt to disentangle causality from simple correlation.

Estimation Technique

Multivariate statistical techniques provide a way to control for many observable factors that may confound the relationship between maternal age and filial incarceration. Given the binary (yes or no) nature of the incarceration outcome, the probit model is a natural technique to choose.

Denote the incarceration variable by I, so $I = 1$ if the respondent is ever interviewed in jail, and $I = 0$ otherwise. Denote the young teen mother dummy by Y; $Y = 1$ if the respondent's mother first gave birth at age 17 or earlier, and $Y = 0$ otherwise. Probit analysis allows one to assess the relationship between I and Y while holding constant the influence of observable, potentially confounding, variables X. The model is motivated by proposing that the probability (P) of ever being interviewed in jail, as a function of maternal age and the background variables, is given by

$$P(I = 1|Y, X) = \Phi(\alpha Y + X\beta)$$

where Φ is the standard normal distribution function. Symbolically, this states that the probability of incarceration is a function of the mother's age at her first birth, a number of background characteristics, and unknown parameters α and β. The larger α is, the stronger is the relationship between maternal age and the risk of filial incarceration.

The characteristics to be included in the variables, X, merit some discussion. Ideally I would include all characteristics of the mother that might affect both the preconceived likelihood that she would become a young mother and the likelihood that her sons eventually would go to jail. Unfortunately, since the NLSY focuses on the respondent rather than his parents, the survey provides little a priori information about the mother.

The variables in X also should capture those characteristics of the respondent that are not under his direct control but that influence his risk of incarceration independently of the age of his mother. Among these characteristics are the respondent's birth order and his age at the beginning of the observation period. Birth order is clearly beyond the respondent's control but may affect his participation in crime. Birth order affects educational attainment, which in turn affects wages (Hanushek 1992). Wages in turn play an important role in young men's decisions to commit crime (Grogger 1996).

The respondent's age may capture differences in crime-proneness. Alternatively, it may control for the fact that different sample respondents are observed over different portions of their criminal careers. The late teens are typically the ages at which young men commit the most crimes. Therefore, the older NLSY respondents may appear to face a lower incarceration risk over the observation period simply because most of their criminal careers are already behind them.

Many other variables are deliberately excluded from the model. Some of these, such as the mother's education and ultimate family size, may themselves be affected by the mother's early fertility (Bronars and Grogger 1994; Grogger and Bronars 1993). Because I exclude these variables from the regression, the probit model estimates the total effect of early fertility, which includes both direct effects and indirect effects that operate through the mother's educational attainment and family size.

I also exclude variables that may reflect the mother's response to early signals about her child's delinquency, which could mask the effect of early fertility. Examples include the mother's employment and marital status during her son's childhood—that is, after he is born but before he is observed in the sample. For example, the mother of a youngster who acts out in school may decide to work part time rather than full time in order to keep closer tabs on her child. Or she may more readily pursue a potential husband in order to provide a male role model for her son.

Both these actions may reduce the child's likelihood of eventual incarceration. However, because they resulted from early, unobservable (to the analyst) behavior on the part of the child (behavior that itself may have stemmed from the mother's early childbearing), the results of this type of action on the part of the mother should not be netted out in measuring the effect of early childbearing. In other words, variables that potentially represent the response of the mother in attempting to mitigate the effects of her early childbearing are endogenous and should not be included in the model.

Estimates with Observable Factors Controlled

I present a number of specifications that include different sets of background characteristics to illustrate the effect of potentially confounding factors on the estimated effect of early fertility (table 8.2). Model 1 is the simplest; the only explanatory variable is the young teen mother dummy.

Table 8.2. Relationship between Male Offspring's Incarceration Risk and Mother's Age at Birth ($n = 5,204$)

Variable	Model 1	Model 2	Model 3	Model 4
Young teen mother	0.511	0.345	0.331	0.320
(17 or younger)	(0.079)	(0.087)	(0.088)	(0.100)
	[0.065]	[0.037]	[0.035]	[0.033]
Mother 18–19 at first birth				0.106
				(0.107)
Mother 23 or older at first birth				−0.105
				(0.098)
Birth order			0.025	0.024
			(0.016)	(0.016)
Respondent's age in 1979		−0.050	−0.049	−0.047
		(0.017)	(0.017)	(0.018)
Black		0.813	0.796	0.776
		(0.076)	(0.076)	(0.080)
Hispanic		0.258	0.242	0.230
		(0.098)	(0.099)	(0.131)
Log likelihood	−947.1	−878.3	−876.9	−874.5

Source: Based on data from the NLSY, 1979–91.

Notes: Estimates are derived from probit models. In addition to the variables shown, all regressions include a dummy for urban residence, for residence in the western census region, and for missing region. Also included in each regression are missing value flags associated with all included regressors. These missing flags take on the value one if data were missing for the associated regressor, and zero otherwise. Missing values of the associated regressor are set to zero. Standard errors, corrected for dependent observations within families, are in parentheses. Average treatment effects are in square brackets.

The probit coefficient of 0.511 on the young teen mother variable is roughly six times the magnitude of its standard error, indicating that it is statistically quite significant. The magnitude of the coefficient itself, however, is difficult to interpret. For this reason, I estimate the "average treatment effect" associated with young teen motherhood in square brackets below the estimated coefficient. This gives the difference in the probability between the children of young teen mothers and the children of older mothers of being observed in jail, holding constant the other variables in the equation.[2] It has the advantage of being directly comparable to the unadjusted difference in incarceration rates between the sons of teen and older mothers. Indeed, for model 1, the average treatment effect is 6.5 percentage points, reflecting (as it should) exactly the same differential in incarceration rates as was obtained by simply cross-tabulating the raw data (table 8.1).

Several background characteristics, including race, the respondent's age in 1979, and indicator variables for the respondent's region of residence and for residence in an urban area,[3] are added to model 2. The coefficients associated with these variables show that older survey respondents are less likely to be observed in jail than their younger counterparts and that blacks and Hispanics are more likely to be incarcerated than whites (the omitted race category). The background variables have a substantial bearing on the estimated effect of early fertility: the probit coefficient is 0.345, and the average treatment effect has fallen to 3.7 percentage points.

The respondent's birth order is added to model 3. Its coefficient indicates that later-born offspring are more likely to be incarcerated than their older siblings, although this effect is only marginally significant. Adding birth order to the model reduces the estimated effect of early childbearing only slightly.

A more general specification of the relationship between the mother's age at her first birth and the likelihood of incarceration on the part of her male children is allowed in model 4. Compared with the omitted base group of children whose mothers first gave birth between the ages of 20 and 22, the children of older teen mothers—18- and 19-year-olds—were only slightly and insignificantly more likely to be incarcerated as young adults. Likewise, the children of the mothers who waited the longest to start their families were only slightly and insignificantly less likely to end up in jail eventually. These estimates suggest that there is an important difference in the jail-proneness of the children of young teen mothers but not of the children born to older teenage mothers.

Two conclusions emerge. First, the qualitative relationship between maternal age and filial incarceration remains significant even after controlling for some important background characteristics. Second, the quantitative association falls a great deal as one controls for more background measures. In particular, the unadjusted 6.52 percentage point differential in incarceration rates grossly overstates the true effect of early childbearing.

Using the Mother's Age at Her First Birth to Control for Unobservable Confounding Factors

Due to the presence of unobservable confounding factors, even the estimates with controls for the broadest set of background characteristics may overstate the true effect of maternal age. Indeed, maternal characteristics that may affect both the age at which a woman first gives birth and the ultimate success of her children are easy to think of but difficult to measure. Emotional maturity and orientation toward the future are two examples.

For this reason, I need to devise an approach that controls for unobserved differences across mothers in estimating the effects of maternal age on filial incarceration. The approach I propose is based on a simple observation: a mother is older at the births of her later children than she is at the births of her earlier children. Put differently, there is necessarily a delay between the birth of one child and the birth of the next. In contrast, a mother's age at her first birth is a fixed trait that does not vary across her children.

These two observations give rise to a simple estimation strategy. I use the young teen mother dummy as a control variable, to account for all unobservable characteristics of the mother that led her to become a young teen mother. I then use the variation in the mother's age at the birth of her various children, controlling for birth order as before, to measure the effects of delaying childbearing.[4]

This approach is appealing for its simplicity, but it warrants some further scrutiny. Recall that I have defined the effect of early fertility on the likelihood of imprisonment as the difference in the likelihood of imprisonment facing a child born to a young mother and the likelihood of imprisonment that same child would have faced if his mother had delayed her childbearing. My approach approximates this unobservable counterfactual by basing an estimate of the effect of early fertility—or equivalently, of the effect of delaying childbirth—on the difference in incarceration outcomes between, say, the first and second children of the same mother, holding constant her age at her first birth. If maternal maturation has the same effect on child outcomes, independent of whether the mother has yet had her first child, then my approach provides a valid estimate of the effect of delay as defined by the counterfactual. If not, then I may either over- or underestimate the effect of interest.

To illustrate this point further, consider an example. I would like to compare the outcome of a child born when his mother was, say, 16 to the outcome that *same* child would have experienced had his mother not had him until she was, say, 20. Instead, I compare two children born to the same mother, one at age 16 the other at age 20. In both cases, the mother matures four years. In the counterfactual case, those four years come before her first birth; in the observable case, they come after her first birth. If maternity enhances the effect of maturation, then four years as a mother reduce the likelihood that the son eventually goes to jail by a greater amount than four prematernal years; in this case, my approach overstates the beneficial effect of maternal maturation on the likelihood of incarceration. If, instead, maternity hinders maturation, then four years of maturation as a mother are less effective in reducing the likelihood of filial incarceration, and my approach underestimates the beneficial effect of maternal maturation on incarceration rates. Unfortunately, the counterfactual nature of the comparison prevents empirical verification of either the presence or magnitude of either of these countervailing effects.

The estimates are presented in table 8.3 for mother's age at respondent's birth as a dummy variable (young teen or not, model 1) and for mother's age as a continuous variable (model 2). In addition to the variables shown, models include all variables included in model 3 of table 8.2.

When mother's age at the respondent's birth is either teen or nonteen, age appears to have little effect on the likelihood that her son eventually goes to jail. When mother's age at the respondent's birth is allowed to vary continuously, it has a negative and significant coefficient, indicating that delaying childbearing reduces the likelihood of the child's eventual incarceration. The latter specification also fits the data better, as indicated by the log likelihood. The linear specification yields a higher value (i.e., a smaller negative number), indicating that it has a greater likelihood of being the model that gave rise to the observed data. As before, however, attaching an intuitive quantitative interpretation to the coefficient is difficult. Because, moreover, the mother's age at the respondent's birth appears in the model linearly, to speak of the average treatment effect associated with delayed childbearing makes no sense.

Table 8.3. Relationship between Incarceration and Mother's Age at Birth, Using the Mother's Age at Her First Birth to Control for Unobservables ($n = 5,204$)

Variable	Model 1	Model 2
Young teen mother (17 or younger at first birth)	0.320	0.216
	(0.095)	(0.097)
Mother under 18 at respondent's birth	0.043	
	(0.197)	
Mother's age at respondent's birth		−0.019
		(0.008)
Log likelihood	−876.8	−873.3

Source: Based on data from the NLSY, 1979–91.

Notes: In addition to variables shown, all regressions include the full set of regressors from model 3 of table 8.2. Standard errors, corrected for dependent observations within families, are in parentheses.

To aid in interpreting these estimates, I provide the results of some simulations based on the coefficient of the mother's age at the respondent's birth from model 2 of table 8.3.

The simulations address the question, "By how much would the likelihood of incarceration fall among all children born to a young teen mother, if the young teen mother were to delay her childbearing?" To answer this question, one must first specify the magnitude of the delay being considered. I present three scenarios. The first asks how these mothers' children would have fared had the mothers delayed the birth of their first child until the age at which their second child actually was born, which on average was age 18.5. The second asks how the children would have fared if the young teen mothers had waited until just beyond their teens, giving birth at age 20.5. The third asks how the children's risk of incarceration would have differed had their mothers waited till age 22.9 to have their first child, where 22.9 is the average age at first birth among all women whose first birth occurred after age 17.[5]

These three scenarios (table 8.4) reflect the benefits that one could expect from policies designed to encourage delayed childbearing, as a function of the effectiveness of those policies. For example, the first scenario is informative about policies that succeed in encouraging young teen mothers to delay their first birth just beyond the young teen threshold. The third scenario depicts the results of a highly effective policy that

Table 8.4. Effect on Incarceration Rates of Delayed Childbearing, Simulation Results

	Change mean age at first birth among young teen mothers from 16.0 to:	Incarceration rate (percent) among sons of young teen mothers falls from 10.32 to:	Percentage change in incarceration rate among sons of young teen mothers	Overall incarceration rate (percent) falls from 4.58 to:	Percentage change in overall incarceration rate
Scenario 1	18.5	9.68	−6.2	4.49	−2.0
Scenario 2	20.5	9.10	−11.8	4.42	−3.5
Scenario 3	22.9	8.56	−17.1	4.35	−5.0

Source: Based on data from the NLSY, 1979–91.

Note: Simulations are based on model 2 of table 8.3 and use the coefficient on the mother's age at the respondent's birth to estimate the effect of delayed childbearing.

succeeds to the extent that women who would have been young teen mothers actually delay their childbearing to the point where, on average, their age at first birth is the same as that of older mothers. The second scenario represents the effects of a policy of intermediate effectiveness.

Delaying the age at first birth from 16 to 18.5 results in an incarceration rate of 9.68 percent among the sons of young teen mothers. This amounts to a reduction of only six-tenths of 1 percentage point, or only 6 percent of the observed incarceration rate of 10.32 percent.

Longer delays have greater effects. A delay in the age at first birth from 16 to 20.5 would result in a filial incarceration rate of 9.10 percent, a reduction of 1.22 percentage points, or 12 percent. If young teen mothers were to delay their childbearing by 6.9 years, so on average their first birth occurred at age 22.9, then the incarceration rate among their sons would fall to 8.56 percent. This 1.76 percentage point differential amounts to 17 percent of the actual incarceration rate.

To simulate the incarceration rate among the entire cohort, I construct a weighted average of the simulated incarceration rate among the sons of young teen mothers and the predicted incarceration rate among the sons of older mothers, using weights that reflect each group's representation in the cohort.[6] Under scenario 1, the overall incarceration rate falls 0.09 percentage points, from 4.58 percent to 4.49 percent, which amounts to a 2.0 percent reduction. Under scenario 2, the overall reduction is 0.16 percentage points, or 3.5 percent of the actual incarceration rate. For the greatest delay, the overall incarceration rate falls to 4.35 percent. This reduction of 0.23 percentage points amounts to 5.0 percent of the actual incarceration rate.

These simulation results show that policies that successfully encouraged young teen mothers to delay their childbearing would reduce the likelihood of incarceration on the part of their sons. Not surprisingly, they also show that policies that encouraged longer delays would have greater effects. I next consider the cost savings associated with these various reductions in incarceration rates.

Costs

We would like to know how the costs of corrections, as borne by state, federal, and local governments, would fall in response to delayed childbearing on the part of young teen mothers. To go from reductions in observed incarceration rates to reductions in correctional costs, however, requires some theoretical work. I first consider what information would be needed to estimate the expected lifetime cost of incarcerating a particular individual as a function of his mother's age at birth. I then discuss how such a lifetime cost measure may be expressed in annual expenditures.

The expected lifetime cost of incarcerating a criminal is the product of the cost per unit of time of keeping him behind bars times the expected total amount of time he spends in jail. His total expected time in jail, in turn, is the product of the probability that he ever goes to jail and the expected number of times he is incarcerated, times the expected length of his jail spells. To express this relationship symbolically, let C denote the lifetime cost of incarcerating a particular individual, let T denote the total amount of time he spends behind bars, and let c be the cost of incarceration per unit of time. Let J denote the event that the individual is ever incarcerated, let N denote the number of times he goes to jail, and let S denote the length of a typical jail spell. Then, conditional on the mother's age at birth, denoted by A, we have

$$C = cE(T|A) \qquad (8.1)$$

where

$$E(T|A) = P(J|A)E(N|A)E(S|A) \qquad (8.2)$$

In equations 8.1 and 8.2, E denotes a mathematical expectation, and $P(\ )$ denotes the probability of an event. The costs of incarceration due to early childbearing are then given by the expression

$$c\left[E(T|\text{early childbearing}) - E(T|\text{later childbearing})\right] \qquad (8.3)$$

Expressions 8.1 through 8.3 show that, to estimate the incarceration-related costs of early childbearing directly, one would need to know the cost per unit of time in jail and be able to estimate the effect of early fertility on the probability of ever going to jail, on the expected number of jail spells, and on the expected length of a jail spell. The annual costs of incarceration are readily available in published reports. The other information, however, is harder to come by. The NLSY, given its sampling scheme, provides data on the likelihood of being observed in jail but not on the likelihood of ever going to jail. Although the two are likely closely related, direct cost estimation requires the more comprehensive measure.

Likewise, the sequences of interviews at which NLSY respondents were observed in jail can be used together with intervening employment histories to count the observed jail spells for each sample member. Again, although observed and actual jail spells are likely to be highly correlated, direct cost estimation requires the actual number. Finally, the NLSY provides only qualitative information about the length of jail spells. If a respondent is observed in jail at two sequential interviews, then I presume that he spent at least one year (the length of time between interviews) behind bars, provided that he was not observed in the labor force in the intervening period. For a jail spell that spans a single interview, however—roughly 60 percent of all observed spells—we know much less about its duration. In some cases, the longitudinal records in the NLSY can be used to determine the maximum amount of time the respondent could have spent in jail. In about half these cases, however, the employment data are largely uninformative.

Thus the NLSY provides only quantitative information about the length of observed jail spells. Specifically, I can classify some of the spells as long (i.e., as lasting a year or more), and I can classify some of the others as short. Although these qualitative indicators are likely correlated with the average length of actual spells, they fall short of the quantitative information required to estimate the average spell length as a function of maternal age.

Because there are such formidable barriers to estimating the incarceration-related costs of early childbearing directly, I take an indirect approach instead. The NLSY data have permitted me to estimate the likelihood that a respondent is observed in jail given that he was born to a young mother, relative to the likelihood of being observed in jail given that he was born to an older mother. Letting I denote the event of being interviewed in jail, as above, this can be expressed symbolically as

$$\frac{P(I|\text{early childbearing})}{P(I|\text{later childbearing})} \tag{8.4}$$

To estimate the incarceration-related costs of early childbearing indirectly, I begin by determining the conditions under which the ratio of total time spent in jail, as a function of maternal age, is equal to the relative probability of ever being interviewed in jail, as a function of maternal age. Symbolically, I provide conditions under which

$$\frac{E(T|\text{early childbearing})}{E(T|\text{later childbearing})} = \frac{P(I|\text{early childbearing})}{P(I|\text{later childbearing})} \tag{8.5}$$

Manipulating equations 8.2 through 8.5, the necessary conditions are

$$(A) \frac{P(J|\text{early childbearing})}{P(J|\text{later childbearing})} = \frac{P(I|\text{early childbearing})}{P(I|\text{later childbearing})}$$

$$(B)\ E(N|\text{early childbearing}) = E(N|\text{later childbearing})$$

$$(C)\ E(S|\text{early childbearing}) = E(S|\text{later childbearing})$$

Condition A says that the odds of actually going to jail given birth to a young mother must equal the odds of being observed in jail given birth to a young mother. Condition B says that on average the number of jail spells served is independent of the age of one's mother's age at birth, and condition C says that the average sentence length must also be independent of maternal age.

Under conditions A through C, the effect of early fertility on the total time an individual spends in jail over his lifetime will equal the effect of early fertility on the probability of being observed in jail. If one also assumes prisons are characterized by constant marginal costs, then a delay in age at birth that brings about a p percent reduction in the likelihood that the son will ever be observed in jail also brings about a p percent reduction in the cost of incarcerating him. If data were available on the lifetime cost of imprisoning a typical criminal, then I could estimate the reduction in lifetime incarceration costs associated with scenarios 1 through 3 above by invoking assumptions A through C, together with the constant cost assumption, and applying the proportionate reductions in observed incarceration rates from the last column of table 8.4.

Such lifetime cost data, however, do not exist. Rather, correctional authorities report the annual expenditures: expenses they incur in order to maintain the current year's prisoners. These annual data are nonetheless useful under a set of three assumptions, which I will refer to as steady state assumptions. If (1) the proportion of births to young teen mothers is constant over time, (2) the effect of early childbearing is likewise constant across cohorts, and (3) the overall incarceration rate does not change over time, then the proportionate reduction in lifetime incarceration costs for a fixed birth cohort that results from a given delay in childbearing can be approximated by the same proportionate reduction in the cost of incarcerating the current year's prisoners. I can do this because, in the steady state, the current behavior of older cohorts is the same as the future behavior of younger cohorts. In other words, in the steady state, a snapshot view of all prisoners at a point in time mirrors a prospective view of a fixed age cohort over the lifetime of its members. Thus, under conditions A through C, the constant cost assumption, and the steady state assumptions 1 through 3, I can estimate the steady-state incarceration cost savings attributable to a given delay in early childbearing on the part of young teen mothers by multiplying the proportionate reduction in observed incarceration rates attributable to that delay by reported annual corrections costs.

Incarceration-Related Costs of Early Childbearing

Correctional expenditures by all levels of government amounted to $24.96 billion in 1990 (U.S. Department of Justice 1992c). In 1994 dollars, that amounts to $28.94 billion. Roughly 90 percent of the budget, or $26 billion, goes to incarcerate men.

A 2.0 percent reduction in this amount, which is the predicted result of young teen mothers delaying their childbearing by 2.5 years (last column of table 8.4), comes to $522 million. Longer delays result in greater savings. If young teen mothers first gave birth at, on average, age 20.5 rather than at age 16, incarceration costs would fall by 3.5 percent, or $920 million. If they waited until age 22.9, the average age at first birth among older mothers, the savings would amount to $1.29 billion.

This general approach also can be used to provide a more detailed breakdown of the incarceration-related costs of early childbearing. The estimated cost savings[7] that would occur if different groups of young teen mothers were to delay their first births by varying amounts (table 8.5) largely reinforce the earlier conclusions: small delays lead to small cost savings, whereas large delays have substantial effects.

These cost figures also implicitly estimate how the prison population would fall in response to delayed childbearing on the part of young teen mothers. The cost of incarcerating one criminal for one year is widely estimated to average $20,000 to $25,000 (DiIulio and Piehl 1991; U.S. Department of Justice 1992b; U.S. General Accounting Office 1991; Zedlewski 1987). Thus a delay in childbearing on the part of young teen mothers of 2.5 years, which is estimated to reduce annual correctional expenditures by $522 million, implies a reduction in the prison population of roughly 21,000 to 26,000 men.[8] At the extreme, if young teen mothers were to delay their first births until age 22.9, the prison population would fall by 52,000 to 65,000 men.

Testing the Assumptions

The population estimates and the corresponding cost estimates are both based on a number of assumptions. Because the estimates are valid only if the assumptions hold, providing at least some indirect evidence on the validity of the assumptions is desirable. I begin with evidence on conditions

Table 8.5. Cost Savings Associated with Various Delays in Childbearing ($ millions a year)

| Age at first birth | Cost Savings if First Birth Had Been Delayed until | | | | |
	Age 16–17	Age 18–19	Age 20–21	Age 22–41	Age 20 or older
15 or younger	162.7	293.5	421.9	727.5	638.0
16–17	NA	240.2	498.8	1,111.3	932.2
Total	162.7	533.7	920.7	1,838.8	1,770.3

Source: Based on data from the NLSY, 1979–91.

Notes: Average ages used in calculated savings are 14.2 for 15 or younger, 16.7 for age 16–17, 18.6 for age 18–19, 20.5 for age 20–21, 25.5 for age 22–41, and 24.0 for age 20 or older. See endnote 7 of the text for a complete discussion. No cost savings are calculated for delays on the part of older teen mothers (i.e., 18- and 19-year-olds) because the estimates reported showed no significant association between births to older teens and higher rates of filial incarceration.

NA = not applicable

A through C. Condition A requires that the odds of a young male ever actually going to jail given a young teen mother must equal the odds of being interviewed in jail given a young teen mother. This will tend to be true if the crimes committed by the sons of young teen mothers are no more likely to result in a jail term than the crimes committed by the sons of older mothers and if, at each conviction, the length of the offender's previous criminal record does not depend on his mother's age at birth.

Robbery is the crime most likely to result in an incarcerative sentence, both because of its severity and because it involves face-to-face contact between the victim and the offender. If, among the youths who commit crime, the sons of young teen mothers commit, on average, a higher proportion of robberies than the sons of older mothers, then the sons of the young teen mothers would be more likely to be incarcerated, all else equal. Using the NLSY 1980 self-reported offending crime module, I can ask whether the fraction of reported offenses that involves robbery depends on maternal age. Likewise, I can determine whether the age at first arrest or age at first conviction, both of which will be correlated with the extent of the offender's arrest record, vary by maternal age.

Condition B requires the number of jail spells to be unaffected by maternal age, whereas condition C requires that the average length of a jail spell be independent of the mother's age at birth. The number of observed jail spells can be used to examine the validity of condition B, and the qualitative data on length of spells provide information about condition C.

The results of a series of regressions provide substantial support for conditions A through C (table 8.6). Each row gives the results of a different regression. In addition to the variables shown, all regressions include all variables from model 3 in table 8.2.[9] I employ the same statistical procedure as above to control for unobservable confounding factors associated with both the mother's early fertility and her son's proneness to crime, using the young teen mother dummy as a control variable and using variation in the mother's age at the births of her children to estimate the effect of delayed childbearing.

None of the coefficients on the mother's age at the respondent's birth are significant. Young teen childbearing is positively correlated with the number of observed jail spells. Given the specification, this provides evidence of confounding factors but not of a causal relationship. The apparent validity of assumptions A through C provides greater confidence in the cost estimates based on those assumptions.

Table 8.6. Early Fertility and Various Criminal Justice Outcomes

Dependent variable	Young teen mother (17 or under)	Mother's age at respondent's birth
1. Robbery rate	−0.002	0.004
(*n* = 3,798)	(0.004)	(0.005)
2. Age at first arrest	−0.296	0.008
(*n* = 807)	(0.229)	(0.016)
3. Age at first conviction	−0.538	−0.005
(*n* = 463)	(0.293)	(0.021)
4. Number of observed jail spells	0.384	−0.003
(*n* = 378)	(0.147)	(0.011)
5. Long jail spell	0.078	0.003
(*n* = 626)	(0.131)	(0.010)
6. Short jail spell	0.035	−0.018
(*n* = 626)	(0.141)	(0.011)

Source: Based on data from the NLSY, 1979–91.

Notes: Each row reports the results of a separate regression. Estimates are based on weighted data. In addition to variables shown, all regressions include the full set of regressors from model 3 in table 8.2. For regressions 5 and 6, the unit of observation is the jail spell rather than the respondent. Standard errors, corrected for dependent observations within families, are in parentheses.

For evidence on the remaining assumptions, I turn to the existing literature. California prisons exhibit roughly constant marginal costs (Block and Ulen 1979). Federal prisons, in contrast, exhibit increasing marginal costs (Schmidt and Witte 1984). The vast majority of the nation's prisoners are held in state rather than federal facilities (U.S. Department of Justice 1992a). To the extent that the California state system is more representative of state prisons generally than are those run by federal authorities, the constant marginal cost hypothesis receives some support.

The evidence is more mixed for the steady state assumptions. The proportion of births to young teen mothers has varied within a fairly narrow band over time. In 1950, the share of all births that women under 18 years old accounted for was 3.7 percent; this rose to 7.6 percent in 1975 and fell again to 4.6 percent in 1989 (National Center for Health Statistics various years).

No evidence whatsoever exists on changes in the intergenerational effect of early childbearing on crime. The only other study on the topic also used the NLSY, albeit the 1980 SRO data (Morash and Rucker 1989).

To determine whether the effect of maternal age on filial crime had changed over time would, however, require studies based on cohorts of different vintages of youths.

Finally, recent data show that the assumption of constant incarceration rates is false. According to the 1980 Census, there were roughly 479,000 prisoners in the United States. By 1990, that figure had risen to 1.1 million, a 130 percent increase. The concomitant growth in population, in contrast, was only 9.8 percent. Recent "three strikes" proposals would reinforce this trend in the future.

The implication of this trend for my cost estimates is clear. As imprisonment increases, prison costs rise, and a given proportionate reduction in prison costs translates to a larger absolute cost savings. Therefore my cost estimates, which are based on the assumption of constant incarceration rates, are conservative.

Conclusions

The results of this study provide evidence that early childbearing and youth crimes are linked. Based on a model that provides controls for unobservable characteristics of the mother that may be correlated with her early age at first birth, I conclude that delayed childbearing on the part of young teen mothers—women under the age of 18 at the time of their first births—would reduce the risk of incarceration on the part of their sons. Specifically, if a young teen mother were to delay her childbearing until just beyond her 18th birthday, then her son's incarceration risk would fall by about 6 percent. If all young teen mothers so delayed their fertility, then the number of men behind bars in the United States would fall by 21,000 to 26,000, and annual corrections budgets could be reduced by roughly $522 million.

Longer delays would have larger effects. If would-be young teen mothers were to delay their first births until they were almost 23 years old—the average age at which other women begin their families—then their sons' incarceration risk would fall by 17 percent. As a result, prison populations would fall by 52,000 to 65,000, and corrections costs incurred by local, state, and federal governments would decrease by $1.29 billion a year.

Because these figures reflect only correctional costs, they almost certainly substantially understate the full crime-related costs of early childbearing. In 1990, correctional expenditures accounted for only one-third of the roughly $75 billion devoted to criminal justice activities by all levels of government (U.S. Department of Justice 1992c). In addition, direct costs to crime victims have been estimated at $17 billion (Klaus 1994). Although this latter figure includes victims' losses due to theft, which constitute social transfers rather than true social costs, it excludes the costs of private security measures and insurance. It also excludes the costs associated with people's fear of being victimized. Thus the total crime-related costs of young teen childbearing may exceed the incarceration-related costs by a great deal.

Nevertheless, even though the crime-related costs of early childbearing may be substantial, early childbearing itself explains only a small fraction of the difference in incarceration rates between the children of young teen mothers and the children of older mothers. The sons of young teen mothers are 2.7 times more likely to be incarcerated at some point during their 20s than the sons of older mothers. Even if young teen mothers were to delay their first birth until age 23, however, their sons would still be 2.2 times more likely to end up in jail than the sons of their older counterparts. Thus even large changes in young teen mothers' age at first birth would have a relatively modest effect on their sons' incarceration risk.

Why is this true? The age of the mother is but one of the differences in the circumstances facing the children of young teen mothers compared with the children of older mothers. Other factors contribute to the risk of delinquency among the children of young teen mothers. These factors in total have greater effects than early childbearing itself. Although the precise definition of these factors is unclear, what is clear is that social policy designed to reduce teen childbearing will have only relatively small effects on youth crime. In order to have large effects, social policy would have to identify and address the other risk factors, as well.

Updated Estimates through 2002

Lauren Sue Scher and Saul D. Hoffman

Grogger explored the relationship between early fertility and rates of male imprisonment and estimated the costs of this phenomenon to society and the economy. He used data from the National Longitudinal

Survey of Youth (NLSY79) to explore this issue by following a cohort of young men age 14–21 as of 1979 until they were age 26 to 33 in 1991. This update uses the same dataset to follow the men until 2002, when they are in their late 30s and early 40s, in order to get a more complete depiction of each respondent's criminal history. It also analyzes total cumulated prison time as well as the probability of ever being in prison.

Similar to Grogger's, this analysis focuses solely on the male population of respondents.[10] The full NLSY79 sample includes 12,696 respondents, 6,403 of whom were male. Of these males, 5,570 had sufficient data regarding mother's age at first birth, and 3,665 had positive sample weights in 2002.

We also followed Grogger's example by focusing on the more objective measure of incarceration. This measure is based on the annual interview information that codes the "type of residence" in which the respondent is located. While specific questions are related to taking part in criminal activities, these are based on self-reports, which have been shown to be less reliable than more objective measures (as discussed in part 1 of this chapter).

As Grogger notes, this more objective measure has one main flaw: it measures only one particular point in time during each year. Therefore, it will likely underestimate incarceration rates due to the loss of information on shorter spells in prison. In addition, it is not possible to determine the length of stay in prison and number of spells. For example, a respondent who is in prison for multiple years has similar data as a different respondent who is in and out of prison for consecutive years. It is possible, however, to calculate the number of years a respondent is interviewed in jail, which is a rough estimate of the number of years spent in jail.

Our analysis therefore includes two main outcomes: (1) ever being interviewed in jail, and (2) the number of years interviewed in jail.[11] Table 8.7 presents basic descriptive statistics for these two main outcomes for all males and separately by race. The first row presents the portion of the full sample that had ever been interviewed while in jail. Compared with the original Grogger analysis, the incidence of being in jail increased 2 percentage points from 1991 to 2002 (ranging from an increase of over 1 percentage point for whites to an almost 5 percentage point increase for blacks). In general, approximately 7 percent of males in this sample have ever been interviewed in jail between 1979 and 2002. Higher proportions of black than white or Hispanic men were in jail at any time, consistent with national statistics.

Table 8.7. Mean Incarceration Outcomes by Race and Ethnicity for Young Men, 1979–2002

	Number of cases	All races	White	Black	Hispanic
Ever interviewed in jail (%)	3,665	6.78	4.35	19.17	9.68
Born to young teen mother (<18)	605	13.92	9.18	24.16	9.47
Born to mother age 18–19	761	8.77	6.26	18.31	13.89
Born to mother age 20–22	1,120	6.19	4.20	18.21	9.33
Born to mother older than 22	1,179	3.76	2.40	14.86	7.29
Amount of time spent in jail (years)	3,665	0.25	0.13	0.89	0.33
Born to young teen mother (<18)	605	0.57	0.30	1.16	0.29
Born to mother age 18–19	761	0.29	0.16	0.80	0.44
Born to mother age 20–22	1,120	0.22	0.11	0.87	0.41
Born to mother older than 22	1,179	0.13	0.08	0.67	0.18

Source: Based on data from the NLSY79, weighted to provide estimates representative of the population of males age 14 to 21 in 1979.

Table 8.7 also shows that men born to mothers who had children before age 18 were more likely to have been in prison at least once, particularly white and black men. Nearly 14 percent of men born to mothers who began having children before age 18 were in jail at least once, compared with less than 4 percent of men born to mothers who began having children after age 22. The bottom rows in table 8.7 provide the average number of times that men were interviewed in jail. The relationship between mother's age at first birth and total incarceration time for sons is quite strong, stronger than the relationship between age at birth and the probability of being ever incarcerated. The sons of early teen mothers spent an average of .57 years in jail, twice as much as the sons of later teen mothers (.29) and more than four times as long as the average for men born to mothers who began having children at age 23 or older.

Analysis

While table 8.7 suggests a correlation between early childbearing and incarceration, we conducted multivariate analyses techniques to get a better sense of the relationship. Since the outcome of ever being interviewed in jail is binary (0 = never interviewed in jail, 1 = interviewed in jail at least once), we use logit models to explore the effects of age of mother at first birth, controlling for various background characteristics.[12] For simplicity and comparability, we chose to include the same background characteristic variables as controls as Grogger used. Since the outcome for the number of times interviewed in jail is count data that have a general Poisson distribution (skewed toward zero, with very few cases above 2), we used Poisson models to explore the relationship between age at first birth and this outcome, controlling for additional background characteristics.

Table 8.8 presents the descriptive statistics for all the key predictor and control variables included in the logit models. The main predictor variables include dummy variables for the age when respondents' mothers began having children.[13] This is broken into four categories: younger than age 18; age 18 to 19; age 20 to 22; and age 23 and older. Approximately 13 percent of the analysis sample was born to mothers under the age of 18, nearly 20 percent was born to mothers between the ages of 18 and 19, 31 percent was born to mothers in their early 20s, and 37 percent was born to mothers who were 23 or older. Background characteristics related to the respondent include birth order of the respondent, age, and race/ethnicity. The sample is approximately 14 percent black and 7 percent Hispanic. Also

Table 8.8. Descriptive Statistics and Covariates Used in Incarceration Analysis ($n = 3,665$)

Variable	Weighted mean	Standard deviation
Mother's fertility		
Born to young teen mother (<18)	0.127	0.270
Born to mother age 18–19	0.192	0.320
Born to mother age 20–22[a]	0.316	0.378
Born to mother older than 22	0.365	0.391
Individual characteristics		
Birth order of respondent	2.870	1.457
Age of respondent in 1979 (years)	17.725	1.796
Nonblack or Hispanic[a]	0.794	0.313
Black	0.140	0.269
Hispanic	0.066	0.192
Northwest	0.167	0.286
Urban residence in 1979	0.772	0.338

Source: NLSY79, 1979–2002.

a. Omitted groups used as comparisons in the multivariate analysis.

included as covariates are more general geographical and contextual variables, such as region of the country and urban residence.

Results

Rather than re-estimate all the models presented by Grogger, we focus on those with a fuller specification of covariates. Table 8.9 presents estimates of Grogger's model 4 (see his table 8.2) for both outcomes we examine—whether ever incarcerated and number of years incarcerated. In both analyses, there is a clear, monotonic relationship between the age of the mother at first birth and incarceration. An early teen birth has a large and statistically significant effect in both models, while a later teen birth has a smaller impact that is not statistically significant at conventional levels. Children of mothers older than 22 have particularly low rates of incarceration and cumulative prison time, even after controlling for other traits. Using the estimated logit coefficient for an early teen birth, the probability of ever being incarcerated would fall from its mean value of 13.92 percent to 9.6 percent with a delay in mother's age at first birth to age 20 or 21, a decline of nearly one-third. Black and Hispanic men have higher rates of incarceration, a result consistent with the unadjusted means in table 8.7 and with other analyses of incarceration (Western 2006). Being a younger child slightly increases the probability of incarceration, while an individual's age reduces it.

In a Poisson model, the marginal effect equals the estimated coefficient times the sample mean. The estimated Poisson coefficient (.381) thus means that a delay to age 20 or 21 in age at mother's first birth would reduce average years incarcerated for these men from .572 to .354. The other covariates have similar impacts and statistical significance as in the logit model.

In table 8.10 we examine the impact of being the son of a teen mother on incarceration by using a mother's age at first birth and her age at the respondent's birth as two distinct covariates to control for unmeasured variables correlated with an early birth and with incarceration. The goal of this exercise is to obtain a conservative estimate of the impact of a teen birth, net of measured and unmeasured individual risk factors. Mother's age at first birth is naturally constant across siblings, but age at respondent's birth will vary. In this specification, the effect of mother's age at respondent's birth is identified by differences in incarceration rates across

Table 8.9. Relationship between Male Child's Incarceration Risk and Mother's Age at Birth ($n = 3{,}665$)

	Whether ever in jail[a]	Years in jail[b]
Main predictors		
Born to young teen mother (<18)	0.422**	0.381**
	(0.128)	(0.059)
Born to mother age 18–19	0.193	0.07
	(0.128)	(0.063)
Born to mother older than 22	−0.378**	−0.441**
	(0.133)	(0.069)
Individual characteristics		
Birth order of respondent	0.038*	0.022**
	(0.02)	(0.009)
Age of respondent in 1979	−0.081**	−0.075**
	(0.021)	(0.01)
Black	1.366**	1.596**
	(0.11)	(0.05)
Hispanic	0.582**	0.648**
	(0.141)	(0.075)
Contextual characteristics		
Urban residence	0.176	0.333**
	(0.125)	(0.066)
Living in western census region	0.470**	0.553**
	(0.123)	(0.058)
Intercept	−1.784**	−0.947**
	(0.399)	(0.197)
−2 log likelihood	−3,316.9	−3,285.9

Source: NLSY79, 1979–2002.

Notes: In cases with missing data, missing variables were set to zero, and a dummy variable for missing characteristics was included in the model. This affected the following variables: birth order of respondent, urban residence, and living in western region. Standard errors are in parentheses.

a. Estimated by logit.

b. Estimated by Poisson.

*significant at the .10 level; **significant at the .05 level

siblings. The specification is equivalent to a family fixed-effect model in which mother's age at first birth is used to capture otherwise unobservable family characteristics.

We follow Grogger's procedures to determine mother's age at respondent's birth. Age of mother at birth of respondent is based on information

Table 8.10. Relationship between Incarceration and Mother's Age at Birth, Using Mother's Age at First Birth to Control for Unobservables ($n = 3,665$)

	Whether Ever in Jail[a]		Years in Jail[b]	
	(1)	(2)	(3)	(4)
Mother age 17 or younger	0.442**	0.288**	0.462**	0.297**
at first birth	(0.119)	(0.120)	(0.054)	(0.055)
Mother age 17 or younger	0.109		0.051	
at respondent's birth	(0.209)		(0.094)	
Mother's age at		−0.032**		−0.033**
respondent's birth		0.010		0.005
−2 log likelihood	−3,325.8	−3,314.8	−3,291.8	−3,267.3

Source: NLSY79, 1979–2002.

Note: All regressions include the full set of regressors from table 8.9. See notes there for further information. Standard errors are in parentheses.

a. Estimated by logit.

b. Estimated by Poisson.

**significant at the .05 level

from the 1979 roster, which includes information on mother's age (month and year) and the respondent's age. If this information was not available, we relied on data from the 1987 and 1988 surveys that asked the age of mother at respondent's birth (in years) and combined this with information on the age of oldest sibling in 1979.

For each outcome, we estimate two models, one with a dummy variable identifying whether the mother was age 17 or younger at the respondent's birth and a second that substitutes a continuous measure of mother's age at the respondent's birth. Both models also include a dummy variable measuring whether the respondent's mother had an early first birth (not necessarily the respondent) plus the individual and contextual variables used in table 8.9. To make the table simpler, we present only the age at birth variables.

Being the son of a young teen mother has a consistent positive effect on the probability of being incarcerated and on years spent incarcerated. In models 1 and 3, the estimated impact of whether the mother was age 17 or younger at the respondent's birth is positive but small and not statistically significant. Grogger also found this result, which may reflect the smaller effective sample size (women with an early birth and two sons) used to identify this effect. The linear term for mother's age at respondent's birth is negative and statistically significant, meaning that a delay in mother's age reduces the probability of incarceration and total time incarcerated. Like Grogger, we find a better fit for the linear model (lower log-likelihood) and on that basis, we choose it as our preferred model.

The estimated impact of being the son of a teenage mother is smaller than in the models analyzed in table 8.9, but it nevertheless has a meaningful quantitative impact. The logit estimate implies that a four and half year delay (age 16.0 to 20.5—the delay considered by Grogger) would reduce the probability of a teen birth by 1.7 percentage points, from 13.9 to 12.2 percent. This is an 11.9 percent decline in the probability of incarceration, about one-third of the impact found in the previous table. The analysis of years of incarceration indicates a slightly larger impact of a teen birth: average years of incarceration would decline by 15 percent from .572 to .486 if a mother was 20.5 at her son's birth rather than 16.

Grogger reported that a delay in age at first birth from 16 to 20.5 would reduce the incarceration rate for the sons from 10.32 to 9.10 percent, a decline of 11.8 percent (see table 8.4). On that basis, he predicted that the overall incarceration rate would decline by 3.5 percent and that the national costs of running the prison system would fall by approximately $920 million in 1994 dollars. Our corresponding estimate of the impact of a 4.5 year delay on the probability of incarceration is virtually identical to his—12.2 percent—although our baseline incarceration rate is higher, consistent with the longer time frame we consider. For assessing cost impacts, the estimate of total years incarcerated is the more useful estimate. We estimate that states spent $29.3 billion in 2004 to house male inmates (approximately 93 percent of prison inmates were men in 2004). After taking account of the incarceration rates for sons of older mothers, we estimate that the overall incarceration rate would decline 4.42 percent if a young teen mother delayed her second son's birth by 4.5 years. This amounts to a decline in costs of $1.3 billion and a decline in the prison population of more than 54,000 inmates.

Summary

Our analysis updates the work of Grogger on the impact of early teen childbearing on incarceration. We use the same data as Grogger—males from the NLSY79—but extend the analysis more than a decade longer when the men are age 37 to 44. We also examine years in prison as well as whether the respondent was ever interviewed in prison. This enables us to construct a better measure of the impact of a teen birth on prison costs.

Like Grogger, we find a young teen birth consistently affects both outcome variables, even after controlling for other risk factors. Our most conservative estimate, based on a family fixed-effect approach, finds that a delay of a teen birth would decrease the probability of incarceration by 10.6 percent and years in jail by 13.4 percent. A less conservative approach, based on mother's age at first birth, rather than at the respondent's birth, implies that delay would reduce the probability of incarceration by almost 33 percent and years in jail by 38 percent. Thus our estimates strongly confirm the impact of a teen birth on the incarceration of sons.

NOTES

1. Source data are from U.S. Department of Justice (1991, 1992b, 1994). The author's calculations are available on request.

2. Formally, the average treatment effect is given by

$$n_{-1} \sum_{i=1}^{n} w_i \left[\Phi\left(\hat{\alpha} + X_i \hat{\beta} \right) - \Phi\left(X_i \hat{\beta} \right) \right]$$

where the hat notation denotes the maximum likelihood estimates, the i subscript indexes individual observations, n is the sample size, and w_i is the sampling weight for the ith observation.

3. The coefficient of the region dummies and the urban dummy are omitted from the table to save space.

4. Formally, I estimate the probit model given by

$$P(I = 1 | Y, A, X) = \Phi(\alpha Y + \gamma A + X\beta)$$

where A denotes the mother's age at the respondent's birth and γ is a parameter to be estimated.

5. The simulated incarceration rate among the sons of young teen mothers is given by

$$\hat{I}_1(\Delta) = n_1^{-1} \sum_{i=1}^{n_1} w_i \Phi \left[\hat{\alpha} Y_i + \hat{\gamma} (A_i + \Delta) + X_i + \hat{\beta} \right]$$

where the summation runs over the n_1 respondents whose mothers' first births occurred before age 18. The term Δ is calculated as the mean difference between the actual age at first birth among the young teen mothers and the target age for the given scenarios. Thus, for the simulations in the first row of table 8.4, $\Delta = 18.5 - 16.0 = 2.5$.

6. The simulated incarceration rate for the entire cohort is constructed as

$$\hat{I}(\Delta) = \pi(\Delta)\hat{I}(\Delta) = \pi\hat{I}(\Delta) + \hat{I}_0$$

where π is the fraction of youths born to young teen mothers ($= 0.1206$ from table 8.1) and $\hat{I}_0$ is the predicted incarceration rate among the sons of older mothers. It is calculated as

$$\hat{I} = {}_0^{-1} \sum_{i=1}^{n_0} w_i \Phi \left[\hat{\alpha} Y_1 + \hat{\gamma} (A_i = \Delta) = X_i \hat{\beta} \right]$$

where the summation runs over the n_0 sample members whose mothers were 18 or older at their first births.

7. The cost savings are based on simulated reductions in overall incarceration rates computed similarly to the manner described in footnote 6. A word on the calculation of Δ is in order, however. In each cell, Δ is equal to the difference between the mean age at first birth among sample mothers in the target age range and the mean age at first birth of the indicated group of young teen mothers. For example, the mean age at first birth among sample mothers who first gave birth at age 15 or earlier was 14.2. Among mothers who first gave birth at age 20 or 21, the mean age at first birth was 20.5. Thus, for the cell in the first row, third column, $\Delta = 20.5 - 14.2 = 6.3$. Mean ages used in calculating Δ for each cell are given in the notes to table 8.5.

8. Strictly speaking, this is a reduction of 21,000 to 26,000 man-years of incarceration.

9. Regressions 1 through 4 are ordinary least squares. Regressions 5 and 6 are probit.

10. While we initially attempted to include female incarceration rates as well, the sample sizes were too small to conduct a valid multivariate analysis.

11. Because interviews took place every other year starting in 1994, some imputations were included to estimate whether a respondent was in jail in the intervening years. The basic rule was: If a respondent was in jail the year prior and the year following and there were no reported hours of work during the intervening period, then he was considered to be in jail in the intervening year. This procedure was followed for 1995, 1997, 1999, and 2001.

12. Our models are estimated using logit, rather than the probit models used by Grogger; results are invariant to this change, and the logit is easier to interpret.

13. Note that this is a measure of the age of respondent's mother at her *first* birth, which may not necessarily be the same as the age of the mother at the respondent's birth. Our analyses examine both mother's age at first birth and her age at the respondent's birth.

REFERENCES

Block, M. K., and Thomas S. Ulen. 1979. "Cost Functions for Correctional Institutions." In *The Costs of Crime,* edited by Charles M. Gray (187–212). Beverly Hills, CA: SAGE Publications.

Blumstein, Alfred, Jacqueline Cohen, Jeffrey A. Roth, and Christy A. Visher. 1986. *Criminal Careers and "Career Criminals."* Washington, DC: National Academy Press.

Bronars, Stephen G., and Jeff Grogger. 1994. "The Economic Consequences of Unwed Motherhood: Using Twin Births as a Natural Experiment." *American Economic Review* 84(5): 1141–56.

DiIulio, John J., Jr., and Anne Morrison Piehl. 1991. "Does Prison Pay? The Stormy National Debate Over the Cost-Effectiveness of Imprisonment." *Brookings Review* 9(4): 28–35.

Freeman, Richard B. 1991. "Crime and the Employment of Disadvantaged Youths." Working Paper 3875. Cambridge, MA: National Bureau of Economic Research.

Geronimus, Arline T., and Sanders Korenman. 1992. "The Socioeconomic Consequences of Teen Childbearing Reconsidered." *Quarterly Journal of Economics* 107(4): 1187–214.

Grogger, Jeffrey. 1996. "Market Wages and Youth Crime." Santa Barbara: University of California Department of Economics. Mimeograph.

Grogger, Jeffrey, and Stephen G. Bronars. 1993. "The Socioeconomic Consequences of Teenage Childbearing: Findings from a Natural Experiment." *Family Planning Perspectives* 25(4): 156–61.

Hanushek, Eric A. 1992. "The Trade-off between Child Quantity and Quality." *Journal of Political Economy* 100(1): 84–117.

Hindelang, Michael J., Travis Hirschi, and Joseph G. Weis. 1981. *Measuring Delinquency*. Beverly Hills, CA: SAGE Publications.

Klaus, Patsy A. 1994. *The Costs of Crimes to Victims*. Washington, DC: U.S. Department of Justice, Bureau of Justice Statistics.

Morash, Merry, and Lila Rucker. 1989. "An Exploratory Study of the Connection of Mother's Age at Childbearing to Her Children's Delinquency in Four Data Sets." *Crime and Delinquency* 35(1): 45–93.

National Center for Health Statistics. Various years. *Vital Statistics of the United States, Vol. I, Natality*. Washington, DC: U.S. Government Printing Office.

Schmidt, Peter, and Ann Dryden Witte. 1984. *An Economic Analysis of Crime and Justice*. Orlando, FL: Academic Press.

U.S. Department of Justice. Bureau of Justice Statistics. 1991. *Census of Local Jails, 1988: Volume I*. Washington, DC: U.S. Government Printing Office.

———. 1992a. *Census of State and Federal Correctional Facilities, 1990*. Washington, DC: U.S. Government Printing Office.

———. 1992b. *Correctional Populations in the United States, 1990*. Washington, DC: U.S. Government Printing Office.

———. 1992c. *Justice Expenditures and Employment, 1990*. Washington, DC: U.S. Government Printing Office.

———. 1994. *National Corrections Reporting Program, 1991*. Washington, DC: U.S. Government Printing Office.

U.S. General Accounting Office. 1991. *Prison Costs: Opportunities Exist to Lower the Cost of Building Federal Prisons*. Washington, DC: U.S. Government Printing Office.

Western, Bruce. 2006. *Punishment and Inequality in America*. New York: Russell Sage Foundation.

Zedlewski, Edwin W. 1987. *Making Confinement Decisions*. Washington, DC: National Institute of Justice.

9

Children of Teen Mothers as Young Adults

EDITORS' NOTE

"Children of Early Childbearers as Young Adults" by Robert Haveman, Barbara Wolfe, and Elaine Peterson examined the impact of a teen birth on three outcomes for young adults: educational attainment, having a teen birth (for young women only), and being economically inactive at age 24. Their analyses found that a teen birth substantially affected each outcome, even after controlling for detailed individual and neighborhood characteristics. The authors based their analysis on a sample of 1,700 children age 1–6 in 1968 who were followed through 1988, when they were age 20–26. The children are representative of births to mothers of all ages that occurred between 1962 and 1968.

The original chapter by Haveman, Wolfe, and Peterson is included here in its entirety, except for its analysis of the monetary benefits of delaying a birth. That material is no longer timely and it superseded by the analysis by Maynard and Hoffman in chapter 10. Saul Hoffman and Lauren Sue Scher update and extend the original Haveman, Wolfe, and Peterson analysis in the second part of this chapter. The data used in 1997 are now dated. The teen births that occurred in the early to mid-1960s were far more likely to be marital than they are today and thus may not be very informative about the current impacts of such births. Additionally, the young adult outcomes are observed as of the mid- to late 1980s, again at least two decades ago.

Hoffman and Scher use data from the NLSY79 Young Adult Sample and observe outcomes through 2002. Using methods and models similar to those used in the original chapter, the authors find stronger impacts of a teen birth on high school graduation and teen fertility of the children than did Haveman, Wolfe, and Peterson.

Consequences of Teen Childbearing for the Life Chances of Children, 1968–88

Robert Haveman, Barbara Wolfe, and Elaine Peterson

Few social issues have attracted so much attention in the popular press as the high level of and rapid increase in the number of births to teenagers—especially those who are not married. The reason for this interest is easy to discern. Children born to teen mothers often do not have an even start in life. They are more likely to grow up in a poor and mother-only family, to live in a poor or underclass neighborhood, and to experience high risks to both their health status and potential school achievement. People who value equal opportunity as a social goal view the high rate of births to teens with great apprehension.

The presence, direction, and magnitude of impacts on the mother of the teen birth itself, as opposed to non-birth-related factors, are the subject of chapter 3. Whether or not early childbearing itself negatively affects the mother's long-term earnings and welfare receipt, it may well adversely affect the family life of the young mother and her approach to and resources for raising her children. And those impacts may well affect her children negatively. This chapter addresses two questions: (1) Do the children of teen mothers experience adverse effects from the teen birth and the accompanying shift in the life path of their mothers? (2) Can these effects be measured some two decades after the mothers' early fertility?

The Mother-Child Outcome Relationship

To answer questions about adverse effects, we consider three models that reflect three different views of the effect on children of having an "early fertility" mother (one who first gave birth when she was very young [15 or younger], a young teen [16 to 17], or an older teen [18 to 19]).

Model 1 presumes that initially, before giving birth, teen mothers are not very different from other girls. Then, when they become mothers at an early age, motherhood interferes with their human capital formation (in terms of schooling and work experience), marriage ability, and general living situation. Their life path then diverges from the trajectory it would have taken if they had delayed childbearing until later in life, especially until their postadolescent years.

If this is the case, we would not expect to observe significant *prebirth* differences between girls who are early-fertility mothers and those who are not. Nevertheless, the *postbirth* life paths of the early-fertility mothers will differ from those of later-fertility mothers, and these life path differences are at least in part attributable to early fertility. These differences may then also affect the early mothers' children's lives, and these intergenerational effects would result from early fertility. Hence, to measure the total effect that having an early-fertility mother has on a particular outcome for children, we estimate a simple equation relating a measure of the outcome for the child to dummy variables (those taking on a value of either zero or one) indicating whether the child was born to an early (or very early) fertility mother.

Model 2 reflects the view that, even in prebirth years, differences exist between early- and later-fertility mothers that are likely to influence the development and attainments of their children. To the extent that such *prebirth* differences are reasonably represented by descriptive characteristics of these mothers, the *total* effect that being born to a teen, or early-fertility, mother has on children's outcomes can be measured by an equation relating some child's outcome measure to a dummy variable indicating whether the child was born to an early-fertility mother, but also including variables to control for prebirth differences in the mother's choices and background. The coefficient on the early-fertility mother dummy variables would then reflect this effect, apart from the other prebirth differences between teen and later-fertility women.

Model 3 suggests not only that the early- and later-fertility mothers might differ in some important *prebirth* ways but that the environments in which the children grow up and reach adolescence also differ in ways potentially related to the policy regimes in effect. Hence, in addition to controlling for differences in the observed prebirth characteristics between teen and later-fertility mothers, we control for selected differences in the policy regimes confronting their children. The coefficients on the early-fertility dummy variables should not change (will be robust) if these policy regimes are truly exogenous (i.e., predetermined outside the model). However, if children of adolescent mothers are at a disadvantage, the coefficients on these variables may give some insight into whether poor outcomes can be mitigated by public policy.[1]

Data

Our estimation is based on a sample of 1,705 persons who were 0 to 6 years old in 1968 and were then surveyed for each of 21 years (through 1988). The data are from the Panel Study of Income Dynamics (PSID) and include background information such as age of the mother when she had her first child. Some retrospective information on when the mother was growing up is available in the PSID; we added data on state welfare generosity and state spending on family planning services, based on where the child lived.[2]

Individuals who did not respond for two consecutive years were excluded from the sample. Observations with missing data were generally assigned values based on an interpolation of their data for the prior and subsequent year. In a few cases, additional dummy variables indicating missing data were also created. Our sample does not include anyone who was incarcerated or died between 1968 and 1988.[3]

We focus on four outcomes: the probability that the teen mother's child will graduate from high school, the probability that her female children will give birth as teenagers, the probability that her female children will give birth out of wedlock as teenagers, and the probability that her child will be economically inactive at age 24. Youth are defined as inactive if they fall into *none* of the following categories: a mother of an infant or of two or more children, one of whom is less than 6 years old; working 1,000 or more hours a year; a full-time student; a part-time student and working at least 500 hours a year; or a part-time student and a mother with one child less than 6 years old.[4]

We use dummy variables to capture alternative definitions of early fertility. Thus, in each model, four dummy variables describing ages of childbearing of 21 years or less are included in the specification:

- childbearing at age ≤ 15
- childbearing at age 16 or 17
- childbearing at age 18 or 19
- childbearing at age 20 or 21

The omitted category is childbearing at age 22 or older. Delineation of these early childbearing categories allows us to explore impacts of early fertility and to simulate the effect that fertility delays of various magnitudes will have on children's outcomes.

Since model 1 presumes that early- and later-fertility mothers are similar in their family backgrounds and the policy environments that influence their childbearing decisions, only dummy variables for the gender of the child and whether the child is firstborn are added to the variables describing the mother's early childbearing experience. Model 2 tests the hypothesis that early- and later-fertility mothers have different observed preadolescent characteristics that might influence their children's attainments and be correlated with (or causal to) their choice of when to first give birth. Because we wish to estimate the total, direct, and indirect effects of adolescent motherhood on the children's eventual outcomes, we omit any variables for the period while the child was growing up that might have been affected by the mother's life path. For model 2, we add the following variables:

- whether the mother lived with both her parents when she was growing up
- whether the mother's father ("grandfather") had a high school education or more
- whether the mother's mother ("grandmother") had a high school education or more
- the mother's score on a sentence completion test (and a dummy variable indicating whether the mother's score is missing)
- whether the mother is black
- whether the mother is Catholic
- the number of times the mother attended religious services each month (based on earliest response available between 1968 and 1972)
- whether the mother grew up in a poor family

Since model 3 tests the hypothesis that early- and later-fertility mothers have different observed preadolescent characteristics and that the two groups may have faced a different policy environment, we add the following variables:

- average adult unemployment rate in the neighborhood in which the child lived from age 6 to 15

- average real maximum state welfare benefits in state where daughter lived from age 15 to 18
- average real public per capita family planning expenditures in state where daughter lived from age 13 to 19[5]

High School Graduation

Early childbearing reduces the chances that the child will graduate from high school (table 9.1). Our estimates for the simplest model (model 1) are in the first column. The coefficients on all three childbearing variables representing early motherhood are negative and statistically significant at the 1 percent level.[6]

As the additional, prebirth characteristics of the mother and the policy environment when the child was growing up are added in models 2 and 3, the magnitude of the impacts of early-fertility variables shrinks, as does the significance level. However, in all cases, the coefficients on the variables for childbearing before age 20 are statistically significant at conventional levels. And in both model 2 and model 3, the set of early childbearing variables passes the log likelihood ratio test, again rejecting the null hypothesis that age of motherhood does not matter.

Being a female child and being firstborn each increase the probability of graduating from high school, and these variables are statistically significant in all models. The firstborn variable also indicates that this is the child born to the teen mother (if the mother gave birth as a teen). The positive coefficient suggests that being born to an early-fertility mother while she was a teen has no additional negative impacts beyond those experienced by all her children.

The control variables indicating the mother's prebirth characteristics are generally as expected and are often significant. If the mother lived with both her parents, had a mother (the child's grandmother) who graduated from high school, is black, or is Catholic, the probability that the child graduates from high school increases and is statistically significant in each case. Although the education of the mother's father (grandfather), the economic status of her family while she was growing up, and the frequency of her attendance at religious services have the expected sign, none of these variables is uniformly statistically significant. The higher the mother's sentence completion score, the higher the probability that the child will graduate high school, and this effect is significant. The policy variable—the unemployment rate in the neighborhood in which the child lives—has a

Table 9.1. Probability That Child Graduated from High School ($N = 1,705$)

	Model 1 coefficient	Model 2 coefficient	Model 3 coefficient
Mother had first birth at age ≤15	0.707 (0.209)***	0.437 (0.222)**	0.421 (0.224)*
Mother had first birth at age 16–17	0.594 (0.150)***	0.373 (0.159)**	0.341 (0.161)**
Mother had first birth at age 18–19	0.415 (0.139)***	0.291 (0.146)**	0.270 (0.147)*
Mother had first birth at age 20–21	0.223 (0.143)	0.140 (0.150)	0.140 (0.150)
Firstborn child	−0.083 (0.126)	0.032 (0.131)	0.033 (0.131)
Mother lived with both her parents		−0.127 (0.112)	−0.104 (0.114)
Maternal grandfather had a high school education or more		−0.325 (0.165)**	−0.305 (0.169)*
Maternal grandmother had a high school education or more		−0.051 (0.133)	−0.036 (0.134)
Mother's sentence completion score		−0.080 (0.039)**	−0.079 (0.039)**
Missing mother's sentence completion score		−0.340 (0.114)***	−0.329 (0.115)***
Mother is black		0.181 (0.121)	0.147 (0.134)
Mother is Catholic		−0.327 (0.166)**	−0.279 (0.171)
Number of times mother attends religious services each month		−0.062 (0.041)	−0.064 (0.041)
Mother grew up poor		0.091 (0.107)	0.106 (0.109)
Average neighborhood adult unemployment rate at child's age 6–15			−0.034 (0.010)***

(continued)

Table 9.1. *(Continued)*

	Model 1 coefficient	Model 2 coefficient	Model 3 coefficient
Constant	1.057	−0.687	−0.425
	(0.083)***	(0.300)**	(0.310)
Log likelihood	−720.65	−670.35	−664.56
Chi-square	41.952	142.56	154.13
Percentage of zeros correctly predicted	0.0	3.7	4.1
Percentage of ones correctly predicted	100	99.4	99.4

Source: Panel Study of Income Dynamics.

Note: Standard errors are in parentheses.

*significant at the .10 level; **significant at the .05 level; ***significant at the .01 level

distinctly negative effect on the probability that the child will graduate high school, and it too is statistically significant.[7]

Giving Birth as a Teenager

The probability that a child will give birth as a teenager is clearly greater for women whose mothers were also teens at their first birth (table 9.2).

In the simple case (model 1), all early-fertility variables indicating a birth before age 19 are statistically significant. The positive signs indicate that early childbearing by the mother increases the probability that her daughter will give birth as a teen. The test statistic for a log likelihood ratio test of the significance of the full set of the early childbearing variables exceeds the critical value at the .01 level, leading to rejection of the null hypothesis that early fertility of the mother has no effect on the outcome of the child.[8]

As additional, prebirth characteristics of the mother and the policy environment when the child was growing up are added in model 2 and model 3, the magnitudes of the coefficients on the early-fertility variables again fall, as does the significance level. However, in all cases, the coefficients on the variables for childbearing before age 20 are statistically significant at conventional levels.[9]

As before, the impact of being born to an early-fertility mother is essentially the same for the first child and for the additional children. The impacts

Table 9.2. Probability That Child Had a Birth at Age <19: Female Sample ($n = 873$)

	Model 1 coefficient	Model 2 coefficient	Model 3 coefficient
Mother had first birth at age ≤15	−0.526 (0.154)***	−0.392 (0.166)**	−0.391 (0.166)**
Mother had first birth at age 16–17	−0.384 (0.113)***	−0.244 (0.121)**	−0.225 (0.122)*
Mother had first birth at age 18–19	−0.273 (0.101)***	−0.206 (0.107)*	−0.219 (0.107)**
Mother had first birth at age 20–21	−0.060 (0.109)	0.002 (0.116)	−0.006 (0.116)
Female child	0.133 (0.075)*	0.135 (0.077)*	0.135 (0.078)*
Firstborn child	0.364 (0.099)***	0.294 (0.103)***	0.296 (0.104)***
Mother lived with both her parents		0.277 (0.083)***	0.260 (0.083)***
Maternal grandfather had a high school education or more		0.144 (0.123)	0.104 (0.123)
Maternal grandmother had a high school education or more		0.411 (0.108)***	0.401 (0.108)***
Mother's sentence completion score		0.104 (0.029)***	0.105 (0.029)***
Missing mother's sentence completion score		0.462 (0.086)***	0.431 (0.087)***
Mother is black		0.337 (0.094)***	0.437 (0.099)***
Mother is Catholic		0.302 (0.116)***	0.287 (0.117)***
Number of times mother attends religious services each month		0.033 (0.030)	0.033 (0.030)
Mother grew up poor		−0.109 (0.082)	−0.140 (0.083)*
Average public family planning expenditures per capita in states child lived at age 13–19			−0.195 (0.153)

(continued)

Table 9.2. *(Continued)*

	Model 1 coefficient	Model 2 coefficient	Model 3 coefficient
Average neighborhood adult unemployment rate at child's age 6–15			0.023 (0.014)
Real average maximum state welfare benefits at child's age 15–18			−0.001 (0.001)
Constant	−1.167 (0.101)***	−0.009 (0.400)	0.259 (0.518)
Log likelihood	−412.67	−387.24	−384.43
Chi-square	23.974	74.852	80.471
Percentage of zeros correctly predicted	100	98.6	98.6
Percentage of ones correctly predicted	0.0	4.2	6.0

Source: Panel Study of Income Dynamics.

Note: Standard errors are in parentheses.

*significant at the .10 level; **significant at the .05 level; ***significant at the .01 level

of the mother's prebirth characteristics are again as expected, though fewer of them are statistically significant than in the case of high school graduation. The mother's test score and the grandfather's education are both negatively related to the probability that the daughter will give birth as a teenager, and in each case the coefficient is statistically significant. The education of the grandmother and whether the mother's family was poor do not have a statistically significant effect, however, although in both cases the signs are as expected. In this case, unlike the results for teen out-of-wedlock childbearing discussed below, none of the policy variables has a statistically significant effect on the probability that the daughter will give birth as a teenager.[10]

Giving Birth Out of Wedlock as a Teenager

The relationship between mother's age at first birth and whether her daughter will give birth out of wedlock as a teenager is less clear than for teen childbirth itself (table 9.3). In the simple model in column 1, all the

Table 9.3. Probability That Child Had an Out-of-Wedlock Birth at Age < 19: Female Sample ($n = 873$)

	Model 1 coefficient	Model 2 coefficient	Model 3 coefficient
Mother had first birth at age ≤15	0.716 (0.221)***	0.391 (0.237)*	0.381 (0.239)
Mother had first birth at age 16–17	0.568 (0.163)***	0.308 (0.176)*	0.252 (0.180)
Mother had first birth at age 18–19	0.437 (0.151)***	0.273 (0.162)*	0.232 (0.165)
Mother had first birth at age 20–21	0.263 (0.156)*	0.179 (0.168)	0.177 (0.169)
Firstborn child	−0.284 (0.145)*	−0.186 (0.154)	−0.182 (0.154)
Mother lived with both her parents		−0.161 (0.122)	−0.120 (0.124)
Maternal grandfather had a high school education or more		−0.174 (0.180)	−0.152 (0.185)
Maternal grandmother had a high school education or more		0.034 (0.146)	0.062 (0.148)
Mother's sentence completion score		−0.128 (0.042)***	−0.129 (0.043)***
Missing mother's sentence completion score		−0.257 (0.124)**	−0.239 (0.127)*
Mother is black		0.501 (0.136)***	0.475 (0.153)***
Mother is Catholic		−0.242 (0.191)	−0.170 (0.197)
Number of times mother attends religious services each month		−0.103 (0.046)**	−0.109 (0.047)**
Mother grew up poor		0.001 (0.119)	0.018 (0.121)
Average public family planning expenditures per capita in states child lived at age 13–19			−0.394 (0.174)**

(continued)

Table 9.3. *(Continued)*

	Model 1 coefficient	Model 2 coefficient	Model 3 coefficient
Average neighborhood adult unemployment rate at child's age 6–15			0.031 (0.015)**
Real average maximum state welfare benefits at child's age 15–18			−0.001 (0.001)
Constant	−1.338 (0.112)***	−0.086 (0.430)	0.695 (0.575)
Log likelihood	−346.54	−313.87	−307.4
Chi-square	24.002	89.343	102.281
Percentage of zeros correctly predicted	100.0	99.3	98.8
Percentage of ones correctly predicted	0.0	4.8	8.8

Source: Panel Study of Income Dynamics.

Note: Standard errors are in parentheses.

*significant at the .10 level; **significant at the .05 level; ***significant at the .01 level

early-fertility variables indicating the mother gave birth before age 19 are statistically significant. The positive sign on these variables indicates that early childbearing by the mother increases the probability that her daughter will give birth out of wedlock as a teen.[11] As before, adding the additional prebirth characteristics of the mother and her environment as she grew up reduces the magnitude of the impacts. They are still statistically significant at the .10 level for model 2 but not for model 3.[12]

Being a firstborn child decreases the probability that the daughter will give birth out of wedlock as a teenager, but this variable has a statistically significant coefficient only in the simplest model (column 1). This again suggests that the impact of being born to an early-fertility mother is essentially the same for the first child and for the additional children. The control variables indicating the mother's prebirth characteristics are again signed as expected, and several are statistically significant. If the mother is black, the probability that her daughter will give birth out of wedlock as a teenager increases, and the coefficient is statistically significant in each specification. The mother's test score and the regularity of her attendance at religious services are both negatively related to the probability that the daughter will give birth out of wedlock as a teenager, and in each case the coefficient is statistically significant. Here, as opposed to the results for high school completion, the education of the mother's parents and whether her family was poor do not have a statistically significant effect on the outcome, although in both cases the signs are as expected.

With respect to the policy variables, an increase in the unemployment rate tends to increase the probability of a teen nonmarital birth, increases in state family planning expenditures tend to reduce the probability, and generosity of state welfare spending has no statistically significant effect.

Being Economically Inactive at Age 24

The relationship between early fertility and being inactive as a young adult is weak (table 9.4). Only for the simple model are all the early-fertility variables indicating a birth before age 19 statistically significant, indicating that early childbearing increases the probability that a mother's child will be economically inactive as a young adult.[13] Being firstborn decreases the probability that the child will be economically inactive as a young adult, but this variable is only statistically significant in the simplest model. Again, adding the additional prebirth characteristics of the mother and her environment as she grows up reduces the magnitude of the relationship between early motherhood and being economically inactive as a young adult, with only one age category variable statistically significant.[14] Most control variables indicating the mother's prebirth characteristics are again signed in the direction expected, though only three are statistically significant. The mother's test score and grandmother's education are both negatively related to the probability that the child will be economically inactive as a young adult, and in each case the coefficient is statistically significant.

The Effects of Delayed Childbearing

The predicted effects of delays in childbearing are shown in tables 9.5 through 9.8. For these simulations, we group the children based on when their mothers first gave birth. We hold constant all the observed characteristics of the mothers who gave birth in each age category, except for the variables indicating when the mother first gave birth. We then use

Table 9.4. Probability of Child Being Economically Inactive at Age 24
($n = 765$)

	Model 1 coefficient	Model 2 coefficient	Model 3 coefficient
Mother had first birth at age ≤15	0.581 (0.213)***	0.362 (0.226)	0.360 (0.226)
Mother had first birth at age 16–17	0.327 (0.158)**	0.190 (0.166)	0.187 (0.166)
Mother had first birth at age 18–19	0.376 (0.134)***	0.276 (0.140)*	0.275 (0.140)**
Mother had first birth at age 20–21	0.038 (0.144)	0.016 (0.148)	0.016 (0.148)
Female child	0.308 (0.144)	0.302 (0.104)***	0.302 (0.104)***
Firstborn child	−0.259 (0.133)*	−0.209 (0.136)	−0.199 (0.137)
Mother lived with both her parents		−0.118 (0.114)	−0.106 (0.115)
Maternal grandfather had a high school education or more		0.101 (0.155)	0.109 (0.155)
Maternal grandmother had a high school education or more		−0.234 (0.138)*	−0.229 (0.138)*
Mother's sentence completion score		−0.089 (0.041)**	−0.088 (0.041)**
Missing mother's sentence completion score		−0.061 (0.115)	−0.052 (0.116)
Mother is black		0.198 (0.127)	0.165 (0.133)
Mother is Catholic		−0.252 (0.152)*	−0.250 (0.152)
Number of times mother attends religious services each month		−0.053 (0.042)	0.052 (0.042)
Mother grew up poor		−0.057 (0.108)	−0.043 (0.110)
Average neighborhood adult unemployment rate at child's age 6–15			0.013 (0.015)

Table 9.4. *(Continued)*

	Model 1 coefficient	Model 2 coefficient	Model 3 coefficient
Constant	−1.015	−0.160	−0.264
	(0.114)***	(0.407)	(0.426)
Log likelihood	−409.36	−397.49	−397.15
Chi-square	29.917	53.663	54.34
Percentage of zeros correctly predicted	100	98.6	98.4
Percentage of ones correctly predicted	0.0	4.8	7.0

Source: Panel Study of Income Dynamics.

Note: Standard errors are in parentheses.

*significant at the .10 level; **significant at the .05 level; ***significant at the .01 level

the previously estimated coefficients to obtain the predicted probability of each outcome (e.g., high school graduation) for each child under alternative childbearing variables and take the weighted average of the newly predicted probabilities for each group. Model 3 is the basis for the simulations.[15]

Delayed childbearing clearly benefits high school graduation rates (table 9.5). The probability of graduating high school for a child born to

text continues on page 340

Table 9.5. Simulations of Impact Delaying Childbearing Has on High School Graduation of the Children: Full Sample

For children of mothers first giving birth while:	Number of observations in group	Estimated Probability for the Child if the Mother Delayed Her First Birth until Age:				
		Original	16–17	18–19	20–21	≥22
Age ≤15	98	.710	.760	.762	.819	.820
Age 16–17	262	.785		.786	.839	.840
Age 18–19	427	.832			.877	.878
Age 20–21	380	.885				.886

Source: Panel Study of Income Dynamics.

Table 9.6. Simulations of Impact Delaying Childbearing Has on Adolescent Childbearing: Female Sample

Age of daughter at childbearing	Age at which mother first gave birth	Number of observations in group	Estimated Probability for the Child if the Mother Delayed Her First Birth until Age:				
			Original	16–17	18–19	20–21	≥22
<18	≤15	50	.185	.169	.143	.142	.129
	16–17	137	.158		.133	.132	.119
	18–19	203	.089			.089	.079
	20–21	203	.090				.080
<19	≤15	50	.279	.255	.234	.200	.166
	16–17	137	.248		.227	.193	.159
	18–19	203	.168			.139	.112
	20–21	203	.141				.113
<20	≤15	50	.358	.291	.305	.255	.222
	16–17	37	.286		.300	.250	.217
	18–19	203	.229			.185	.157
	20–21	203	.189				.161

Source: Panel Study of Income Dynamics.

Table 9.7. Simulations of Impact Delaying Childbearing Has on Adolescent Out-of-Wedlock Childbearing: Female Sample

Age of daughter at out-of-wedlock childbearing	Age at which mother first gave birth	Number of observations in group	Original	Estimated Probability for the Child if the Mother Delayed Her First Birth until Age:			
				16–17	18–19	20–21	≥22
<18	≤15	50	.142	.116	.116	.128	.102
	16–17	137	.098		.098	.110	.085
	18–19	203	.060			.068	.051
	20–21	203	.070				.053
<19	≤15	50	.205	.175	.171	.160	.126
	16–17	137	.164		.159	.148	.116
	18–19	203	.104			.095	.071
	20–21	203	.095				.071
<20	≤15	50	.234	.200	.205	.189	.164
	16–17	37	.193		.197	.181	.156
	18–19	203	.130			.117	.098
	20–21	203	.116				.097

Source: Panel Study of Income Dynamics.

Table 9.8. Simulations of Impact Delaying Childbearing Has on Economic Inactivity at Age 24 or Older

For children of mothers first giving birth while:	Number of observations in group	Estimated Probability for the Child if the Mother Delayed Her First Birth until Age:				
		Original	16–17	18–19	20–21	≥22
Age ≤15	45	.376	.314	.345	.258	.253
Age 16–17	108	.262		.290	.212	.207
Age 18–19	187	.242			.171	.167
Age 20–21	173	.171				.167

Source: Panel Study of Income Dynamics.

a mother who gave birth at age 15 or younger is about 71 percent. If her mother had delayed childbearing until age 16–17, the probability would rise to 76 percent, an increase of 5 percentage points. If her mother had delayed childbearing until age 18–19, the probability that the child would graduate high school would rise to 76.2 percent. Delay until age 20–21 or after age 22 would increase the probability to 82 percent.[16]

For the daughters' probability of adolescent childbearing, the results are equally clear (table 9.6). If the mothers with the earliest fertility delayed their childbearing until age 22 or older, for example, the probability of their daughters having an adolescent birth would drop by over 11 percentage points. The patterns are similar for those who give birth under age 18 and under age 20. For the daughters' probability of adolescent out-of-wedlock childbearing, the effects are similar but somewhat smaller (table 9.7). If mothers with the earliest fertility delayed their childbearing until they were age 22 or older, for example, the probability of their daughters having an adolescent out-of-wedlock birth would drop by 7.9 percentage points.

Delays in childbearing also reduce the probability of the child being economically inactive at age 24 (table 9.8). If the mothers with the earliest fertility delayed childbearing until age 22 or older, the probability of their children being economically inactive would drop by about 12.3 percentage points. In this table, uncertainty as to the relative magnitude of the effects of early fertility at age 16–17 leads to a strange result. A one- to two-year delay in childbearing by mothers who had their first child while age 16–17 appears to increase the probability of their children being economically inactive. This suggests that the most reliable estimates in this table are those based on the statistically significant estimated coefficient for the children of mothers who first became mothers at age 18–19. For this group, delayed childbearing by the mothers is estimated to decrease the probability of the child being economically inactive by about 7.5 percentage points.[17]

Conclusion

Having a mother who first gave birth as a teen has negative consequences for her children. This is so even after taking into account differences in the backgrounds of these mothers compared with later-fertility mothers. Statistically, the impact is more significant for the child's education level than for the daughter's fertility behavior or the child's economic inactivity at age 24. If teenagers could be convinced to postpone childbearing, their children (and hence society) would have improved life chances and outcomes.

If teenagers who give birth before age 15 could be induced to postpone their first births to age 16–17, for example, the probability that their children would graduate high school would increase by about 7 percent, from .71 to .76. Similarly, the probability that their daughters would give birth by age 19 would be decreased by about 9 percent. We estimate an even larger decrease, about 16 percent—the biggest estimated impact—in the probability that the daughters would give birth out of wedlock by age 19. We also expect that the probability of children being economically inactive as young adults would decrease by about 16 percent.

If teenagers who are currently having their first birth between the ages of 16 and 17 could be induced to postpone that birth until they are 18 to 19, the expected increase in the probability of their children graduating high school is quite small. However, postponement until age 20 or later leads to sizable expected increases of about 7 percent, from .785 to .839. In the case of subsequent early fertility for the daughters born to these teenage mothers, a one- to two-year postponement of the age when the mother first gave birth (from 16–17 to 18–19) is not expected to affect her daughter's probability of giving birth as a teen; however, a shift to age 20 or older again has a much larger expected impact.

The characteristics of early-teen mothers differ from women who first give birth at later ages. Nevertheless, a policy to postpone their initial age at first birth would be expected to have sizable impacts on the future attainments of their children. Beyond this, if young teens do not give birth at these young ages, they may change their life course in other ways as well (e.g., increase their own levels of schooling and job opportunities). Such changes could have additional positive impacts on the well-being of their children.

Consequences of Teen Childbearing for the Life Chances of Children, 1979–2002

Saul D. Hoffman and Lauren Sue Scher

Haveman, Wolfe, and Peterson's estimates of the consequences of teenage childbearing for children as young adults examined the impact of a teen birth on four outcomes for young adults: educational attainment; having a teen birth (for young women only); having a teen out-of-wedlock birth (for young women only); and being economically inactive at age 24, where inactivity meant that an individual was neither working, attending school, nor raising young children.[18] Their analyses found substantial impacts of a teen birth on each of these outcomes.

The data for their analysis came from the Panel Study of Income Dynamics. Their sample included approximately 1,700 children age 0 to 6 in 1968, who were followed through 1988, when they were age 20 to 26. The children are representative of births to mothers of all ages that occurred between 1962 and 1968. As such, it was an appropriate dataset to test the impact of a teen birth on the outcomes.

The inherent weakness of this study now is its dated sample. The births themselves are four decades old and represent an era when teen births, in particular, were quite different than in the 1990s and 2000s. For example, between 1962 and 1967 approximately 85 percent of teen births were marital births, compared with just 20 percent currently. Median age at first marriage for women was 20.5 in 1964 and median age at first birth was just 22; most recently these median ages have risen to 25.0 and 24.8, respectively (National Center for Health Statistics 2005).[19] Additionally, the young adult outcomes themselves are observed as of the mid- to late 1980s, again at least two decades ago. It seemed clear that updating the relationship between a teen birth and young adult outcomes would be helpful. This section offers such an update, using data from the NLSY79 Young Adult Sample.

Data and Methods

We have followed the general approach of Haveman, Wolfe, and Peterson (hereafter HWP), using data from the National Longitudinal Survey of Youth, 1979 Young Adult sample in place of the PSID. NLSY79 is a sample of more than 13,000 adolescents and young adults, age 14 to 21 in 1979. The young adult sample includes all children of the NLSY79 sample members. We use data through 2002 and limit the sample to young adults who were at least age 21 in 2002—that is, young adults born no later than 1981. These young adults were born between 1970 and 1981, roughly 8 to 13 years later than in HWP. During this time, approximately 45 percent of teen births were nonmarital, substantially above the figure for the HWP analysis but still well below the current figure.

Unlike HWP, the sample we use is not fully representative of mothers of all ages at their first birth. The oldest mothers were age 23 at their first birth—21-year-olds in 1979 who had a first birth in 1981. But our sample is representative of births to women at ages 20 and 21, which is the comparison group we are interested in.

We adopt the general research approach of HWP. We focus on two of the outcomes they examined: whether a young adult graduated from high school and whether a young woman had a teen birth herself. We do not examine economic inactivity at age 24 because some of our sample is not yet old enough,[20] especially children of older mothers. Our models are estimated using a logit model, rather than the probit model used in HWP; the results are invariant to this change and the logit is easier to interpret. We follow their model specification as fully as possible, except we combine all births to teens age 17 and younger and do not further distinguish births to mothers at age 15 or younger, and we do not include measures of neighborhood quality.[21] These neighborhood variables had almost no impact on estimates of teen birth effects in HWP.[22] Because these variables were not available in the same way in the NLSY79, we opted to estimate simpler models that exclude these variables. This should have little or no effect on our estimates. All estimates are based on weighted data.

Our sample consists of 1,461 adolescents who were born to members of the original NLSY79 sample and ranged in age from 21 to 31 years.

The female-only sample, which was used to explore whether the teen had a birth, consisted of 719 young adults. Table 9.9 presents descriptive statistics for the three main outcomes explored in this analysis, the main predictor variables of interest (whether the young adult was born to a teen mother), and the covariates used as statistical controls. As this table shows, 84 percent of our analysis sample of young adults reported grad-

Table 9.9. Sample Characteristics, NLSY79 Young Adult Dataset, Persons Age 21–31 in 2002

	N	Weighted mean	Standard deviation
Outcome variables			
Graduated from high school[a]	1,466	0.84	0.39
Had a birth at age <19 (female sample only)	719	0.23	0.44
Number of years of education completed	1,450	12.40	2.00
Predictor variables[b]			
Mother had first birth at age ≤17	1,461	44.1%	NA
Mother had first birth at age 18–19	1,461	32.7%	NA
Mother had first birth at age 20–21	1,461	23.1%	NA
Additional covariates			
Female	1,466	0.46	0.50
Firstborn child	1,466	0.70	0.46
Mother lived with both biological parents at age 14	1,463	0.64	0.50
Maternal grandfather had at least a high school education	1,117	0.48	0.48
Maternal grandmother had at least a high school education	1,335	0.43	0.47
Mother's AFQT percentile	1,406	33.95	22.43
Mother is black	1,466	0.25	0.50
Mother is Catholic	1,457	0.27	0.46
Number of times mother attended religious services in 1979	1,464	2.91	1.62
Mother's family received welfare payments in 1979	1,447	0.23	0.47

Sources: NLSY79 and NLSY79-YA (young adult) datasets.

NA = not applicable

a. Includes receipt of a high school diploma or a GED.

b. Age of mother at first birth, not at birth of the young adult respondent.

uating from high school (with an average of 12.4 years of schooling completed), and 23 percent of the females reported having a child before the age of 19.

Because of the nature of our sample, a larger proportion of the young adults in our analysis come from higher-risk families than would be expected in a nationally representative sample of young adults. For example, over three-quarters of the young adults were born to mothers who started having children by age 19 or younger. The average age at first birth for mothers of these young adults is 18, compared with the national average for the full NLSY sample of 24. In addition, this sample over-represents children born to black mothers (25 percent versus a national average of 14 percent) and children born to mothers who grew up in homes receiving welfare payments (23 percent versus a national average of 9 percent). Our analyses attempt to control for these differences in background characteristics as a way of isolating the effect of having a mother who was a teen when she first gave birth versus having a mother who delayed childbearing until her early 20s.

Analysis

Our estimates of the impact of a teen birth on high school graduation are presented in table 9.10. Model 1 controls only for mother's age at first birth plus dummy variables for gender (female = 1) and firstborn child. Model 2 adds family background measures, including whether the mother lived in a single-parent family at age 14, education of the mother's parents, the mother's AFQT score, whether the family was poor in 1979, and dummy variables for race (black = 1) and religion (Catholic = 1). All these variables were used by HWP, except for the AFQT score, which we use in place of the sentence completion score available in the PSID. The AFQT score is arguably a better measure of cognitive ability than the sentence completion score.

As shown in the model 1 results, an early birth has a statistically significant negative effect on the probability of completing high school. A later teen birth (age 18 to 19) has no effect; this is not surprising, given the age of the birth and the usual age of high school graduation. Girls are more likely to graduate than boys and firstborn children are more likely to graduate than later-born children. The quantitative impact is very large—delaying a teen birth to age 20 to 21 would increase the graduation rate for these chil-

Table 9.10. Logit Estimates of Probability That Child Graduated from High School (*N* = 1,461)

	Model 1	Model 2
Mother had first birth at age ≤17	−0.677**	−0.338*
	(0.17)	(0.18)
Mother had first birth at age 18–19	−0.129	−0.042
	(0.18)	(0.18)
Female	0.274**	0.32**
	(0.12)	(0.13)
Firstborn	0.279**	0.361**
	(0.13)	(0.14)
Mother lived with both her parents		0.174
		(0.14)
Maternal grandfather had a high school education or more		0.407**
		(0.15)
Maternal grandmother had a high school education or more		0.027
		(0.15)
Mother's AFQT score		0.017**
		(0.00)
Mother is black		0.178
		(0.16)
Mother is Catholic		0.149
		(0.15)
Number of times mother attended religious services in 1979		0.015
		(0.04)
Mother's family received welfare payments in 1979		−0.165
		(0.15)
Constant	1.045**	−0.015
	(0.18)	(0.29)
−2 log likelihood	1,664.946	1,588.73

Sources: NLSY79 and NLSY79-YA datasets.

Note: Standard errors are in parentheses.

*significant at the .10 level; **significant at the .05 level

dren from 66 percent to 79.2 percent. Equivalently, the dropout rate would decline from 33 percent to 20 percent.

Controlling for background variables reduces the impact of a teen birth (model 2), but it remains substantial and statistically significant. Holding other risk factors constant, a mother's early teen birth reduces the probability that her child will complete high school by about 7 percentage points, about half the quantitative effect of the simpler model. Other risk factors that have a statistically significant impact include grandfather's education and mother's AFQT score, along with being female and firstborn.

We also examined the impact of a teen birth on total years of schooling (see table A.9.2 for coefficient estimates). Because the younger members of the sample have not had the opportunity to complete college, we truncate completed education at 14 years and use a tobit model to account for this censoring. In this model, we find that an early teen birth reduces accumulated educated by .7 years with no control except whether female and whether firstborn and by .229 years with control for background variables; the former estimate is statistically significant at conventional levels, while the latter is just short of significance at the 10 percent level on two-tailed tests.

It is useful to contrast this result with the logit result on completion of high school. The logit model indicates that a delayed birth would increase the absolute proportion of students completing high school by 7 percentage points. The tobit estimate of an average gain for the entire sample of .229 years then implies that these 7 percent complete more than three additional years of schooling or, more realistically, that there are also educational effects on those students who would complete high school even if they were the child of a teen mother.

Table 9.11 presents the corresponding analysis of the impact of a teen birth on a daughter's risk of having a teen birth herself. The analysis sample includes 719 women, age 21 to 31, of whom 189 (23 percent weighted) had a birth at age 19 or younger. As seen in the results for model 1, an early teen birth has a large, positive, and statistically significant impact on a daughter's early fertility compared with daughters whose mothers had their first birth in their early 20s. A later teen birth also has a positive effect, but its coefficient is smaller and it is not quite statistically significant at the 10 percent level. Delaying an early teen birth to age 20 to 21 would reduce the proportion of daughters with a teen birth from nearly 33 percent to just over 10 percent, while delaying a later teen birth to that age would reduce the proportion with a teen birth from 17 percent to 10.5 percent. In this model, being a firstborn child has no effect on the probability of having a teen birth.

This intergenerational teen birth effect remains large and statistically significant, even after controlling for family background. The coefficient estimates of the impact of a teen birth fall 10 to 20 percent. With control for other risk factors, delaying a mother's early teen birth would reduce

Table 9.11. Logit Estimates of Probability That Child Had a Birth at Age <19 (Female Sample) (*N* = 719)

	Model 1	Model 2
Mother had first birth at age ≤17		
Mother had first birth at age 18–19	1.437**	1.137**
	(0.315)	(0.330)
Female	0.541	0.481
	(0.340)	(0.349)
Firstborn	0.105	0.091
	(0.204)	(0.221)
Mother lived with both her parents		−0.067
		(0.213)
Maternal grandfather had a		0.167
high school education or more		(0.243)
Maternal grandmother had a		0.108
high school education or more		(0.236)
Mother's AFQT score		−0.017**
		(0.006)
Mother is black		−0.189
		(0.259)
Mother is Catholic		−0.051
		(0.233)
Number of times mother attended		−0.142**
religious services in 1979		(0.063)
Mother's family received welfare		0.581**
payments in 1979		(0.232)
Constant	−2.2173**	−1.403**
	(0.337)	(0.469)
−2 log likelihood	689.941	658.049

Sources: NLSY79 and NLSY79-YA datasets.

Note: Standard errors are in parentheses.

**significant at the .05 level

her daughter's probability of having a teen birth to 13.5 percent (compared with 10.4 percent without controls) and delaying a later teen birth would reduce the daughter's probability from 17 percent to 11.1 percent (compared with 10.5 percent without controls). Other statistically significant risk factors include mother's AFQT score, frequency of mother's attendance at religious services as a youth, and whether the family was poor in 1979 (the first year of the survey). Interestingly, none of the other risk factors, including race and mother's and grandparents' education, have significant impacts. The mother's AFQT score is the only risk factor besides mother's age at birth that was a statistically significant predictor of both high school graduation and having a teen birth.

Conclusion

Table 9.12 summarizes our estimates for young adults in 2002 and those of HWP for young adults in 1988. Separately for mothers who had a first birth at age 17 or less or at age 18–19, the table shows the baseline proportions of children who graduated from high school and of daughters who had a teen birth, along with the corresponding predicted proportions if the birth had been delayed to age 20 or 21. The predicted proportions are taken from tables 9.10 and 9.11, model 2 of this section and tables 9.5 and 9.6 of HWP. The HWP results shown are a weighted average of results shown separately there for births to mothers age 15 or younger and those age 16 to 17.

HWP find higher proportions who are high school graduates for both groups. The impacts of a teen birth for the children of younger teen

Table 9.12. Estimated Impacts of a Teen Birth on Probability of High School Completion and Probability of Having a Teen Birth from Parts 1 and 2 of Chapter 9

Mother's age at first birth	Child Graduated from High School		Daughter Had a Birth as a Teenager	
	HWP	HS	HWP	HS
Age ≤17				
Baseline	0.764	0.660	0.305	0.328
If delay birth to age 20–21	0.833	0.731	0.251	0.135
Age 18–19				
Baseline	0.832	0.775	0.229	0.168
If delay birth to age 20–21	0.877	0.783	0.185	0.111

HWP = Haveman, Wolfe, and Peterson, estimates from PSID, 1988 for young adults age 20–26.

HS = Hoffman and Scher, estimates from NLSY79-YA, 2002 for young adults age 21–31.

mothers are very similar in the two analyses—6.9 percentage points in HWP and 7.1 percentage points in HS. HWP find a larger impact for the children of older teen mothers—4.5 percentage points versus 0.8 percentage points.

For a teen birth, our impacts are consistently larger than the ones HWP found. For children of a young teen mother, our estimate of the impact is three and a half times as large as theirs. In our sample, fewer daughters of older teen mothers had a teen birth themselves, but the impact of a teen birth is still larger than in HWP—5.7 percentage points versus 4.4 percentage points. Since the baseline proportion is lower in our analysis, the proportionate impact of being the daughter of an older teen mother is far larger than in their analysis.

Both analyses strongly confirm the intergenerational impact of a teen birth on outcomes for young adults, even after controlling for other risk factors. Especially strong impacts are found for children of young teen births (a birth at age 17 or younger) for both high school completion and, even more so, the probability of having a teen birth.

Table A.9.1. Means and Standard Deviations of Variables Used in Estimation

A. Full-Sample Statistics ($N = 1{,}705$)

Variable	Mean	Standard deviation
Mother had first birth at age ≤15	0.06	0.23
Mother had first birth at age 16–17	0.15	0.36
Mother had first birth at age 18–19	0.25	0.43
Mother had first birth at age 20–21	0.22	0.42
Mother lived with both her parents	0.70	0.46
Maternal grandfather had a high school education or more	0.20	0.40
Maternal grandmother had a high school education or more	0.29	0.46
Mother's sentence completion score	8.56	1.20
Missing mother's sentence completion score	0.70	0.46
Mother is black	0.43	0.49
Mother is Catholic	0.19	0.39
Number of times mother attends religious services each month	1.95	1.29
Mother grew up poor	0.46	0.50
Average public family planning expenditures per capita in states child lived at age 13–19	1.06	0.36
Firstborn child	0.23	0.42
Female child	0.51	0.50
Child graduated from high school	0.84	0.36
Average neighborhood adult unemployment rate at child's age 6–15	7.08	4.08
Real average maximum state welfare benefits at child's age 15–18	$353.95	$78.45

Source: Panel Study of Income Dynamics.

Table A.9.1. *(Continued)*

B. Female Sample Statistics (*N* = 873)

Variable	Mean	Standard deviation
Mother had first birth at age ≤15	0.06	0.24
Mother had first birth at age 16–17	0.14	0.35
Mother had first birth at age 18–19	0.24	0.43
Mother had first birth at age 20–21	0.23	0.42
Mother lived with both her parents	0.71	0.45
Maternal grandfather had a high school education or more	0.19	0.39
Maternal grandmother had a high school education or more	0.28	0.45
Mother's sentence completion score	8.54	1.22
Missing mother's sentence completion score	0.67	0.47
Mother is black	0.43	0.49
Mother is Catholic	0.19	0.40
Number of times mother attends religious services each month	1.94	1.23
Mother grew up poor	0.47	0.50
Average public family planning expenditures per capita in states child lived at age 13–19	1.14	0.39
Firstborn child	0.21	0.40
Female child	0.54	0.50
Child graduated from high school	0.86	0.35
Average neighborhood adult unemployment rate at child's age 6–15	6.64	3.72
Real average maximum state welfare benefits at child's age 15–18	$371.59	$83.11
Child had a birth at age <20	0.24	0.43
Child had a birth at age <19	0.19	0.39
Child had a birth at age <18	0.13	0.33
Child had out-of-wedlock birth at age <20	0.18	0.38
Child had out-of-wedlock birth at age <19	0.14	0.35
Child had out-of-wedlock birth at age <18	0.10	0.30

Source: Panel Study of Income Dynamics.

Table A.9.1. *(Continued)*

C. Sample Age ≥24 in 1988 Statistics (*N* = 765)

Variable	Mean	Standard deviation
Mother had first birth at age ≤15	0.06	0.23
Mother had first birth at age 16–17	0.16	0.36
Mother had first birth at age 18–19	0.23	0.42
Mother had first birth at age 20–21	0.23	0.42
Mother lived with both her parents	0.70	0.46
Maternal grandfather had a high school education or more	0.19	0.40
Maternal grandmother had a high school education or more	0.29	0.45
Mother's sentence completion score	8.52	1.20
Missing mother's sentence completion score	0.71	0.46
Mother is black	0.45	0.50
Mother is Catholic	0.18	0.39
Number of times mother attends religious services each month	1.97	1.27
Mother grew up poor	0.48	0.50
Average public family planning expenditures per capita in states child lived at age 13–19	1.07	0.36
Firstborn child	0.21	0.41
Female child	1.00	0.00
Child graduated from high school	0.86	0.35
Average neighborhood adult unemployment rate at child's age 6–15	7.14	4.10
Real average maximum state welfare benefits at child's age 15–18	$354.07	$77.15
Child economically inactive at age 24	0.24	0.43

Source: Panel Study of Income Dynamics.

Table A.9.2. Tobit Estimates of Determinants of Years of Education ($N = 1,461$)

	Model 1	Model 2
Mother had first birth at age ≤17	−0.729**	−0.229
	(0.15)	(0.15)
Mother had first birth at age 18–19	−0.191	−0.034
	(0.16)	(0.15)
Female	0.466**	0.502**
	(0.11)	(0.11)
Firstborn	0.356**	0.393**
	(0.13)	(0.13)
Mother lived with both her parents		0.338**
		(0.12)
Maternal grandfather had a high school education or more		0.402**
		(0.13)
Maternal grandmother had a high school education or more		−0.023
		(0.13)
Mother's AFQT score		0.023**
		(0.00)
Mother is black		0.316**
		(0.15)
Mother is Catholic		0.136
		(0.13)
Number of times mother attended religious services in 1979		0.054
		(0.03)
Mother's family received welfare payments in 1979		−0.181
		(0.14)
Constant	12.37**	10.72
	(0.17)	(0.26)
Sigma	2.09**	1.986
	(0.05)	(0.05)
−2 log likelihood	−2,673	−2,598

Sources: NLSY79 and NLSY79-YA datasets.

Note: Standard errors are in parentheses.

**significant at the .05 level

NOTES

1. We also considered a model in which important unobserved pre-motherhood differences between adolescent and older mothers would make the outcomes of the children differ. Because of the difficulty of determining why some mothers become early-fertility mothers and others do not, however, our estimations were not satisfying. Hence, we cannot rule out the possibility that unobserved characteristics are the true cause of both the mother's early fertility and the children's subsequent disadvantages. Further details, including the estimates of our two-stage estimation procedure, are available from the authors upon request.

2. Data on state welfare generosity were obtained from Robert Moffitt. Data on state spending for family planning services come from *Family Planning Perspectives* (see Gold and Guardado 1988; Gold and Macias 1986; Gold and Nestor 1985; Nestor 1982; Orr and Brenner 1981; Torres and Forrest 1983; and Torres, Forrest, and Eisman 1981). State population and price index data come from the *Statistical Abstract of the United States* (see U.S. Bureau of Census 1987, 1993, and 1994).

3. Appendix table A.9.1 presents the means and standard deviations for the variables we use.

4. Because each of the outcomes is a limited dependent variable taking on the values of zero and one, we fit the models using maximum likelihood probit estimation.

5. The maximum state welfare benefits and per capita family planning expenditure variables are included only in specifications for the teen childbearing and teen out-of-wedlock childbearing outcomes.

6. As a set, these early childbearing variables are statistically significant at the .01 level, when a log likelihood ratio test of the null hypothesis of no significant effect of early childbearing is tested. The critical value for the log likelihood ratio test at the .01 level is 13.28; the test statistic equals 21.8.

7. For the model 2 and model 3 results, tests of structural differences in the parameters for these equations and estimates based on subsamples of blacks and nonblacks could not reject the null hypothesis of no structural difference. The chi-square test statistics for these equations are 15 and 13, and the .1 critical values are 25 and 26.

8. The critical value for the log likelihood test at the .01 level is 13.28; the test statistic equals 22.99.

9. In model 2, the set of early childbearing variables passes the log likelihood ratio test, again rejecting the null hypothesis that age of motherhood does not matter. The log likelihood ratio test statistic for whether the four estimated coefficients on the early-fertility dummy variables are statistically different from zero for model 2 is 8, and the .1 critical value is 7.78. The test statistic for model 3 is 6.7, statistically significant only at the .15 level.

10. However, for the results in model 3 of table 9.2, a test of structural difference in the parameters for this equation and estimates based on subsamples of blacks and nonblacks rejected the null hypothesis of no structural difference. The chi-square test statistic for the third model is 31.98 (versus only 19.38 for the second model, which doesn't include the policy variables) and so rejects the null hypothesis at the .05 level, for which the critical value is 25. In the estimates based on nonblacks, an increase in the unemployment rate tends to increase the probability of a teen birth; in the estimates based on blacks, increases in state family planning expenditures tend to reduce the probability. The generosity of state welfare spending appears to have no statistically significant effect on this outcome in any of the estimations.

11. The test statistic for a log likelihood ratio test of the significance of the early child-bearing variables exceeds the critical value at the .01 level, leading to rejection of the null hypothesis that early fertility of the mother has no effect on the outcome of the child. The critical value for the log likelihood test at the .01 level is 13.28; the test statistic equals 18.95.

12. As a set, the log likelihood ratio test indicates rejection of the null hypothesis at the .05 level. We also estimated several variants of these models. We considered variants using out-of-wedlock childbearing by the daughters when they were ≤ 19 and ≤ 17 as the dependent variables and variants using one dummy variable for early maternal fertility based on whether the mother had her first child while ≤ 19, ≤ 18, and ≤ 17. In addition, we considered each variant for the full sample and for separate subsamples of nonblacks and blacks. Tests for structural differences in the parameters for these equations and estimates based on subsamples of blacks and nonblacks rejected the null hypothesis of no structural differences. The chi-square test statistics for the second and third models are 26.5 and 37.25 and so reject the null hypothesis at, respectively, the .05 and .01 levels. The .05 critical value for model 2 is 25, and the .01 critical value for model 3 is 35. From these we learned that the relationship between the mother's early fertility and adolescent out-of-wedlock childbearing for the daughter is strongest for nonblacks. For example, we found the early-fertility dummies jointly statistically significant from zero for all three models when looking at out-of-wedlock childbearing at age ≤ 18 (with significance levels of .05, .05, and .04) and at age ≤ 17 (with significance levels of .012, .015, and .013). When one dummy variable for having an early-fertility mother is used in these equations, the estimated coefficient is also statistically significant. Estimates for out-of-wedlock childbearing at < 19 are jointly significantly different from zero only for the full sample using the first model, although for nonblacks several estimated coefficients on the dummy variables are individually statistically significant in each of the three models. For the subsample of blacks, the estimated coefficients on the dummy variables for early maternal fertility are not statistically significant in any of these estimations.

13. The test statistic for a log likelihood ratio test of the significance of the full early childbearing variables exceeds the critical value at the .01 level, leading to rejection of the null hypothesis that early fertility of the mother has no effect on the outcome of the child. The critical value for the log likelihood test at the .01 level is 13.28; the test statistic equals 15.07.

14. As a set, the log likelihood ratio test does not indicate rejection of the null hypothesis for model 2 or model 3. The log likelihood ratio test statistics for models 2 and 3 are both 5.9 and so would only be significant at the .2 level.

15. The weights on the PSID are intended to represent proportions of the U.S. population. Even though some coefficients are not statistically significant, they are our best predictor of the likely impact on children of the mother postponing her first birth. Nevertheless, the lack of significance reduces the confidence one should place on some of these results. One further caveat also applies: although we include a broad set of background factors of the mother, unobserved factors may still play a role. To the extent this is the case, our simulations may over- or underestimate the expected change caused by delay in childbearing.

16. Mothers who first gave birth while less than 15 years old tended to have other characteristics that put their children at a disadvantage. Hence, although delaying childbearing increases the probability of the children graduating, it does not mean the children will have as great a chance of graduating as the children of mothers in the other groups. For example, although delaying childbearing until age 20 or 21 raises the probability of mothers' children graduating from high school by 10.9 percentage points, this is less than the 17.5 percentage point difference in the probabilities of graduation for children in the different groups.

17. The simulated results for both blacks and nonblacks were also estimated based on equation estimations on these subsamples but are not shown here. Most of the coefficients relevant for simulating these results are not statistically significant for blacks, which may be attributable to small sample sizes in many of the age-at-first-birth categories.

18. See part 1 of this chapter for further details.

19. See also U.S. Census Bureau, Current Population Survey, March and Annual Social and Economic Supplements, 2005 and earlier, table MS-2, September 21, 2006, accessed at http://www.census.gov/population/socdemo/hh-fam/ms2.pdf.

20. More than half our sample is between 21 and 24 years old.

21. Havemen and colleagues use three measures: the average neighborhood adult unemployment rate, average state welfare benefits, and average public per capita family planning expenditures.

22. When neighborhood variables are included in the analysis of high school completion, the effect of a birth at age 15 or younger changes from −.392 to −.391, the effect of a birth at age 16–17 changes from −.244 to −.225, and the effect of a birth at age 18–19 changes from −.206 to −.219. For the analysis of a teen birth, the corresponding coefficient changes are .437 to .421, .373 to .341, and .291 to .270.

REFERENCES

Gold, Rachel Benson, and Sandra Guardado. 1988. "Public Funding of Family Planning, Sterilization and Abortion Services, 1987." *Family Planning Perspectives* 20(5): 228–33.

Gold, Rachel Benson, and Jennifer Macias. 1986. "Public Funding of Contraceptive, Sterilization and Abortion Services, 1985." *Family Planning Perspectives* 18(6): 259–64.

Gold, Rachel Benson, and Barry Nestor. 1985. "Public Funding of Contraceptive, Sterilization and Abortion Services, 1983." *Family Planning Perspectives* 17(1): 25–30.

National Center for Health Statistics. 2005. *Vital Statistics of the United States, 2002, Volume I, Natality.* Hyattsville, MD: National Center for Health Statistics. http://www.cdc.gov/nchs/datawh/statab/unpubd/natality/natab2002.htm.

Nestor, Barry. 1982. "Public Funding of Contraceptive Services, 1980–1982." *Family Planning Perspectives* 14(4): 198–203.

Orr, Margaret Terry, and Lynne Brenner. 1981. "Medical Funding of Family Planning Clinic Services." *Family Planning Perspectives* 13(6): 280–87.

Torres, Aida, and Jacqueline Darroch Forrest. 1983. "Family Planning Clinic Services in the United States, 1981." *Family Planning Perspectives* 15(6): 272–78.

Torres, Aida, Jacqueline Darroch Forrest, and Susan Eisman. 1981. "Family Planning Services in the United States, 1978–1979." *Family Planning Perspectives* 13(3): 132–41.

U.S. Bureau of the Census. 1987. *Statistical Abstract of the United States 1987.* 107th ed. Washington, DC: U.S. Government Printing Office.

———. 1993. *Statistical Abstract of the United States 1993.* 113th ed. Washington, DC: U.S. Government Printing Office.

———. 1994. *Statistical Abstract of the United States 1994.* 114th ed. Washington, DC: U.S. Government Printing Office.

10

The Costs of
Adolescent Childbearing

Rebecca A. Maynard and Saul D. Hoffman

Previous chapters in this book have focused on specific facets of the behavior, social circumstances, and economic transactions associated with adolescent childbearing. This chapter builds upon the earlier ones to examine the measurable costs attributable to adolescent childbearing—costs that could be avoided if all would-be teen parents delayed childbearing. Although this work builds on the estimates of the other studies in the volume, it does not represent a consensus view of the cost implications of the findings from these other studies. Rather, this chapter analyzes and interprets those findings independently.

Why include a cost chapter in a volume like this? The findings of the contributing authors for the preceding chapters speak for themselves about the important consequences of adolescent childbearing and the potential benefits of successful prevention efforts. This chapter summarily assesses the consequences of teen childbearing in terms that are easy for the public and for policymakers to understand and use. Policymakers and the public want to know how much adolescent childbearing and parenting is costing and, thus, what level of investment in prevention is warranted on economic grounds. Chapter 11 complements the findings in this chapter by showing how successful various common prevention strategies are likely to be.

When confronted with proposals for new programming to prevent adolescent parenting or to mitigate its consequences, policymakers in particular want some idea of the savings that could be achieved though such expenditures. Even practitioners are asking for summative data to answer such questions as the following: How much is the decision to have a baby as a teenager costing these women? Are teenagers making large financial sacrifices when they chose to have babies or do they actually make out financially? For completeness, the chapter also estimates the aggregate costs of teen childbearing from the broader social welfare perspective. How much is adolescent childbearing costing the nation as a whole—the teen parents and the rest of society combined?

There is no single "best" answer to these questions. However, this chapter provides the most complete picture of the costs (and, sometimes, benefits) of adolescent childbearing from various possible perspectives, given available data. To the extent possible, these estimates reflect the costs of adolescent childbearing itself, not costs attributable to other correlated factors, such as poverty.[1]

Deriving a comprehensive inventory of the costs of adolescent childbearing is an intricate enterprise. It depends on having reliable estimates of both observed outcomes for teen parents along many dimensions of their lives and what these outcomes would have been had the women delayed childbearing for some predefined period or until some specified age. This analysis focuses on the consequences of adolescent childbearing in four broad domains: economic productivity of the mothers, the fathers, and the children when they become adults; private transfers and taxes; public assistance from various sources; and other consequences, including children's health, welfare, and criminal behavior. In each case, the analysis judges the consequences of adolescent childbearing by comparing observed outcomes for teen mothers (as well as their spouses, the fathers of their children, and their children) with predicted outcomes assuming that these mothers delayed childbearing until age 20 to 21.

The particular consequences of adolescent childbearing are estimated from the perspectives of the teen parents, taxpayers, and society as a whole. Then, these individual cost components are aggregated following an analytic framework commonly applied in benefit-cost evaluations. This framework applies clearly defined assumptions about the period over which costs are measured, the rate of time preference or discounting, and the costs (or shadow prices) associated with various consequences of adolescent childbearing not measured directly in dollars.

As the preceding chapters make evident, estimating the myriad consequences of adolescent childbearing is complex, constrained by available data, and sensitive to assumptions about the alternative life courses for would-be teen parents if they delayed childbearing. How long would they delay? Under what circumstances would the delays occur? Would they delay childbearing but otherwise experience no changes in life circumstances or would the delay in childbearing be accompanied by improvements, for example, in perceived educational and career options or in the social and economic support available to them?

The main analysis relies on well-defined assumptions about these issues to produce benchmark estimates of the cost of adolescent childbearing. The benchmark cost estimates manipulate outcome estimates reported in the preceding chapters only as necessary to fit them into the cost accounting framework. They do not, for example, reflect omission of results for outcomes that failed standard tests for statistical significance. Nor are they adjusted upward or downward for possible biases due to limitations of the data or study methodologies. In order to judge the sensitivity of the analysis to these underlying assumptions, and even to some of the estimated impacts of adolescent childbearing that flow from the analysis reported in the earlier chapters, costs are re-estimated varying five key assumptions of the analysis, one at a time.

There are, of course, some potentially very important consequences of adolescent childbearing that cannot be readily measured or quantified. These include, for example, elevated risks of poor academic skills, social pressures associated with raising children as a single parent, and numerous developmental, educational, and social consequences for the children. The discussion includes commentary on the many consequences of adolescent childbearing identified in the *Kids Having Kids* research that are not explicitly included in the cost analysis. However, readers are left to make their own judgments regarding the significance of such outcomes in the context of the cost analysis findings.

Background

The framework for the analysis was shaped by an understanding of the major public concerns about adolescent childbearing: concern about poor educational outcomes for mothers and children, concern about single parenthood and self-sufficiency, and concern about child welfare. Judging by the data on observed outcomes for teen mothers and their children, these concerns are well founded.

Outcomes for Teen Parents and Their Children

Nearly half of all teen mothers never earn a high school diploma, and 30 percent do not even earn a General Education Development (GED) certificate. Only about 10 percent complete a two- or four-year college program by middle adulthood (table 10.1). By the time their oldest child is age 15, teen mothers will have had another 1.36 children, on average, despite the fact that they will have spent about 40 percent of these years as a single parent.

These young mothers have very low earnings, averaging just under $6,500 annually over their first 15 years of parenthood. Further, given the limited number of years they are married and their choice of marriage partners, their access to income from spouses is modest—averaging just under $12,000 annually. These combined factors mean that, on average, teen mothers are dependent on public assistance for about a third of their parenting years (an average of 4.7 of their first 15 years of parenthood). In addition, they rely heavily on noncash assistance—food stamps, public housing, and (not shown) medical assistance.

One great source of concern over adolescent childbearing relates to the young mothers' success as parents—a concern supported by the evidence of poor outcomes for children born to teen mothers. Twenty percent of the children of teen mothers are reported to have chronic health conditions, 10 percent are obese by their early teen years, and 14 percent of the girls will have a baby by age 18. Further, it is estimated that there will be 56 foster care placements for every 1,000 teen parents and that, on average, children of teen parents spend .93 years in prison.

In nearly all cases, outcomes for teenagers who have their first child before age 18 are considerably worse than are outcomes for those who have their first child at age 18 or 19 (table 10.1, columns 1 and 2). Not surprisingly, the most striking difference is in the educational attainment levels of younger and older teen parents and in the average number of years they spend as a single parent. Less than 40 percent of those who have their first child before age 18 earn a high school diploma, compared with 62 percent of those who have their first child at age 18 or 19, for example. And, younger teen parents spend an average of 8 of their first 15 years of parenthood single, compared with only 5 years for older teen parents. Not surprisingly given the differences in single parenthood and education between younger and older teen mothers, younger teen mothers are considerably more dependent on public assistance than are older teen mothers. Most

Table 10.1. Outcomes for Teen Parents and Predicted Outcomes if They Had Delayed Childbearing until Age 20 to 21

	Observed Outcomes for Teen Parents, by Age at First Birth			Predicted Outcomes if Delayed Childbearing until Age 20–21, by Age at First Birth		
	Under age 18	Age 18–19	Total under age 20	Under age 18	Age 18–19	Total under age 20
Education (15 years following first birth)						
High school diploma	39%	62%	54%	53%	72%	65%
High school diploma or GED	62%	74%	70%	61%	74%	69%
Completed two-year college	7%	10%	9%	15%	20%	18%
Completed four-year college	2%	3%	2%	4%	7%	6%
Household composition (15 years following first birth)						
Number of children	2.37	2.35	2.36	1.97	2.45	2.27
Years as single parent	8.12	5.17	6.28	6.79	5.05	5.70
Earned income (average annual over 15 years following first birth)						
Mother's earnings	$5,884	$6,773	$6,439	$7,762	$6,109	$6,729
Spouse's earnings	$9,070	$13,653	$11,932	$8,536	$16,022	$13,211
Public assistance (15 years following first birth)						
Years on cash assistance	5.91	3.95	4.69	6.40	4.66	5.31
Cash assistance (average annual)	$2,076	$1,310	$1,598	$2,418	$1,609	$1,913
Years on food stamps	4.74	3.40	3.90	5.86	4.54	5.04

(continued)

Table 10.1. *(Continued)*

	Observed Outcomes for Teen Parents, by Age at First Birth			Predicted Outcomes if Delayed Childbearing until Age 20–21, by Age at First Birth		
	Under age 18	Age 18–19	Total under age 20	Under age 18	Age 18–19	Total under age 20
Food stamp benefits (average annual)	$743	$533	$612	$919	$712	$790
Years in public housing	1.80	1.19	1.42	1.58	1.41	1.47
Outcomes for children						
Chronic health condition	21%	20%	20%	19%	19%	19%
Obesity (age 12–16)	9%	11%	10%	13%	13%	13%
High school completion	66%	78%	73%	73%	81%	78%
Birth by age 18	13%	15%	14%	9%	9%	9%
Foster care placements per 1,000 teen mothers	73.87	44.82	55.73	40.68	40.66	40.67
Years adolescent and adult male children are incarcerated	1.35	0.67	0.93	0.98	0.66	0.78
Births to teenagers (2004)[a]						
Total	140,761	281,282	422,043	140,761	281,282	422,043
First births	126,471	210,312	336,783	126,471	210,312	336,783

Sources: These data are based on the results reported in chapters 3 through 9 and on special tabulations prepared by the authors of those chapters. The predicted outcomes had the teen mothers delayed childbearing until age 20 to 21 are based on multivariate estimation models that control for demographic and background characteristics of the mothers.

Notes: Outcomes for teen parents are unadjusted means. Consult the individual chapters for the details regarding databases and analytic methods used to generate the estimates and for descriptions of the control variables included in the estimation models.

a. Data are from Martin et al. (2006), table 2.

striking of all are the large differences in the foster care placement rates and years of incarceration for children born to women who begin childbearing before age 18 compared with those who have their first child at age 18 or 19. Children of young teen parents spend twice as much time in prison (1.35 versus .67 years) and are 1.6 times more likely to be placed in foster care than are children born to women who begin childbearing at age 18 or 19.

Predicted Outcomes if Childbearing Is Delayed until Age 20 to 21

If all would-be teen mothers could be induced to delay childbearing until their early 20s, they and their children still face outcomes that are less than optimal, albeit considerably better along many dimensions than those experienced by teen mothers (table 10.1, columns 4–6). Only 65 percent of these mothers are expected to complete high school, a rate 11 percentage points higher than that observed for teen mothers. Although only 6 percent will complete a four-year college education, this is three times as large as the observed rate among teen mothers. Mothers who delay childbearing would spend over a third of their first 15 years of parenthood single, living with combined average annual earnings from their labor and that of their spouse of about $20,000. While slightly better off than they would be as teen parents, the mothers still will be highly dependant on public assistance. In fact, it is predicted that if these mothers delayed childbearing until their early 20s, they would draw down more, not less, public assistance than they would have had they given birth as teens.

In virtually all areas examined, the predicted outcomes for children of would-be teen mothers who delay childbearing are better than those observed for children of teen mothers. However, some outcomes are still problematic. Nearly 20 percent of children have chronic health conditions, 13 percent are obese in adolescence, and less than 80 percent will graduate from high school. There will be an estimated 41 foster care placements per 1,000 mothers among this group, and their children can expect to experience a combined average of .78 years in prison.

Notably, as was the case with observed outcomes, the predicted child outcomes tend to be substantially worse among would-be younger teen mothers—those who first give birth before they turn 18. In several cases, most of the overall difference between the observed outcomes for teen parents and the predicted outcomes had they delayed childbearing comes from differences in the observed and predicted outcomes for younger teen mothers. For example, if women who have their first child at age 18 to 19 were induced to delay childbearing until their early 20s, it is predicted that they would have slightly more children and spend slightly more time on public assistance, and their children would be expected to spend about the same amount of time in prison. In contrast, if those who have children before age 18 were induced to delay childbearing until their early 20s, on average, they would be expected to have substantially fewer children (1.97 versus 2.37), spend less time in public housing (1.6 versus 1.8 years), and with few exceptions witness better outcomes for their children—higher graduation rates (73 versus 66 percent), lower teen birth rates (9 versus 13 percent), and less time incarcerated among males (.98 versus 1.35 years).

Who Bears the Costs of Adolescent Childbearing

The economic costs of adolescent childbearing are borne by the taxpayers and by the rest of society, not by the teen mothers themselves.[2] Over their first 15 years of parenthood, women who give birth before age 18 can expect to have net incomes from all sources (including various forms of public assistance) that average just under $1,700 more annually than would be expected if they delayed childbearing until age 20 to 21. In contrast, those who become parents at age 18 or 19 have average net incomes that are just over $300 more a year than would be expected if they delayed childbearing (figure 10.1).

In a steady state with the annual number of first-time teen mothers mirroring the 2004 level of 336,783, the average annual cost to U.S. taxpayers of teen childbearing is an estimated $7.3 billion annually or $1,445 per teen mother (figure 10.2).[3] A major source of these costs is the forgone income and consumption taxes resulting from the lower earnings of the teen mothers and the fathers of their children ($3 billion). However, even larger costs are associated with the poor social and economic outcomes for children born to teen mothers. As a result of their lower productivity, children born to teen parents contribute an estimated $2.5 billion less annually in income and consumption taxes than if their mothers delayed childbearing. In addition, teen childbearing results in an estimated $1.58 billion more annually in taxpayer expenditures for medical assistance of children, $2 billion more to support foster care costs, and $1.84 billion more to build and maintain prisons.

Figure 10.1. Economic Consequences of Adolescent Childbearing over the First 15 Years of Parenthood (average annual economic resources, $2004)

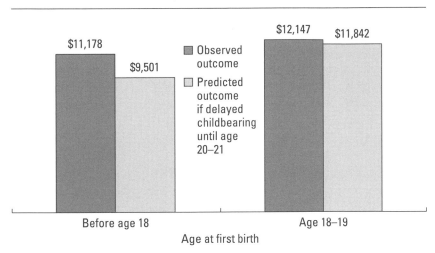

Source: Authors' calculations based on data from chapters 3–9, this volume.

Figure 10.2. Aggregate Annual Costs (or Benefits) of Adolescent Childbearing to Taxpayers and to Society (billions of $2004)

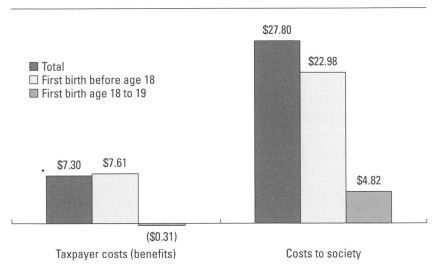

Source: Authors' calculations based on data from chapters 3–9, this volume.

The costs to society are estimated to be nearly four times as large as those borne by taxpayers—$5,502 per teen mother a year. This means that, in a steady state, if all would-be teen mothers would delay childbearing until their early 20s, society would have nearly $28 billion annually to direct to other uses (figure 10.2). Most (about 80 percent) of this sum would derive from the higher productivity of fathers of the children born to teen mothers and the higher productivity of the children themselves. However, the mothers' productivity also would be higher, and fewer resources would be diverted for children's health care needs, foster care, and incarceration of juvenile and adult offenders.

Analytic Approach to Measuring the Costs

The cost analysis rests on three key sets of assumptions and design decisions. One set relates to the particular measured economic consequences of adolescent childbearing considered. These are bounded by the scope of the core studies reported in previous chapters. The second set concerns the question: from whose perspective are costs and benefits measured—that of teen parents, that of taxpayers, or that of society as a whole? The third set of assumptions relates to the particular counterfactual condition against which the outcomes for the teen parents are judged. For example, if a would-be teen mother delays childbearing, what do we assume about her future? Does it look like that of the average mother or that of a typical young woman who gives birth at a particular older age, such as 20 or 21? Does the analysis assume that childbearing is delayed but that nothing else changes, or does it assume that the same policies that induced a delay in childbearing also would address other sources of poor outcomes for teen mothers?

The Measured Economic Consequences

The measured economic consequences of adolescent childbearing fall into three broad categories.[4] The first relates to the productivity of the mothers, their spouses (who often are not the fathers of mothers' first children), the fathers of their children (whether or not they are married to the mothers), and their children in adulthood. The studies measure directly the effects of adolescent childbearing on income from employment and productivity of the mothers, their spouses, and the fathers of their babies (see chapter 3, part 2, and chapter 4 in this volume). However, the consequences of adolescent childbearing on the productivity of children during their adult years are based on the predicted impacts of teen parenthood on the educational attainment of children (chapter 9, part 2 in this volume) combined with estimates of the predicted lifetime earnings for workers with different educational attainment levels.[5] These estimated effects on earnings then provide the basis for estimating the impacts of adolescent childbearing on private transfers (child support) and consumption and other taxes.[6]

The second category of economic consequences is public assistance received by the mothers for themselves and their children. The study measures directly the value of cash and near-cash assistance programs, like Temporary Assistance for Needy Families (TANF) and food stamps (chapter 3, part 2). Families receiving cash assistance through TANF also tend to receive considerable other support, including employment and support services such as child care and transportation. In fiscal year 2002, for every dollar of cash assistance, 8.4 cents were spent under TANF on employment-related services such as child care and transportation.[7] The number of years parents lived in public housing was estimated directly from national survey data. The cost of public housing subsidies was computed based on these estimates and published data on the approximate dollar value of the average subsidy level.[8]

Estimates of the consequences of adolescent childbearing on health care subsidies for children were estimated using the Medical Expenditure Panel Survey data (chapter 6 in this volume). These costs include the per child estimated costs paid through public programs, primarily Medicaid and the State Children's Health Insurance Program (SCHIP).[9] In estimating the net costs of adolescent childbearing on public expenditures for children's health care, we adjusted the data to reflect the observed and predicted fertility rates of mothers (see table 10.1).

The administrative costs of public assistance are estimated from national budget information for the TANF, Food Stamp, and Medicaid programs. Published data indicate that, for every dollar of TANF benefits, 10.1 cents are spent administering the program; for every dollar spent on food stamp benefits, 11.6 cents are spent on administration; and for every dollar of medical assistance through Medicaid, 5.1 cents are spent on administration.[10]

The third category of outcomes includes three other important consequences of adolescent childbearing: (1) out-of-pocket costs of children's health care, (2) costs associated with foster care placement of children, and (3) costs of incarcerating adolescent and adult offenders.

Adolescent childbearing affects both the mother's fertility and the health of her children, thereby affecting both overall use of medical care and the allocation of those costs between taxpayers (primarily Medicaid) and parents (out-of-pocket costs). The per child consequences of teen childbearing for out-of-pocket health care costs for children are measured directly (chapter 6 in this volume). These estimates are combined with estimated effects of adolescent childbearing on fertility (table 10.1) to generate estimated child health–related costs of adolescent childbearing and to allocate those costs between teen parents and taxpayers.

As noted above, adolescent childbearing substantially elevates the likelihood that children will be placed in foster care. The cost analysis uses estimates of the consequence of teen childbearing on the likelihood of a foster care placement for children born in Illinois between 1989 and 1998 (chapter 7 in this volume) combined with estimates of changes in family size (table 10.1) and published data on the average annual cost of supporting foster children to calculate an estimate for the total foster care costs associated with teen childbearing.[11]

The cost of incarceration is estimated based on the estimated net effect of adolescent childbearing on the number of years male children of teen mothers spend in jail (chapter 8, part 2 in this volume) and the costs per inmate of building and maintaining prisons. It is not possible to estimate directly the impact of teen parenting on prison time for female children because of their low representation among the prison population (about 7 percent). In recognition of this, the unit cost applied to the incarceration results for males is the ratio of total annual costs of building and maintaining prisons to the number of male inmates ($23,940).[12] By applying this figure to estimates of the incarceration years estimated for males, the resulting total cost estimate pertains to males and females, assuming that adolescent childbearing affects the incarceration time of male and female children proportionally.

Accounting Perspectives

These various outcome measures have been arrayed in a framework that makes it possible to aggregate the costs and compare them across the three perspectives (table 10.2). The framework indicates whether a positive measured difference between the predicted outcome if would-be teen mothers

Table 10.2. Analytic Framework for the Cost Analysis

	Impact of a Positive Difference between the Predicted Outcome if Adolescent Childbearing Were Delayed and the Observed Outcome for:		
	Teen mothers	Taxpayers	Society
Productivity			
Mother's earnings	Gain	Neutral	Gain
Spouse's earnings	Gain	Neutral[a]	Neutral
Father's earnings	Neutral	Neutral	Gain
Earnings of young adult children	Neutral	Neutral	Gain
Private transfers and taxes			
Child support	Gain	Neutral	Neutral
Mother's income and consumption taxes	Loss	Gain	Neutral
Spouse's income and consumption taxes	Loss	Neutral[a]	Neutral
Father's income and consumption taxes	Neutral	Gain	Neutral
Income and consumption taxes of adult children	Neutral	Gain	Neutral
Public assistance			
Cash assistance	Gain	Loss	Neutral
Employment and support services	Neutral	Loss	Loss
Food stamp benefits	Gain	Loss	Neutral
Rent subsidies	Gain	Loss	Neutral
Medical assistance for parents	Gain	Loss	Neutral
Medical assistance for children	Neutral	Loss	Loss
Administrative costs of public assistance programs	Neutral	Loss	Loss
Other consequences			
Out-of-pocket cost of children's health care	Loss	Neutral	Loss
Foster care of minor children	Neutral	Loss	Loss
Incarceration of adolescent and adult children	Neutral	Loss	Loss

[a]This framework assumes that changes in spouses' earnings, as distinct from those of fathers of children born to teen mothers, represent shifts in the allocation among families rather than net changes in the productivity and tax revenues. That portion of the spouses' earnings difference that is linked to productivity effects associated with teen childbearing is assumed to be picked up in the estimated changes to the fathers' earnings and taxes.

delayed childbearing and the observed outcome should be viewed as a gain, a loss, or neutral from the particular perspective—that of teen mothers themselves, that of taxpayers, or that of society at large. The component costs and benefits are organized into four clusters: (1) productivity effects as measured by earnings of mothers, their spouses, the fathers of their children (who often are not married to them), and their children; (2) private transfers and taxes, including child support paid by noncustodial fathers and income and consumption taxes associated with the productivity effects; (3) public assistance, including cash assistance, food stamps, rent subsidies, and medical assistance; and (4) other consequences, including out-of-pocket costs of children's health care, costs of foster care for minor children, and incarceration costs for adolescent and adult children.

This framework does not incorporate various consequences of adolescent childbearing that are less easily measured in dollars but are important for the health and well-being of individuals and of society. Some of these were discussed above, and others are reported in several preceding chapters in this book. Further, the chapter does not look at the *overall* economic consequences from the perspectives of the fathers of children born to teen mothers, the mothers' spouses, or the children themselves. Yet, these other outcomes are clearly important and should be considered in conjunction with the cost analysis results reported below.

Measuring the Component Costs (or Benefits) for Teen Mothers

The economic consequences of adolescent childbearing for teen mothers span all four categories (table 10.2). The central factors relate to their own earnings and those of their spouses. These earnings, in turn, drive their tax liabilities and their entitlement to and receipt of public assistance, including cash assistance, food stamps, public housing, rent subsidies, and health care subsidies for the mother and her children.[13] In addition, to the extent that adolescent childbearing affects earnings of the fathers and the likelihood that birth parents live apart from one another, child support enters the calculus.[14] Finally, adolescent childbearing affects the out-of-pocket costs of children's health care through its effects on the mothers' fertility rates, health care needs of children, and children's eligibility for medical assistance.

This framework ignores some potentially important consequences of adolescent childbearing for the parents. It largely ignores possible impacts on their access to educational and training resources, such as student financial aid and publicly funded job training. Only the small amount of such assistance directly linked with cash assistance is incorporated into the estimates (see further below). The framework also ignores adverse social consequences of teen childbearing, including those generally associated with measured outcomes, such as lower school completion rates, higher proportions of time spent in single parenthood, and larger family sizes (see table 10.1). Then, too, it ignores the social and psychological costs associated with the poorer home environments and developmental outcomes for children (see chapter 5, both parts of chapter 8, and both parts of chapter 9 in this volume). It also could be argued that this framework ignores social-psychological benefits of teen parenthood to the mothers. For example, if having a baby brings joy and love to an otherwise unhappy or lonely young woman, there may be important personal pleasures associated with teen childbearing.[15]

There are three steps in measuring the average economic costs of adolescent childbearing for mothers. The first is to estimate the difference between the outcomes observed for teen mothers over the first 15 years of parenthood and the predicted outcomes for these same women had they delayed childbearing until age 20 to 21. The second step is to discount these costs to the year of the first child's birth. Future costs and benefits are discounted at 5 percent annually for the main analysis. The third step is to sum the component costs.

Measuring the Costs to Taxpayers

The taxpayers' costs of adolescent childbearing are affected by tax revenues, public assistance liabilities, and costs of child welfare and criminal justice. To the extent that adolescent childbearing affects the productivity (as measured by earnings) of teen mothers, the fathers of their children, and the adult children themselves, it is expected to have similar proportional effects on income and consumption tax receipts to federal, state, and local governments.[16] Similarly, adolescent childbearing is expected to affect both the economic needs of families (for example, by affecting family size and medical care needs) and the ability of families to meet these needs through their own earnings. As a result, teen parenting also will affect the level of public assistance to families and costs to taxpayers of administering the programs. Finally, taxpayers bear the economic costs associated with adverse developmental and social consequences for children born to teen parents, particularly those that necessitate intervention by child welfare (foster care) and criminal justice (incarceration).

The framework ignores certain potentially relevant costs to taxpayers that either were not measured in the *Kids Having Kids* research or do not lend themselves to conversion to dollar values. For example, changes in the demand for secondary education and publicly funded higher education are not considered. So, too, the higher levels of learning disabilities and social problems among children of teen mothers have implications for educational and social service costs that are not captured by this framework (see chapter 5). Beyond the direct costs of foster care placement and incarceration, the analysis ignores financial and social costs to taxpayers associated with social deviance and child abuse and neglect.

Measuring the Costs to Society

The costs of adolescent childbearing to society include only those consequences that represent real changes in the resources available for consumption by the population at large. These include changes in the productivity of the teen mothers, the fathers of their children, and their adult children; changes in the level of resources devoted to administering public assistance (but not public assistance costs themselves); changes in the costs of employment and support services; and changes in the level of medical care provided to children. They also include those child welfare and criminal justice costs associated with higher foster care and incarceration rates for children born to teen mothers. Changes that are purely distributional, such as cash assistance and food stamps, affect who benefits from society's resources but not the overall resources available for sharing.

The framework ignores several potentially important social cost factors. Most notably, it ignores the costs of child welfare services other than foster care and the costs of property damage and personal injuries likely to accompany the higher incarceration rates among children of teen mothers.

The Comparison Scenario for the Analysis

This analysis includes estimated costs (and benefits) for all teen mothers. In 2004, there were 140,761 births to mothers younger than age 18. Of these births, nearly all resulted from unintended pregnancies, more than 90 percent were to unmarried women, and 90 percent were first births (chapter 2 in this volume). In this same year, there were 281,282 births to 18- or 19-year-olds, of which about 66 percent were unintended, 80 percent were to unmarried women, and 75 percent were first births.

The analysis reports separately the results for those having their first child before age 18 and for those having their first child at age 18 or 19. The reasons relate to differences in the physical and emotional maturity of younger and older teens, differences in the social support systems for these two groups of parents, differences in whether these young women would have had an opportunity to complete high school, and differences in the nature of prevention service options for the two groups

For both younger and older teen mothers, the comparison scenario (counterfactual) for the analysis is teens with similar background characteristics who delayed childbearing until age 20 or 21. The younger group averages 16.5 years old when they have their first children, which means that the cost estimates assume an average delay in childbearing of about four years. In contrast, for 18- to 19-year-old mothers, the cost estimates assume an average delay of only two years.

This common comparison scenario balances the goal of using a counterfactual condition with social significance and one that is potentially achievable through public policies. Age 20 to 21 is three to four years younger than the current average age of first birth and two to four years older than the average age of first births among teen mothers. Aspiring to achieve longer delays in childbearing seems unrealistic, even through extreme strategies. However, given the importance of education (including both high school completion and some type of postsecondary training) for economic success, it seems a reasonable aspiration. Also, in light of the fact that birth rates among teenagers have been trending downward for more than a decade, such a goal may be within reach.

The results reported in this chapter reflect the best estimates of the measured costs (or benefits) of having a child before age 18 or between age 18 and 19 relative to delaying childbearing until age 20 or 21. They account for the fact that certain characteristics and life circumstances of would-be teen mothers are unlikely to be affected through policies aimed at delaying their childbearing. For this reason, the analysis focuses on the question: what are the costs of teen childbearing relative to a world in which all would-be teen parents had their first child at age 20 or 21 and nothing else changed in their lives? The statistical models underlying these estimates do the best job possible through observational research of isolating the impacts of adolescent childbearing from other factors that may account for the observed outcome.[17] As such, results reported seem reasonable estimates of the gains expected from policies that delay childbearing through abstinence promotion or contraceptive education and access initiatives. The results likely underestimate the potential benefits to policies or programs that delay childbearing through more complex, comprehensive interventions that potentially would improve the home, school, and community environments of children.

Other Basic Assumptions of the Cost Analysis

Two other sets of assumptions went into the cost estimates. The first set pertains to the time frame for the analysis and the cohort size. The second set concerns the discount rate and the use of longitudinal estimates to generate current-year estimates for various cohorts of adolescent mothers.

The Cohort Size and Time Horizon

The analysis projects forward from the present assuming that, in the absence of significant policy shifts, future cohorts of adolescent parents will be the same size as that projected for 2004. This assumption predicts 336,783 new teen mothers annually—38 percent of whom are younger than 18 when they have their first child.

In measuring the costs from the perspective of the teen mothers, the analysis uses a 15-year time horizon, beginning with the birth of the first child.[18] The decision to focus on a 15-year time horizon was driven, in part, by the fact that several key studies (especially those measuring outcomes for the mothers and the health care costs for the children) have limited or no data beyond this time frame. However, the first 15 years of parenthood also are arguably the most important for the developmental well-being of the children of teen parents. Appendix table A.10.1 reports the discounted outcomes and the estimated impacts that feed into the estimated costs for teen mothers.

When measuring costs from the perspective of taxpayers and society, in contrast, the analysis refers to aggregate costs in a given calendar year, 2004. These annual aggregate estimates assume a steady-state world in which cohort size, birth rates to teenagers, and the marginal consequences of adolescent childbearing are constant over time. The estimates include the current-year costs for the cohort of first-time teen mothers, their spouses, and the fathers of their children; the second-year costs for a similarly sized cohort who first gave birth a year ago; and so forth for 15 cohorts.

In addition, the taxpayer and social costs include the current-year costs associated with outcomes for children born to teen mothers. These include costs of incarcerating adolescent and young adult children born to women who had their first child as a teenager, the costs associated with the lifetime lower work productivity of adult children born to mothers who began childbearing as teens, and the costs associated with higher numbers of children in foster care in their first 18 years.[19] Appendix table A.10.2 presents the average annual value (undiscounted) of outcomes and estimated impacts that feed into the cost analysis for taxpayers and for society at large.

Discount Rate

Throughout this analysis, we assume that the teen mothers discount future income and costs at a rate of 5 percent annually. However, discounting is not relevant for the taxpayer and social costs estimates. Rather, steady-state cost estimates for taxpayers and for society are generated by multiplying the average cumulative undiscounted cost (benefit) associated with outcomes by the annual number of first-time teen mothers. For example, the difference between the 15-year total undiscounted value of earnings observed for the average teen mother and the predicted values for her had she delayed childbearing until age 20 to 21 is equivalent to the estimated current-year loss in productivity for the average teen parent in each of 15 cohorts: the teen parent who had her first child in 2004, the teen parent who had her first child in 2003, and so forth, up to the average teen mother who had her first child in 1990. Similarly, the aggregate (undiscounted) productivity loss for adult children over a 43-year work life is used to represent current year's productivity loss associated with adult earnings for children of 43 teen mothers, each in a different year of parenthood. Finally, the aggregate 18-year costs per teen mother associated with higher foster care placements and incarceration rates can be viewed as representing the current-year costs for 18 teen mothers, each in a different year of parenthood.[20]

Costs and Benefits for the Mothers

On average, the net present value of measured income to teen parents from all sources is very low. For both younger and older teen mothers, it is higher than predicted for these same mothers had they delayed childbearing until their early 20s (table 10.3). Teen parents who have their first child before age 18 have measured economic resources over their first 15 years of parenthood of just over $167,000 or an average of $11,178 a year. For their counterparts who delay childbearing until age 18 or 19, the picture is only slightly better. The net present value for them over 15 years of parenthood is $182,205 or an average of just over $12,000 a year.[21] Both groups of teen mothers are predicted to lose slightly if they delay childbearing—younger teens by an average of $1,677 a year and older teens by an average of $305 a year.

For younger teen mothers, their own earnings are slightly lower than expected had they delayed childbearing ($3,883 compared with $4,369 a year). However, their access to earnings of spouses is an estimated $1,300 more per year ($6,210 versus $4,913). The pattern for older teen mothers is the opposite: their own earnings are higher than if they delayed childbearing ($4,161 versus $3,454 a year), and their spouses' earnings are slightly lower than predicted had they delayed childbearing ($8,720 versus $9,177 a year).

There are very modest differences in private transfers and taxes. So, too, the net present value of public assistance benefits teen parents receive is small in absolute size ($2,000 to $3,000 annually) but a sizeable portion of their total income. Finally, the poorer quality of their children's health does not add to their economic burden. The net present value of out-of-pocket health care costs for their children averages only about $553 a year for younger teen mothers and $730 for older teen mothers. For both groups, if they were to delay childbearing, they would incur slightly higher out-of-pocket costs—an estimated $5 a year in the case of the younger teen mothers and an average of $74 a year for the older mothers.

There is considerable room for teen mothers to improve their economic well-being. However, the evidence presented in this volume suggests that delaying childbearing alone is not the way for these women to advance their position.

Importantly, other consequences of teen childbearing may adversely affect mothers. Notably, the children of younger teen mothers consistently experience worse outcomes than would be expected if their mothers had delayed childbearing until their early 20s. For example, children are more likely to experience poor academic outcomes, engage in risk-taking behaviors, become a teen parent, and become incarcerated (chapter 5 and chapter 8, part 2 in this volume).

Table 10.3. Economic Outcomes for Teen Mothers and Predicted Outcomes if They Delayed Childbearing until Age 20–21 (discounted to the first year of parenthood)

	First Birth before Age 18 ($2004)			First Birth Age 18–19 ($2004)		
	Observed outcome	Predicted outcome if delayed	Cost of teen childbearing	Observed outcome	Predicted outcome if delayed	Cost of teen childbearing
Productivity (average annual value total)	10,092	9,282	(810)	12,881	12,631	(250)
Mother's earnings	3,883	4,369	486	4,161	3,454	(707)
Spouse's earnings	6,210	4,913	(1,296)	8,720	9,177	457
Private transfers and taxes (average annual value total)	5,232	3,378	(1,854)	2,462	1,909	(553)
Child support	199	170	(29)	266	611	344
Mother's income and consumption taxes	(905)	(1,018)	(113)	(970)	(805)	165
Spouse's income and consumption taxes	(1,448)	(1,145)	302	(2,033)	(2,139)	(106)
Public assistance (average annual value)	3,792	2,771	(1,021)	2,732	2,427	(306)
Cash assistance	1,497	861	(636)	1,404	967	(437)
Food stamp benefits	542	548	5	355	429	74
Medical assistance for parents	1,123	911	(213)	588	611	23
Rent subsidies	629	452	(178)	385	420	35
Other consequences (average annual value)						
Out-of-pocket cost of children's health care	(553)	(558)	(5)	(730)	(882)	(152)
Net present value per parent						
Average annual value	11,178	9,501	(1,677)	12,147	11,842	(305)
Value over 15 years of parenthood	167,674	142,516	(25,158)	182,205	177,631	(4,574)

Source: Component cost estimates are reported in appendix table A.10.1. The sources and methods used to calculate them are detailed in appendix A.10.

Notes: Negative numbers are in parentheses. Positive values of the observed and predicted outcomes denote income to the teenage mother and negative values for the observed and predicted outcomes represent outlays. Positive differences in the two "cost to teen parent" columns denote economic costs to the mothers associated with adolescent childbearing, whereas negative differences denote net benefits to the mothers as a result of having children at a young age.

Costs for Taxpayers

The net taxpayer (public) expenditures attributable to adolescent child-bearing for services to current and former teen parents total roughly $7.3 billion annually (table 10.4). This amounts to an average cost of just under $1,500 per teen mother a year.

Table 10.4. Estimated Annual Costs (or Benefits) to Taxpayers of Adolescent Childbearing, by Age at First Birth (billions $2004, except where noted)

	Age at First Birth		
	Under age 18	Age 18–19	Total
Private transfers and taxes (total annual value)	4.40	1.07	5.46
Mother's income and consumption taxes	0.83	(0.49)	0.34
Father's income and consumption taxes	1.54	1.08	2.62
Income and consumption taxes of adult children	2.03	0.47	2.50
Public assistance (total annual value)	(0.15)	(1.85)	(2.00)
Cash assistance	(0.65)	(0.94)	(1.59)
Employment and support services	(0.05)	(0.08)	(0.13)
Food stamp benefits	(0.33)	(0.56)	(0.90)
Rent subsidies	0.20	(0.34)	(0.14)
Medical assistance for parents	(0.05)	(0.47)	(0.52)
Medical assistance for children	0.85	0.73	1.58
Administrative costs of public assistance	(0.11)	(0.19)	(0.30)
Other consequences (total annual value)	3.36	0.48	3.83
Foster care of minor children	1.65	0.34	2.00
Incarceration of adolescent and adult children	1.71	0.13	1.84
Total	7.61	(0.31)	7.30
Average per teen parent per year (2004$)	4,010	(98)	1,445

Sources: The undiscounted average annual costs and benefits per teenage parent are reported in appendix table A.10.2. The sources and methods used for generating these component cost estimates are described in appendix A.10.

Notes: Positive values denote net costs associated with adolescent childbearing; negative values, which are in parentheses, denote net benefits associated with adolescent childbearing. Earnings-related outcomes, health care costs, and costs of incarceration reflect current-year aggregated costs over 15 cohorts of teen mothers. Foster care costs are aggregated costs over 18 cohorts; costs related to employment and earnings of children of teen mothers are aggregated over 43 cohorts.

Importantly, however, all the taxpayer burden of adolescent childbearing derives from costs incurred on behalf of women who have their first child before age 18; there is a small net benefit ($.31 million annually) to taxpayers associated with early childbearing among older teen mothers. Childbearing before age 18 is estimated to result in more than $4 billion a year in lost tax revenue because of the lower economic productivity of mothers, the fathers of their children, and the children themselves when they reach adulthood. The lost tax revenues that result from lower earnings of mothers who have children before 18 total an estimated $830 million a year; losses associated with lower productivity of the fathers of their children total $1.54 billion a year, and losses associated with lower productivity of their adult children total $2.03 billion. The aggregate impact on public assistance expenditures of young adolescent childbearing is modest—only $150 million annually—for cash assistance, employment and support services, food stamps, medical assistance, and program administrative costs. Finally, nearly half the net costs to taxpayers of young teen childbearing is associated with the added costs associated with the higher number of children in foster care and the net impact on the prison population. According to the study results, an estimated $1.65 billion in foster care costs and $1.71 billion in criminal justice–related costs could be avoided each year in a steady state, if there were a way to induce all would-be young teen parents to delay childbearing until they reached age 20 or 21.

Based on the findings reported in previous chapters, encouraging would-be older teens to delay childbearing until their early 20s will have no benefit to taxpayers. The modest tax revenue gains from higher productivity by fathers and adult children are partially offset by productivity losses by mothers. And, the modest sums associated with reductions in foster care placements and prison terms for adolescent and adult children would be more than offset by higher public assistance costs.

Costs for Society

Society at large is predicted to incur large costs associated with adolescent childbearing, whether the mothers begin having children before age 18 or after. On average, society is estimated to incur over $5,500 in costs annually for each teen parent, or nearly $28 billion annually (table 10.5). The vast majority (over 80 percent) of the costs are associated with the 38 percent of teen mothers who have their first child at age 18 or younger. In

Table 10.5. Estimated Annual Costs (or Benefits) to Society of Teenage Childbearing, by Age at First Birth (billions $2004, except where noted)

	Age at First Birth		
	Under age 18	Age 18–19	Total
Productivity (total annual value)	18.85	4.58	23.43
Mother's earnings	3.56	(2.10)	1.47
Father's earnings	6.60	4.65	11.25
Earnings of adult children	8.69	2.02	10.71
Public assistance (total annual value)	0.80	0.59	1.38
Employment and support services	0.05	0.05	0.10
Medical assistance for children	0.85	0.73	1.58
Administrative costs of public assistance programs	(0.11)	(0.19)	(0.30)
Other consequences (total annual value)	1.62	(0.48)	1.14
Out-of-pocket cost of children's health care	(0.03)	(0.82)	(0.86)
Foster care of minor children	1.65	0.34	2.00
Incarceration of adolescent and adult children	1.71	0.13	1.84
Total	22.98	4.82	27.79
Average per teen parent per year (2004$)	12,112	1,527	5,502

Sources: The undiscounted average costs and benefits per teenage parent a year are reported in appendix table A.10.2. The sources and methods used for generating these component cost estimates are described in appendix A.10.

Notes: Positive values denote net costs associated with adolescent childbearing; negative values, which are in parentheses, denote net benefits associated with adolescent childbearing. Earnings-related outcomes, health care costs, and costs of incarceration reflect current-year aggregated costs over 15 cohorts of teen mothers. Foster care costs are aggregated costs over 18 cohorts; costs related to employment and earnings of children of teen mothers are aggregated over 43 cohorts.

addition, most of the costs (80 percent) derive from the productivity losses of fathers of the children born to teen mothers and of the children themselves.

For younger teen mothers, their lost productivity adds about $3.56 billion to the total annual costs, foster care costs add $1.65 billion a year, costs associated with the higher rates of incarceration among adolescent and adult children add $1.71 billion a year, and higher medical care usage for children adds over $850 million to the costs.

Society benefits from higher productivity levels among teen mothers than would be expected if they delayed childbearing—a result that appears to derive from these mothers entering the workforce earlier in their parenting years than would be expected if they delayed childbearing. Total consumption of health care for children is only slightly higher for older teen mothers than if they delayed childbearing. However, having a child at age 18 or 19 relative to delaying until age 20 or 21 means that the parents incur higher medical care costs out of pocket for care of their children. Consistent with the fact that adolescent childbearing has smaller impacts on foster care placements and rates of incarceration for children of older teen mothers than for younger teen mothers, the estimated foster care and incarceration costs to society associated with childbearing among older teens is substantially smaller—$340 million and $130 million, respectively.

Sensitivity Analysis

Because no two analysts would have chosen the same assumptions in generating cost estimates like this, it is useful to examine the sensitivity of the bottom-line estimates to various alternative assumptions.[22] Specifically, the costs are re-examined under the following alternative assumptions:

1. The productivity effects for mothers, fathers, spouses, and children are only half those estimated. Productivity effects are relevant to the cost estimates for all three reference groups—teen parents, taxpayers, and society. All four sets of productivity estimates are generated from models that may not have fully controlled for selection effects. In addition, the results for fathers of children born to teen mothers could not be re-estimated using more recent data than those used in the 1997 edition of this book.

2. Teen mothers discount future income at 7.5 percent annually, rather than the 5 percent used in the benchmark estimates. For this study, the discount rate affects only the outcomes from the mothers' perspective. Arguably, teen mothers, as with all youth, might have higher discount rates that the 5 percent rate commonly used in benefit cost analyses.

3. Total criminal justice–related costs are twice as high as the direct costs of incarceration, which are the only crime-related costs included in our benchmark estimates. Examples of other costs include those associated with things like policing, property damage, probation, and parole.

4. Only the first 15 years of productivity gains for adult children born to adolescent children matter. Projected productivity gains for 43 cohorts of adolescent parents include costs incurred well beyond a time frame of relevance for all but the most patient policymakers.

Not surprisingly, the cost estimates are sensitive to these assumptions, although the qualitative conclusions are not greatly affected (table 10.6). Only the first two assumptions affect the estimated costs from teen parents' perspective. If only half of the productivity effects are realized, the economic benefits of teen parenting are reduced by nearly a third for younger teen parents (to $1,027 a year) and increased by about a third for older teen parents (to $458 a year). Under all the alternative assumptions, we find that the economic consequences for teen parents themselves are modest—between a $300 and $2,000 average annual gain over the first 15 years of parenthood.

The estimated costs borne by taxpayers range from $5 billion to $9 billion annually—that is from 25 percent below to 37 percent above the $7.3 billion benchmark estimate reported in table 10.4 and repeated in the top row of table 10.6. The larger figure includes estimates for some of the unmeasured costs, such as criminal justice costs other than prison costs. The lowest figure reduces the estimated productivity gains predicted for delaying childbearing until age 20 or 21 for mothers, the fathers, and the children by 50 percent.

The estimates of social costs are similarly sensitive to changes in the underlying assumptions, with the alternative estimates ranging from 7 percent below to 47 percent above the $27.79 billion baseline estimate. The estimates under the various assumptions range between $16.08 and $29.63 billion annual losses to society in a steady-state world. The largest estimate assumes that incarceration costs capture only half of all crime and crime prevention–related costs associated with teen childbearing. The lowest estimate assumes that the productivity gains are only half as large as estimated based on the results reported in chapters 3, 4, and 9.

Conclusion

Each year, 760,000 women under the age of 20 become pregnant and 422,000 give birth—80 percent of them for the first time. Roughly 38 percent of these first-time parents are younger than 18 when they have their

Table 10.6. Sensitivity of the Estimated Costs of Teenage Childbearing to Alternative Assumptions, by Perspective ($2004)

	Teen Mothers' Perspective, by Age of First Birth[a] (average per year)		Taxpayers' perspective (billions)	Society's perspective (billions)
	Under age 18	Age 18–19		
Benchmark assumptions	(1,677)	(305)	7.30	27.79
Cost estimate specified change in assumptions:				
Productivity effects are only half those estimated	(1,027)	(458)	4.57	16.08
Teenage mothers discount future income at 7.5 percent, not 5 percent	(2,108)	(659)	—	—
Incarceration costs capture only half of all crime- and crime prevention–related costs	—	—	9.14	29.63
Only the first 15 years of productivity gains of children matter	—	—	5.67	20.82
Change in estimate from benchmark assumptions, given specified change in assumptions:				
Productivity effects are only half those estimated	650	(153)	(2.73)	(11.71)
Teenage mothers discount future income at 7.5 percent, not 5 percent	(431)	(354)	—	—
Incarceration costs capture only half of all crime- and crime prevention–related costs	—	—	1.84	1.84
Only the first 15 years of productivity gains of children matter	—	—	(1.63)	(6.98)

Source: Benchmark assumptions for the three perspectives are those reported in tables 10.3, 10.4, and 10.5.

Note: In computing the alternative estimates and the change in estimates, only the one assumption listed was modified from those used in the benchmark estimate.

—The assumption being changed is not relevant to the particular cost estimate.

a. Costs from the teen mothers' perspective are discounted to the birth of the first child.

first child. There are myriad consequences for these young mothers and their children, most of which are not easily measured in dollars and cents. The economic costs for the mothers, for example, are small to nonexistent. Rather, the consequences for them are largely nonmonetary and often not observable for several to many years following the birth of their first child. Teen mothers, especially those who have their first child before age 18, spend more of their early years of parenthood single and, when they do marry, their spouses have relatively low earnings.

The research consistently supports the conclusion that adolescent childbearing has significant adverse consequences for the children that cost them, the taxpayers, and society dearly. The children of teen mothers have poorer health, are more likely to be subjected to abuse and neglect and therefore end up in foster care, and have poorer social and academic outcomes that ultimately lower their economic productivity and increase their likelihood of incarceration. Children of teen parents are also more likely than if their mothers delayed childbearing to become teen parents, thereby perpetuating the cycle of disadvantage and its associated costs.

The costs of childbearing among those under age 18 in particular are sufficient to warrant serious investment in prevention. Yet, as illustrated in chapter 11, prevention is not easy. Simply increasing spending on family planning services or expansion of abstinence education is unlikely to succeed.[23] It seems prudent to continue support for the more expansive, multipronged efforts that have been instituted over the past decade— efforts that include research and public communications by the National Campaign to Prevent Teen Pregnancy, targeted community-based youth services, and medically accurate and developmentally appropriate health and sex education programs offered in both school and community settings. In a world where the United States is spending $5 to $10 billion of taxpayers' money annually and forgoing more than $30 billion in aggregate social welfare as a consequence of adolescent childbearing, substantial investment in teen pregnancy prevention and its attendant ills is worth serious consideration.

Sources of the Estimated Outcomes for Adolescent Parents and of the Consequences of Delaying Childbearing

Earnings-Related Outcomes

Earnings of Mothers and Spouses

All estimates taken from chapter 3, part 2

Data source: National Longitudinal Survey of Youth, 1979 cohort, for 1979–2000.

Method: Estimates of gross impacts are based on ordinary least squares estimation of a model that controls only for a teen birth, age and/or age squared, and interactions between a teen birth and age and/or age squared. The control variables used in the estimation models are listed in table 1.2. Estimates of net impacts are based on an instrumental variables estimation that uses a teen miscarriage as an instrument for a teen birth. Age/age^2 and age/age^2 × teen birth interactions are included and are used to construct age profiles for each of the outcome variables.

Outcomes for teen childbearers: Average values over the 15 years beginning with the birth of mother's first child. Separate 15-year averages were computed for those who had their first child before age 18 and those who had their first child at age 18 or 19.

Predicted outcomes if delayed childbearing until age 20 to 21: Average values over 15 years of the predicted outcomes for a woman with the characteristics of the relevant age group of teen parents (under 18 and 18–19, respectively), assuming they have their first child at age 20 to 21 rather than as a teen.

Earnings of Fathers of Children

Data reported in chapter 4

Data sources: National Longitudinal Survey of Youth, 1979 cohort, for 1979–92; Vital Statistics; National Maternal and Infant Health Survey

Method: Multivariate statistical models to predict fathers' earnings over the 18 years after fathering a child with a first-time mother, controlling for the age of the mother at the birth of the child, marital status, and other background factors listed in table 1.2. Results are reported for groups of fathers defined by the age of mother at the birth of the first child, race, and marital status (table 4.6).

Outcomes for fathers of children born to teen parents: Compute weighted average annual discounted earnings over a 15-year period for fathers of children born to teen mothers under age 18 and age 18–19, respectively. Estimates reported by Brien and Willis in chapter 4 were weighted using 2004 statistics on the distribution of births between married and unmarried mothers and their distribution by age and race/ethnicity (Martin et al. 2006). The discounted values are then scaled by a factor of 1.44 to convert them to undiscounted values, which is the equivalent to the inverse of an average annual 5 percent discount rate over 15 years.

Predicted outcomes for fathers if mothers delayed childbearing until age 20 to 21: These are weighted averages of the predicted median earnings of fathers assuming the mothers of the focal children delayed childbearing until age 20–21 but retained all other measured characteristics of their reference teen parent group. In computing these predicted outcomes, we assumed that the proportion married was two-thirds of the way between the national rate for the reference teenage parent group (age < 18, age 18–19) and 20- to 21-year-old first-time parents.

Earnings of Adult Children of Teen Parents

Chapter 9, part 2, and authors' calculations

Data sources: National Longitudinal Survey of Youth 1979–young adult sample, which includes children of the original NLSY79 sample of young women age 14–21 in 1979; and U.S. Census Bureau, "Table 9a. Earnings in 2003 by Educational Attainment of Workers 18 and Over, by Age, Sex, Race Alone or in Combination, and Hispanic Origin: 2004," http://www. census.gov/population/www/socdemo/education/cps2004.html (created March 15, 2004).

Methods: Lifetime current dollar earnings were estimated by weighting the teen parent population with different levels of educational attainment by the average lifetime (43-year) cumulative earnings estimates based on national data reported in U.S. Census Bureau 2004, table 9. Earnings are a weighted average of male and female earnings for workers age 25–64, after adjusting for labor force participation. Logit models were used to estimate high school completion rates by age of mother at first birth. Control variables included in the model are listed in table 1.2 in this volume.

Outcomes for adult children of teen mothers: These are based on the educational attainment for two groups of teen mothers—those who had their first child before age 18 and those who had their first child at age 18 or 19.

Predicted outcomes for adult children if mothers delayed childbearing until age 20 to 21: Predicted outcomes for children if the mothers delayed childbearing are based on the estimates of the children's educational attainment. In applying the estimates to the earnings data, it was assumed that 80 percent of the additional years of education children complete as a result of their mothers delaying childbearing were in high school and the remaining 20 percent were in some type of postsecondary school.

Private Transfers and Income and Consumption Taxes

Child Support

Chapter 3, part 2, and authors' calculations

Data source: National Longitudinal Survey of Youth, 1979 cohort

Method: Child support payments were computed using the same methodology described for estimating earning of teen mothers and for predicting what their earnings would have been had they delayed childbearing until age 20–21 (see above).

Income and Consumption Taxes

Authors' calculations

Data sources: U.S. federal income tax schedule for 2004. For state sales tax data, see "Tax Facts: State," http://www.taxpolicycenter.org/TaxFacts/tfdb/TFTemplate.cfm. For state income tax rates, see "State Individual Income Tax Rates, 2000–2008," http://www.taxfoundation.org/taxdata/show/ 228.html.

Method: Taxes are estimated to equal 23.31 percent of earned income in 2004 dollars. This rate reflects a federal marginal tax rate of 15 percent and an average state income and sales tax rate of 8.31 percent.

Public Assistance

Cash Assistance, Food Stamps, and Housing Subsidies

Chapter 3, part 2, and authors' calculations

Data sources: National Longitudinal Survey of Youth, 1979 cohort; U.S. Department of Housing and Urban Development Voucher Management System data on Section 8 housing expenditures, provided courtesy of the Center for Budget and Policy Priorities; and U.S. Department of Agriculture, Food and Nutrition Service, "Characteristics of Food Stamp Households: Fiscal Year 2004 Summary," available at http://www.fns.usda.gov/oane/MENU/Published/FSP/FILES/Participation/2004CharacteristicsSum.pdf.

Method: Outcomes were computed using the same multivariate methods described for estimating earning of teen mothers and for predicting what their earnings would have been had they delayed childbearing until age 20–21 (see above). Cash assistance payments were estimated based on survey respondents' direct reports. Food Stamps and housing subsidies are based on the estimated number of years teen parents received benefits and the predicted number of years they would have received them had they delayed childbearing. The average value of food stamps per recipient household a year is $2,353 in 2004 dollars, and the average value of public housing is $7,249 per recipient year in 2004 dollars.

Employment and Support Services

Authors' calculations

Data source: National Longitudinal Survey of Youth, 1979 cohort; data on federal and state expenditures for cash assistance and related support services from U.S. Department of Health and Human Services, Office of Family Assistance, *Temporary Assistance for Needy Families (TANF), Sixth Annual Report to Congress*, chapter 2, table A, available at http://www.acf.hhs.gov/programs/ofa/annualreport6/chapter02/chap02.htm.

Method: Apply the national average expenditures for employment and support services to cash assistance recipients. In 2004, an average of 8.41 cents were spent on such services for every dollar of cash assistance, using the least inclusive definition of such services.

Medical Assistance for Children

Chapter 6 and authors' calculations

Data source: 2002 Medical Expenditure Panel Survey

Method: Multiple regression analysis of health status, medical visits, and expenditures, controlling for background characteristics of the mothers. Control variables are reported in table 1.2. Net cost estimates are taken from table 6.9, model 2. These estimates allow child health to adjust when age at first birth is delayed. Cost estimates account for the predicted impact of a delay in childbearing on total fertility over the first 15 years of motherhood.

The undiscounted estimates are simply the average annual medical care costs reported for adolescent and later mothers under the various assumptions regarding the counterfactual circumstances (Wolfe and Rivers) weighted by Maynard's and Hoffman's estimates of the average number of children in the family. Discounted values were computed using the average annual medical care costs paid by others in society (through social insurance or CHAMPUS) for children born to mothers who were under age 18 and those who were age 20 to 21 when they had their first child. The costs were used to create average annual expenditures over the first 15 years of childhood that conformed to these overall averages but reflected age-specific expenditures per child that were proportional to the age-specific average number of medical care visits. We then created a 15-year series of per child medical care expenditures for each child in the household, using the authors' estimates of the number of children born to mothers during their first 15 years of parenthood. Second children were assumed to be born in year three of parenthood, and third children were assumed to be born in year five of parenthood. Costs were discounted at 5 percent annually beginning with the second year of parenthood.

Administrative Costs of Public Assistance Programs

Authors' calculations

Data sources: U.S. Department of Health and Human Services, Office of Family Assistance, *Temporary Assistance for Needy Families (TANF), Sixth Annual Report to Congress*; Tritz (2005); Fremstad (2003); and Logan, Rhodes, and Sabia (2006).

Method: From the above sources we calculated that for every dollar spent on cash assistance, 10.1 cents are spent on administration; for every dollar spent on Food Stamps, an estimated 11.6 cents are spent on administration; and for every dollar spent on Medicaid, an estimated 5.1 cents are spent on administration. To estimate the administrative costs associated with these outcomes, we simply multiplied our estimated benefit levels for cash assistance, Food Stamps, and medical assistance for adults and children by these factors. The administrative costs of housing subsidies are built into the subsidy estimates.

Other Consequences

Out-of-Pocket Medical Care for Children

Chapter 6 and authors' calculations (number of children)

Data sources: National Medical Care Expenditure Survey 2002 and National Longitudinal Survey of Youth, 1979 cohort.

Method: See discussion of medical assistance estimation methods above. We applied estimates of the proportion of total expenses that are borne privately to the overall estimates of medical care costs to estimate the out-of-pocket costs borne by parents.

Foster Care

Chapter 7 and authors' calculations (number of children)

Data sources: Illinois Integrated Database on Children and Family Services; Illinois birth certificate data; and National Longitudinal Survey of Youth, 1979 cohort

Method: Multivariate models to predict the incidence of foster care placements for children using data from the Illinois Integrated Database on Children and Family Services and Illinois birth certificate data. Impact estimates are based on logit models that estimate average foster care placement rates and abuse/neglect reports in the first five years after birth, controlling for the age of mother at first birth and other characteristics of the mother (see the control variables in table 1.2). Simulations of the impact of a delay in age at first birth hold all characteristics of the mother except age at first birth constant. The estimates assume that, if one child in a family is placed in care, the average child years in care for the family equals 0.5 times the maximum child years of placement possible during the first 18 years following the birth of the first child. Cost estimates adjust for foster care placements after the first five years following the approach in Maynard (1997). Data on foster care costs per placement were derived from published tables in Scarcella and colleagues (2006).

Incarceration

Chapter 8, part 2

Data source: National Longitudinal Survey of Youth, 1979 cohort–young males sample

Methods: Net impact estimates are based on a model that controls separately for mother's age at first birth and mother's age at the birth of the respondent child. In this specification, the impact of a teen birth on the probability that a son will be incarcerated is estimated conservatively from the difference in siblings' probabilities of incarceration. Impact estimates of the probability of ever being incarcerated are derived from logit models. Impact estimates of total years in prison are derived from Poisson models. Cost estimates are based on total years in prison. Data on incarceration are from Harrison and Beck (2005). Prison costs for 2001 are from Stephan (2004); 2001 costs are adjusted to 2004 prices. Cost estimates adjust for the undercounting of short prison spells inherent in the data and the unobserved life cycle from age 40 to end of life.

Table A.10.1. Average Discounted Annual Economic Outcomes
for Teen Mothers and Predicted Outcomes Had Teen Mothers Delayed
Childbearing until Age 20–21 ($2004)

	First Birth before Age 18		
	Mean outcome	Predicted mean if delayed	Difference
Productivity (average annual value)			
Mother's earnings	3,883	4,369	486
Spouse's earnings	6,210	4,913	(1,296)
Father's earnings	14,954	17,372	2,418
Productivity of adult children	50,241	51,619	1,378
Private transfers and taxes (average annual value)			
Child support	199	170	(29)
Mother's income and consumption taxes	905	1,018	113
Spouse's income and consumption taxes	1,448	1,145	(302)
Father's income and consumption taxes	3,486	4,050	564
Income and consumption taxes of adult children	11,712	12,033	321
Public assistance (average annual value)			
Cash assistance	1,497	861	(636)
Employment and support services	126	72	(54)
Food stamp benefits	542	548	5
Rent subsidies	629	452	(178)
Medical assistance for parents	1,123	911	(213)
Medical assistance for children	1,016	680	(337)
Administrative costs of public assistance	189	165	(24)
Other consequences			
Out-of-pocket costs of children's health care	553	558	5
Total			
Average per year	97,972	100,213	2,241
Total for first 15 years of parenthood	1,469,583	1,503,193	33,610

Source: The sources for the various estimates are detailed in appendix A.10.

Notes: These estimates are used in calculating the average annual outcomes over 15 years of childrearing. Negative consequences of delaying childbearing are denoted by parentheses. Undiscounted values are presented in appendix table A.10.2. All data have been discounted at 5 percent annually.

First Birth Age 18–19			Total		
Mean outcome	Predicted mean if delayed	Difference	Mean outcome	Predicted mean if delayed	Difference
4,161	3,454	(707)	4,057	3,798	(259)
8,720	9,177	457	7,777	7,576	(201)
16,751	17,777	1,026	16,077	17,625	1,548
65,167	65,360	193	59,562	60,199	638
266	611	344	241	445	204
970	805	(165)	946	885	(60)
2,033	2,139	106	1,813	1,766	(47)
3,905	4,144	239	3,748	4,109	361
15,192	15,237	45	13,885	14,034	149
1,404	967	(437)	1,439	927	(512)
118	81	(37)	121	78	(43)
355	429	74	425	474	48
385	420	35	477	432	(45)
588	611	23	789	724	(65)
1,051	836	(215)	1,038	777	(261)
107	118	11	138	136	(2)
730	882	152	663	760	97
121,066	122,048	981	112,394	113,848	1,454
1,815,994	1,830,714	14,720	1,685,907	1,707,721	21,814

Table A.10.2. Average Undiscounted Annual Economic Outcomes for Teen Mothers and Predicted Outcomes Had Teen Mothers Delayed Childbearing until Age 20–21 ($2004)

	First Birth before Age 18		
	Mean outcome	Predicted mean if delayed	Difference
Earnings-related outcomes (average annual value)			
Mother's earnings	5,884	7,762	1,878
Spouse's earnings	9,070	8,536	(534)
Father's earnings	21,513	24,991	3,479
Productivity of adult children	167,072	171,654	4,582
Private transfers and taxes (average annual value)			
Child support	305	318	14
Mother's income and consumption taxes	1,372	1,809	438
Spouse's income and consumption taxes	2,114	1,990	(124)
Father's income and consumption taxes	5,015	5,826	811
Income and consumption taxes of adult children	38,948	40,016	1,068
Public assistance (average annual value)			
Cash assistance	2,076	2,418	342
Employment and support services	175	203	29
Food stamp benefits	743	919	176
Rent subsidies	868	763	(105)
Medical assistance for parents	1,495	1,520	26
Medical assistance for children	1,391	942	(449)
Administrative costs of public assistance	389	448	59
Other consequences (average annual value)			
Out-of-pocket cost of children's health care	756	773	17
Foster care of minor children	1,939	1,068	(871)
Incarceration of adolescent and adult children	3,235	2,335	(900)

Source: The sources for the various estimates are detailed in appendix A.10.

Notes: These estimates are used in calculating the net benefits and costs over 15 years of adolescent childrearing to teens. Negative consequences of delaying childbearing are denoted by parentheses. Discounted values are presented in appendix table A.10.1.

First Birth Age 18–19			Total		
Mean outcome	Predicted mean if delayed	Difference	Mean outcome	Predicted mean if delayed	Difference
6,773	6,109	(665)	6,439	6,729	290
13,653	16,022	2,369	11,932	13,211	1,279
24,098	25,573	1,475	23,127	25,355	2,228
216,707	217,348	641	198,068	200,189	2,121
455	1,106	651	398	810	412
1,579	1,424	(155)	1,501	1,569	68
3,183	3,735	552	2,782	3,080	298
5,618	5,962	344	5,391	5,911	519
50,519	50,668	149	46,174	46,668	494
1,310	1,609	299	1,598	1,913	315
110	135	25	134	161	26
533	712	179	612	790	178
575	682	106	685	712	27
867	1,016	149	1,103	1,205	102
1,402	1,171	(231)	1,398	1,085	(313)
249	310	61	301	362	60
974	1,235	261	892	1,062	169
1,177	1,068	(109)	1,463	1,068	(395)
1,609	1,567	(41)	2,219	1,856	(364)

NOTES

1. The previous edition of this book reported gross differences in outcomes between teenage mothers and women who first gave birth in their 20s or later. However, in so far as such estimates clearly overstate the consequences of teenage childbearing, the editors decided not to include such estimates in this updated version and, instead, to devote greater attention to breaking down the results for younger and older teen mothers.

2. In addition to being based on updated analyses that use more recent data, the estimates reported in this chapter differ from those reported in Maynard (1997) in that they include estimated costs for all teen parents, rather than only those who have their first child before age 18.

3. Hoffman (2006) estimates that teen childbearing cost the public sector $9.1 billion in 2004. His estimate is based on most of the same underlying analyses and data, but it makes some different assumptions in translating those analyses into national cost estimates. Hoffman's analysis does not include private or social costs. It also assumes a higher number of births each year.

4. Appendix A.10 provides additional details on the measurement of the various outcomes included in the framework.

5. Estimates of earnings of workers by age, gender, and education level are based on data from the U.S. Census Bureau, "Table 9a: Earnings in 2003 by Educational Attainment of the Population 18 Years and Over, by Age, Sex, Race Alone or in Combination, and Hispanic Origin: 2004" (http://www.census.gov/population/www/socdemo/education/cps2004.html). The 1997 estimates (from chapter 9, part 1 in this volume) use a conceptually similar estimation procedure. Haveman and colleagues estimate productivity loss by applying estimates of impacts on educational attainment to estimates from the Children's Defense Fund (1995) on the average productivity gain associated with an additional year of school.

6. Taxes on earnings are computed at a 23.1 percent rate that reflects a federal marginal tax rate of 15 percent and an average state income and sales tax rate of 8.31 percent. For state sales tax rates, see the Tax Policy Center, "Sales Tax Rates 2000–2008" (http://www.taxpolicycenter.org/TaxFacts/TFDB/TFTemplate.cfm?Docid=411); for state income tax rates, see The Tax Foundation, "State Individual Income Tax Rates, 2000–2008" (http://www.taxfoundation.org/taxdata/show/228.html Year: 2005).

7. This estimate is based on U.S. Department of Health and Human Services (HHS), Office of Family Assistance (OFA), *Temporary Assistance for Needy Families (TANF) Sixth Annual Report to Congress,* chapter 2, table A, available at http://www.acf.hhs.gov/programs/ofa/annualreport6/chapter02/chap02.htm. Total TANF and other state and federal support for such services consumes an estimated 45 cents for every dollar of cash assistance; the figure rises to 64 cents per dollar of cash assistance if transfers in the form of refundable tax credits and individual development accounts are included. This latter estimate is close to the estimate of 64 cents for every dollar of cash assistance computed based on data from U.S. House Ways and Means (2004), table K-4.

8. Public housing cost estimates are based on the annual average cost per Section 8 housing voucher for FY 2005 as reported by the U.S. Department of Housing and Urban Development Voucher Management Information System. Data were provided by the Center for Budget and Policy Priorities, Washington, D.C.

9. Because of recent expansions in health care coverage for children, the estimates reported here may over- or understate the child health–related costs of teen childbearing. See "State Children's Health Insurance Program (SCHIP) Section 1115 Demonstration Projects as of September 21, 2007," available at http://www.cms.hhs.gov/LowCostHealth InsFamChild/.

10. In 2002, the nation spent $25 billion on basic cash assistance under TANF and $2.62 billion on program administration (HHS, OFA, *Temporary Assistance for Needy Families (TANF) Sixth Annual Report to Congress*). In this same year, it spent $18.3 billion on food stamp benefits and $2.4 billion administering the program (U.S. Department of Agriculture, Food and Nutrition Service "Characteristics of Food Stamp Households: Fiscal Year 2004 Summary," available at http://www.fns.usda.gov/oane/MENU/Published/FSP/FILES/Participation/2004CharacteristicsSum.pdf; Logan et al. 2006). The corresponding figures for Medicaid benefits in fiscal 2003 are $261.8 billion for direct services and $13.5 billion for state and federal administrative costs (Tritz 2005, table 2).

11. In 2004 dollars, the costs of foster care nationally totaled $23 billion to serve 532,000 children (Scarcella et al. 2006), resulting in an average annual cost per child of $43,756.

12. This estimate is derived from Bureau of Justice Statistics (Stephan 2004). Total costs of building and maintaining state prisons in 2001 were $27.4 billion, which equals $29.3 billion in 2004 dollars. During this same year, there were a total of 1.22 million male prisoners.

13. In the absence of empirical evidence to the contrary, this analysis assumes that health care subsidies for children are primarily compensating for poorer health status of the children and so are not a net benefit to the mother. This seems like a reasonable assumption, given the results Wolfe and Rivers report in chapter 6.

14. The way child support was estimated implicitly accounts for differences in the marriage and divorce rates.

15. For example, numerous studies document the joy parenthood brings to teen mothers (Edin and Kefalas 2005; Edin and Reed 2005; Luker 1996; Musick 1993; Polit 1992; Quint and Musick 1994). However, some of these studies also highlight many negative social-psychological aspects of early motherhood, such as those that come with the responsibility of parenthood, family tensions around childbearing practices, and painful relationships with the fathers of the babies.

16. The analysis assumes that 23.1 cents of every dollar earned is spent on income or consumption taxes (see footnote 6).

17. The control variables used in the various analyses are reported in chapter 1, table 1.2.

18. Another strategy would have been to focus the analysis on mothers' late adolescence and young adulthood. This would treat the mothers similarly by chronological age but differently across critical stages of their life cycle. For example, during late adolescence, some mothers would be parents and others not; during their late 20s, the teen mothers would tend not to have preschool-age children, while most of the later mothers would still have young children.

19. Productivity outcomes for adult children are estimated over a 43-year time horizon. One sensitivity analysis reports the results on including productivity losses for children over only their first 15 years of employment.

20. By using 18 cohorts for the foster care and incarceration costs, the results encompass the entire "risk" period only for the oldest child.

21. The 2004 poverty guideline for a family of four in the 48 contiguous states and the District of Columbia is $15,670. See *Federal Register* 69, no. 30 (February 13, 2004): 7736–38 or HHS, "The 2004 HHS Poverty Guidelines," http://aspe.hhs.gov/poverty/04poverty.shtml.

22. Detailed worksheets supporting the sensitivity analyses can be obtained from the lead author, Rebecca Maynard.

23. See Scher (chapter 11) for a review of the scientific evidence on the effectiveness of targeted pregnancy prevention programs. Very few programs have reduced teen births, and those few programs do not exhibit characteristics that clearly delineate them from programs that have not shown evidence of success.

REFERENCES

Children's Defense Fund. 1995. *Wasting America's Future.* Washington, DC: Children's Defense Fund.

Edin, Kathryn, and Maria Kefalas. 2005. *Promises I Can Keep: Why Poor Women Put Motherhood before Marriage.* Los Angeles: University of California Press.

Edin, Kathryn, and Joanna M. Reed. 2005. "Why Don't They Just Get Married? Barriers to Marriage among the Disadvantaged." *Future of Children* 15(2): 117–37.

Fremstad, Shawn. 2003. "Falling TANF Caseloads amidst Rising Poverty Should Be a Cause of Concern." Washington, DC: Center on Budget and Policy Priorities. http://www.cbpp.ort/9-4-03tanf.htm.

Harrison, Paige M., and Allen J. Beck. 2005. "Prisoners in 2004." Bureau of Justice Statistics Bulletin. NCJ #210677. Washington, DC: Bureau of Justice Statistics, Office of Justice Programs, U.S. Department of Justice.

Hoffman, Saul D. 2006. *By the Numbers.* Washington, DC: National Campaign to Prevent Teen Pregnancy.

Logan, Christopher, William Rhodes, and Joseph Sabia. 2006. *Food Stamp Program Costs and Error Rates, 1989–2001.* Contractor and Cooperator Report CCR 15. Washington, DC: Economic Research Service, U.S. Department of Agriculture. http://www.ers.usda.gov/Publications/CCR15/.

Luker, Kristin. 1996. *Dubious Conceptions: The Politics of Teenage Pregnancy.* Cambridge, MA: Harvard University Press.

Martin, Joyce A., Brady E. Hamilton, Paul D. Sutton, Stephanie J. Ventura, Fay Menacker, and Sharon Kirmeyer. 2006. "Births: Final Data for 2004." National Vital Statistics Reports 55(1). Hyattsville, MD: National Center for Health Statistics.

Maynard, Rebecca A., ed. 1997. *Kids Having Kids: The Economic Costs and Social Consequences of Teen Pregnancy.* Washington, DC: Urban Institute Press.

Musick, Judith S. 1993. *Young, Poor, and Pregnant: The Psychology of Teenage Motherhood.* Hartford, CT: Yale University Press.

Polit, Denise. 1992. "Barriers to Self-Sufficiency and Avenues to Success among Teenage Mothers." Princeton, NJ: Mathematica Policy Research, Inc.

Quint, Janet C., and Judith S. Musick, with Joyce A. Ladner. 1994. *Lives of Promise, Lives of Pain: Young Mothers after New Chance.* New York: Manpower Demonstration Research Corporation.

Scarcella, Cynthia Andrews, Roseana Bess, Erica H. Zielewski, and Rob Geen. 2006. *The Cost of Protecting Vulnerable Children V.* Washington, DC: The Urban Institute.

Stephan, James J. 2004. "State Prison Expenditures, 2001." Special report. JCJ #202949. Washington, DC: Bureau of Justice Statistics, Office of Justice Programs, U.S. Department of Justice.

Tritz, Karen L. 2005. "Medicaid Expenditures, FY2002 and FY2003." CRS Report for Congress. Washington, DC: Congressional Research Service. http://www.opencrs.com/document/RS21071.

U.S. House of Representatives. Committee on Ways and Means. 2004. *2004 Green Book: Background Material and Data on the Programs within the Jurisdiction of the Committee on Ways and Means.* Washington, DC: U.S. Government Printing Office. http://waysandmeans.house.gov/Documents.asp?section=813.

11

What Do We Know about the Effectiveness of Programs Aimed at Reducing Teen Sexual Risk-Taking?

Lauren Sue Scher

As society has become more aware of the negative consequences of early nonmarital childbearing, policymakers, practitioners, and researchers have tried to determine what can be done to reduce rates of adolescent pregnancies and sexual risk-taking behaviors. Recently, a number of studies have examined whether and how changes in specific teen behaviors account for declines in pregnancy and childbearing rates since the early 1990s (Darroch and Singh 1999; Flanigan 2001; Santelli et al. 2004; Ventura et al. 2001). In general, these authors have concluded that pregnancy rate declines are the result of increases in the number of adolescents delaying initiation of sexual activity and in sexually active adolescents' use of more effective contraceptive methods; there has been little change in sexual activity rates among sexually active youth. The next logical question is to determine why adolescents have been delaying sexual activity, and why sexually active adolescents choose to use contraceptives.

These behavioral changes may be attributed to several factors, such as increased national focus on early teen childbearing (including the formation of the National Campaign to Prevent Teen Pregnancy as well as various federal, state, and local and media initiatives aimed at bringing national attention to this issue); improved contraceptive technologies and access; fear of HIV and other sexually transmitted infections; changing norms and attitudes around teen sex and marriage; and changes in the economy, including recent economic expansion and changes in welfare reform requirements. In addition, persistently high rates of sexual activity, pregnancy rates, and births among teens in the United States have led to a wide range of programmatic initiatives aimed at reducing teen pregnancy and birth rates (Sonfield and Gold 2001; U.S. Department of Health and Human Services 2000). Policymakers and researchers have questioned whether and to what extent these programs have contributed to reductions in teen pregnancies and childbirths. This chapter highlights the diverse efforts under way and seeks to assess what, if any, targeted interventions might effectively promote delays in teen childbearing.

Programs and Policies Aimed at Reducing Sexual Risk-Taking

Several specific programmatic efforts are aimed at reducing sexual risk-taking and early childbearing. Some of these programs focus specifically on reducing pregnancies, others concentrate on reducing transmission of HIV and other sexually transmitted infection rates, while others are aimed at reducing multiple risk behaviors (including drug and alcohol use, delinquency and violence, and so on). Some programs serve broad populations of adolescents, while others target particular higher-risk subgroups. Some programs are intensive and costly, while others are one-time or short-term interventions. This section briefly summarizes the variety and diversity of current efforts. The following sections discuss the available evidence concerning whether these programs effectively reduce adolescent sexual risk-taking.

Clinic-Based Programs

Clinics and health centers across the country are diverse and serve different populations. Most clinics provide services to all ages, while a subgroup (often located in school wellness centers or community centers) focuses its efforts on adolescents. Clinics often provide general reproductive services including check-ups and distribution of contraceptives. Specific adolescent HIV or pregnancy prevention clinic-based interventions are often short term. These "one-time" consultations tend to last no longer than an hour, are provided by health care practitioners (physicians, physician's assistants, or nurses), are often tailored specifically to the needs and sexual backgrounds of the participating adolescents, and often tend to target higher-risk and sexually active adolescents. These programs often go beyond simply dispensing contraceptives to adolescents and include a specific, targeted counseling component.

Sex Education Programs

Sex education programs take different forms, serve adolescents of different ages, and take place in schools or in community-based organizations. Sex education is nearly universal in this country. Nearly all adolescents receive such education at some point during their secondary schooling (Kaiser Family Foundation 2000). Depending on the curriculum and time constraints, sex education programs vary in duration. Many curricula are based on approximately 10 classroom sessions, but some sex education programs are quite short (five hours or less). Others are more intensive and can take place over multiple years. Researchers and policymakers often distinguish two separate categories of sex education programs: abstinence-focused programs and "comprehensive" programs.

Abstinence-focused sex education programs explicitly or implicitly focus on abstinence (refraining from any sexual activity) and do not provide information on contraception. Often, such programs are called "abstinence only" programs. Some interventions within this category include virginity or abstinence pledges, where adolescents pledge not to engage in sexual activity (often until marriage). Programs often focus on decision-making, self-esteem, and refusal skills, and they provide information about the ramifications of engaging in sexual activity (including pregnancies, sexually transmitted infections, and contraceptive failure rates). Some programs are more intensive and include multiple components such as youth development and community service activities. Abstinence-focused programs have grown tremendously across the nation over the past decade (Darroch, Landry, and Singh 2000), largely because of federal support from the Department of Health and Human Services with matching state funds.

Nearly all sex education programs explicitly mention that abstinence is the safest method for avoiding unwanted pregnancies and sexually transmitted infections. However, many also encourage contraception use among those who choose to become or remain sexually active. Often called *comprehensive sex education,* or "abstinence plus," these programs vary in the prominence and nature of their contraception component.

For example, one sex education program may include only one lesson on contraception use (for example, an untitled HIV prevention program cited in Blake et al. 2000), while another may emphasize abstinence and contraception use equally (for example, Project BART, cited in St. Lawrence et al. 1995). In addition, these programs vary widely in the youth they serve and their program characteristics (for example, ages served, curricular focus, duration, and whether the program is based on social cognitive or related theories and/or focused on specific cultures or gender). Comprehensive sex education programs also often incorporate several characteristics of abstinence-focused programs including concentrating on decisionmaking and refusal skills and engaging in role-playing activities.

Multicomponent and Youth Development Programs

These programs generally aim to reduce various risky behaviors (for example, sexual behaviors, alcohol/drug use, life planning), incorporate multiple components, collaborate with multiple networks, or provide youth with development-focused activities. Therefore, promoting abstinence or responsible sexual behavior is often only one goal of such programs. Most multicomponent/youth development programs are more costly and intensive than basic pregnancy and HIV prevention education programs. Many entail over 50 hours (often more than 100 hours) of program-related activities for participating youth. Often these hours include paid work or community service. Most programs target youth at elevated risk (for example, based on school counselor or social service referrals), while others serve broader populations of adolescents (but who are often living in areas where most of the population is considered "at risk"). These programs can operate in community-based organizations or in schools. All offer diverse activities that may include one or more of the following: volunteer experiences, paid work experiences, mentorship programs, life skills classes, academic support and remediation, and contraception education and/or services.

Comprehensive Community-Based Programs

This category of program is the most intensive effort aimed at reducing adolescent sexual risk-taking. In the past decade, whole communities have mobilized to combat early childbearing (for example, see Walker and Kotloff 1999 or Doniger et al. 2001). Such comprehensive community-based efforts bring together multiple stakeholders across communities (for example, schools, community and faith-based institutions, housing developments) and institute multiple strategies toward a shared goal (including implementing various program-based interventions mentioned above). In addition, comprehensive community-based programs institute media campaigns that include advertisements, bulletin boards, and public service announcements.

What Do Prior Reviews of the Evidence Say?

Reviews of evidence on the effectiveness of teen pregnancy prevention programs conducted over the past decade generally yield inconsistent conclusions.[1] The reviews differ in their criteria for including studies and how they analyze the results of included studies. One important difference among reviews is whether they include findings of randomized controlled trials only, both randomized control trials and quasi-experimental design studies, or all studies (including those with no matched control group).

Another important difference is whether the studies describe findings or whether they include statistical meta-analyses. Narrative reviews are useful to researchers and practitioners because they provide evidence about programs that have been studied and highlight cases where individual interventions have found positive program effects. However, although authors of narrative reviews often attempt to pool together the evidence to form general conclusions, the pooling methods are less precise than when evidence is combined more systematically using statistical meta-analysis. In statistical meta-analysis, a researcher pools outcomes from multiple studies of similar programs to overcome the issue of lack of statistical power among studies with small sample sizes and to more precisely estimate the average impact of an intervention or intervention type.

In general, among the more recent reviews that narratively pool studies, there is a growing consensus that certain programs and program components are effective. For example, Kirby's 2001 review of both experimental and quasi-experimental studies in North America concludes that certain programs and program models reduce sexual risk-taking.[2] The review specifically lists ten "components of effective sex education programs" and suggests that multicomponent and youth development programs show particular promise in changing adolescent behaviors (Kirby 2001).

Solomon and Card (2004) list effective program models based on evidence from four separate research syntheses or lists of effective programs. This study provides specific advice to practitioners, recommending that programs be based on curricula that have been shown effective in prior studies, particularly in cases where populations served and the settings that the study took place are similar. Solomon and Card provide the caveat that replication may not be entirely possible when the adolescents or the environment are different.

DiClemente and Crosby (2006) focus solely on experiments and quasi experiments of adolescent HIV prevention programs published since 2000. This analysis states that there is no "one size fits all" method for reducing sexual risk behaviors, and it notes that replicating effective curricula does not guarantee program effectiveness. Instead, the authors suggest that program operators invest significantly in program quality through enough resources, support, and staff training to ensure adequate replication and implementation.

While the most recent narrative reviews focus on the fact that certain programs and program models appear effective, no consistent meta-analytic results published to date have validated these claims. Seven meta-analyses have been published that pool the evidence of programs aimed at reducing adolescent sexual risk-taking. Three of these reviews focus on HIV prevention and find significant effects in programs reducing the incidences of unprotected sexual activity. However, there is less consensus on the effects of programs in delaying sexual initiation and reducing rates of sexual activity and pregnancies. Five of the seven meta-analytic reviews include a combination of experimental and quasi-experimental designs, and the remaining two focus solely on results from experiments. Notably, three studies have found that quasi-experimental study results systematically are more likely to show program effects than randomized experiments (Guyatt et al. 2000; Kim et al. 1997; Scher, Maynard, and Stagner 2006).

DiCenso and colleagues (2002) meta-analyze the effects of only experimental studies of programs aimed at reducing sexual risk-taking. This review uses clear inclusion criteria and is based on a thorough literature search. DiCenso and authors find no evidence that pregnancy prevention programs reduce sexual initiation, improve contraception use, or reduce pregnancies. They conclude that "we do not have a clear solution to the problem of high pregnancy rates among adolescent in countries such as the United States, the United Kingdom, and Canada" (2002, 7). Thus, the results from this review run counter to the much more optimistic conclusions reported in more recent narrative reviews of quasi-experimental and experimental interventions.

An Updated Review of the Evidence

This section summarizes the results from a research synthesis undertaken by Lauren Sue Scher, Rebecca Maynard, and Matthew Stagner. This review builds upon the results from prior syntheses and explains the discrepancies in conclusions. It was conducted and approved under the auspices of the Social Welfare Coordinating group of the Campbell Collaboration (C2), an international nonprofit organization dedicated to preparing, maintaining, and disseminating systematic reviews of studies and interventions.[3] The Scher and colleagues review focuses solely on randomized experiments of interventions aimed at reducing sexual risk-taking. However, unlike DiCenso and colleagues, it applies higher standards for inclusion rather than simply relying on study design. For example, it excludes studies that provide outcome information for less than 60 percent of their original samples. Also, this review includes studies that report outcomes by gender or for both males and females, while the DiCenso and colleagues review only includes outcomes in the meta-analysis if they were available separately by gender.

In contrast to other reviews, rather than trying to answer whether specific programs "work" or "do not work," this review first assesses whether there is adequate information to determine whether specific intervention types work. When possible, it then highlights the average effect size of relatively similar interventions. In addition to pooling studies meta-analytically, this review therefore notes when it is not statistically appropriate to pool together diverse programs and discusses the relative benefits of focusing on pooled effects versus focusing on individual study outcomes.

A broad-based, thorough literature search was conducted for this review in fall 2002; this search was updated in spring 2006. The search strategy used electronic databases, hand searching of journals, Internet searches, and personal contacts. A total of 286 abstracts was reviewed. Of these, 84 were randomized controlled trial studies. After excluding studies due to lack of behavioral outcomes, inappropriate samples, methodological flaws, too short follow-up periods, or lack of sufficient data to calculate effect sizes, 31 remained. Of these, 4 were "one-time consultations,"

3 were abstinence-focused sex education programs, 18 were sex education programs with a contraception component, and 7 were multicomponent or youth development programs.[4] Appendix table A.11 lists these 31 studies, sorted by intervention type. A more detailed description of each of these studies is available in appendix A of the complete Campbell Collaboration report (Scher et al. 2006).

This review analyzes findings for three outcomes: sexual experience, pregnancy risk, and pregnancy.

- *Sexual experience:* The percent of youth in the program and control groups who reported in their follow-up surveys having ever had vaginal sexual intercourse. In total, 40 independent estimates of program impacts on sexual experience rates were reported in 21 separate studies.
- *Pregnancy risk:* The percent of youth who, at follow-up, reported engaging in sexual intercourse but not using an effective method of contraception.[5] Primary studies often assess contraception use only for the subsample of adolescents who are sexually active at follow-up. This measure may have confounding effects if the program changed youth's decisions regarding sexual experience. The "pregnancy risk" measure considers all non-sexually active youth as *not* at pregnancy risk. There are 34 independent estimates of program impacts on pregnancy risk from 24 studies.
- *Pregnancy:* The percent of female sample members who, at follow-up, reported that they had ever experienced a pregnancy or the percent of male sample members who reported causing a pregnancy. There are 25 independent estimates of program impacts from 13 separate studies.

In total, this review presents findings based on more than 37,000 youth who were the subjects of 31 studies that reported on 38 randomized trials of interventions aimed at reducing teen sexual activity and pregnancy. Appendix table B.11.1 describes the sample and intervention characteristics of included studies, and appendix table B.11.2 describes each study's methodological characteristics and outcomes.[6] Like DiCenso and colleagues, when all the effect sizes are combined, there is no statistically significant evidence that programs delay sexual initiation, reduce pregnancy risk, or prevent teen pregnancy. However, because of the diversity in the programs offered and populations served, pooling all programs aimed at reducing adolescent sexual risk taking is statistically inappropriate and does not provide particularly useful evidence.[7] Therefore, it is more appropriate to explore the effects of interventions by program type.

Estimated Impacts on Experience with Vaginal Sexual Intercourse

This analysis does not find consistent evidence that specific programs or program types evaluated rigorously reduce sexual experience rates. Figure 11.1 shows that rates of sexual experience vary widely across program types (due largely to differences in the populations served across program types), but when looking within intervention type, the rates appear to be nearly identical for treatment and control groups. After adjusting for clustering within groups, no pooled impacts within program types are statistically significant.[8]

Estimated Impacts on Pregnancy Risk

Pregnancy risk is defined as unprotected sexual intercourse versus either intercourse with contraceptives or abstinence. Among the subgroups of programs with more similar impact estimates, the one statistically significant pooled effect on pregnancy risk is for multicomponent/youth development programs (figure 11.2). Across these three studies, there was an estimated 6.0 percentage point decline in rates of unprotected sexual intercourse. At least one statistically significant effect was found in each of these three studies.

The pooled impact for neither one-time consultations nor sex education with an abstinence focus is statistically significant. For one-time consultations, which are primarily focused on reducing unprotected sexual intercourse, the pooled effect was a statistically insignificant 3.7 percentage point reduction in pregnancy risk. Sex education programs with an abstinence focus do not cover issues concerning contraception use, and thus, we would not expect increases in contraception use. However, such programs could reduce pregnancy risk by decreasing the number of adolescents engaging in sexual intercourse. The pregnancy risk measure incorporates both of these issues into its calculation.[9] Thus, there is a chance that abstinence-focused programs could reduce (or possibly increase) pregnancy risk. Based on the limited information currently available, there is no evidence that these programs either increase or decrease pregnancy risk.

Figure 11.1. Intervention and Control Group Sexual Experience Rates for All Programs and by Program Type

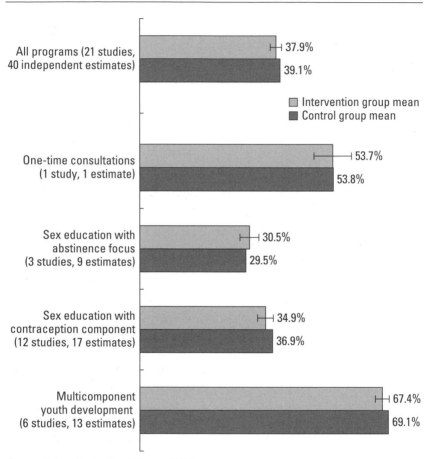

Source: Scher, Maynard, and Stagner (2006).

The pooled impact estimate of 0.5 percentage points favoring the control group has a confidence interval three times as large.

The most variation in impact estimates occurs for studies of sex education programs with a contraception component, making it imprudent to interpret the pooled effects on pregnancy risk. The average effect—1.6 percentage points—is not statistically significant, but it is not particularly telling because of the variation across studies within this intervention type.[10] Five of the 19 estimates for sex education programs with a contra-

Figure 11.2. Estimated Impacts on Pregnancy Risk Rates for All Programs and by Program Type

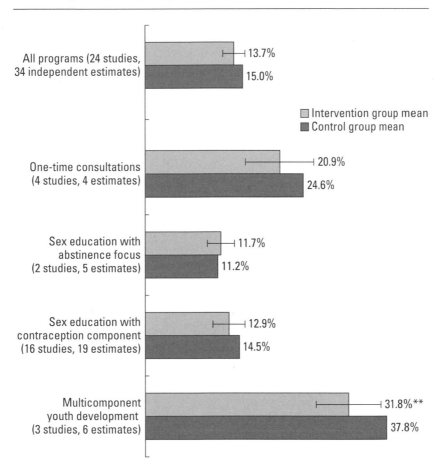

Source: Scher, Maynard, and Stagner (2006).

** Difference between intervention group and control group is significant at the *p* < .05 level.

ception component are statistically significant, four favoring the treatment group and one favoring the control group. Three of the four programs that found statistically significant positive program effects were theory-based and culturally sensitive HIV prevention programs serving primarily black adolescents, characteristics highlighted in prior narrative reviews of the evidence (for example, Kirby 2001 and Solomon and Card 2004).

Estimated Impacts on Pregnancy Rates

Figure 11.3 shows that among the one one-time consultation study and the seven studies of sex education, less the 5 percent of sample members (treatment or control) reported pregnancies, whereas more than 20 percent of the sample of adolescents who participated in studies of multicomponent programs reported pregnancies. Given the diversity of settings and

Figure 11.3. Estimated Impacts on Pregnancy Rates for All Programs and by Program Type

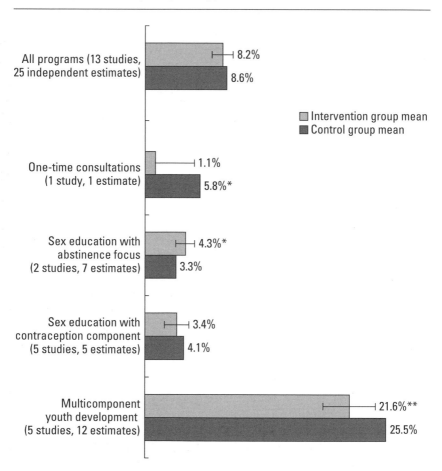

Source: Scher, Maynard, and Stagner (2006).

* Difference between intervention group and control group is significant at the *p* < .10 level.

** Difference between intervention group and control group is significant at the *p* < .05 level.

variability of impacts across intervention types, the near zero (−0.4 percentage points) overall pooled impact estimate is not particularly telling.

Although small sample sizes limit the power of the test, there is no evidence of heterogeneity in the pooled pregnancy rate impacts once studies are grouped by intervention type. The point estimate of effects for the single study of a one-time consultation was statistically significant favoring the treatment group (−4.7 percentage points). Among the two sex education intervention types, the magnitude of the pooled impacts is small. However, it is notable that the pooled estimate from two studies of sex education programs with an abstinence focus (six of seven impacts from one study) is statistically significant favoring the control group (1 percentage point). While all five studies of sex education programs with a contraception component favor the treatment group, none are statistically significant after adjusting for clustering, and the pooled impact is near zero (−.7 percentage points).

Multicomponent/youth development programs showed the greatest evidence of favorable impacts on pregnancy rates. The pooled estimate for the five studies (12 estimates) is moderate (−3.9 percentage points) and statistically significant.

Summary of Review Findings

This review includes a thorough search of the literature and screens out studies with weak sample designs and studies with improper sample maintenance. Appendix B.11 presents aggregate and study-specific results for each of three outcomes in order to provide both a sense of the average impacts and the variability in the effectiveness across studies and implementation settings. The best available rigorous evidence suggests the following conclusions:

- *One-time consultations* (4 studies): There is not currently enough evidence available to determine whether these programs are effective in reducing sexual risk-taking. The only outcome for which it is possible to pool more than one effect size is for the pregnancy risk outcome, and this pooled effect favors the treatment group but is not statistically significant.
- *Abstinence-focused sex education programs* (3 studies): There has recently been a rise in the number of intensive, abstinence-only sex education programs that often use various methods to emphasize an

"abstinence until marriage" message. Only three interventions met the criteria for inclusion in this review, and while they focus on an abstinence message and do not include contraception information, they are not representative of this pool of newer programs that have recently emerged. None of these interventions took place within the past decade. Further, all three programs offered a relatively limited intervention, in two cases between 2 and 10 hours of instruction and in the third between 11 and 30 hours. Among the evaluations included in this review, there is no evidence that, as a group, these programs have changed the likelihood that youth will initiate having sex or that they will be more or less likely to have sex without using contraception. The results suggest a very small impact (1 percentage point) on pregnancy rates favoring the control group.[11]

- *Sex education programs with a contraception component* (18 studies): There is no consistent overall evidence that sex education programs evaluated rigorously altered the likelihood that youth would initiate sex, risk pregnancy, or become (or get someone) pregnant. However, some individual studies have found positive program effects, particularly related to increased contraception use, and have been considered by advocates as models to be replicated (Solomon and Card 2004). Notably, the nature of the programs included within this category varies greatly, as do the size, direction, and statistical significance of the impact estimates for the various programs. This diversity of interventions within this program type suggests that pooling these studies may not be appropriate for determining program effectiveness. As more replication study results become available, it will be possible to pool more similar programs to assess systematically the overall cross-study effects of particular program models.

- *Multicomponent youth development programs* (7 studies): The most promising results are for the more intensive multicomponent youth development programs serving higher risk adolescents, particularly related to reducing pregnancy risk and pregnancy rates.[12] Moreover, within this category, the results tend to be most favorable for females. However, there is a paucity of rigorous evaluations of such programs, and further replication and evaluation is warranted.

Prior narrative reviews have suggested that some programs effectively reduce sexual risk-taking. The results presented above find this to be true, but to a lesser degree. One major difference in these results is related to the fact that most narrative reviews include quasi-experimental studies that inflate impact estimates. Also, after adjusting for clustering within groups and accounting for full sample measures, many program impacts that originally seem to be statistically significant are no longer significant. In the case of sexual initiation, there is little to no evidence that programs evaluated rigorously have succeeded in reducing overall sexual experience rates. However, there is evidence that certain programs reduce pregnancy risk through a combination of improved contraceptive use and reduced sexual activity, and, for multicomponent programs in particular, there is evidence of reductions in pregnancy rates.

Some prior meta-analyses suggest that programs do not effectively reduce sexual risk-taking. Indeed, after combining the available data using meta-analysis, there are very few statistically significant effects. However, pooling dissimilar programs is not a statistically appropriate mechanism for assessing program effects. The overall null differences found when pooling all program types for sexual experience, pregnancy risk, and pregnancy rate outcomes therefore do not necessarily mean that programs are unsuccessful. Instead, it is more instructive to explore pooled impacts within program type. In the case of multicomponent/youth development programs, once only these programs are pooled together, the combined effect size is statistically significant, suggesting that these programs may effectively reduce pregnancy risk and pregnancy rates. Unfortunately, there is limited evidence from which to judge pooled effectiveness once studies are separated by program type, particularly for one-time consultations and abstinence-focused sex education programs. There are a large number of sex education programs with a contraception component, and the pooled effect sizes provide no evidence that these programs reduce sexual initiation or pregnancy rates. However, these programs and program impacts, particularly when looking at the pregnancy risk outcome, are quite varied. This suggests even further refinement within this category of programs in order to get a better pooled estimate of program effects for more similar types of sex education programs.

Discussion

Clearly, a variety of societal, technological, and economic factors have played significant roles in influencing adolescent sexual risk-taking behaviors and ultimately the rates of teen pregnancy and childbearing.

Although there is evidence that some programs reduce sexual risk-taking, a large number of rigorously evaluated programs fail to find program effects, particularly related to sexual initiation rates. It is therefore conceivable that declines in rates of sexual initiation, pregnancies, and births to teens may be the result of more global changes in social norms around sexual activity, education about and access to contraceptives, and improvements in contraceptive technologies. Indeed, one of the reasons that targeted interventions sometimes show little effectiveness may be due to the rise in the prevalence and change in the content of health and sex education nationally.[13]

Since some programs have influenced changes in sexual risk-taking behaviors and since there is generally universal support for education-based programs, it is reasonable to continue pursuing program-based pregnancy prevention interventions. However, the current body of evidence does not provide clear prescriptions of "what works." The most rigorous body of evidence does not yield clear conclusions regarding which programs are the most effective across broad populations. It is also still unclear whether particular program models can be replicated successfully in different settings.

Additional research and evaluation is therefore necessary, including studying programs that have not yet been evaluated rigorously and programs that have been replicated and are serving new populations of adolescents in different communities. Nearly all reviews of the evidence, whether they consider programs effective or ineffective, highlight the fact that no "one size fits all" program will achieve positive results. Therefore, program operators must carefully consider their individual setting when determining the best fit for them, and they must evaluate whether programs are effective for their particular population.

Future research should be mindful to consider both methodological and substantive decisions when framing research studies. Whenever possible, rigorous experimental studies should be conducted. Researchers have found that pregnancy prevention programs evaluated using quasi-experimental designs tend to be more likely to show program effects. In cases where experiments are not possible (for example, when studying comprehensive community-based initiatives), then advanced statistical analyses such as interrupted time series analyses should be undertaken. In addition, care should be taken to follow up with the largest sample possible for as lengthy a period as is feasible. In cases where groups of intervention and control groups are compared, then proper statistical adjustments need to account for this clustering.

Substantively, researchers should also increase the breadth of evaluations to estimate more routinely program impacts for key subgroups of youth defined by such factors as age, gender, and family background. Once a larger body of more similar programs has been evaluated rigorously and reported consistently, then it will be possible to pool the evidence to make more concrete conclusions regarding program efficacy. Having access to solid information about whether particular types of interventions are effective, as well as information regarding *for whom* programs are effective and ineffective, will help policymakers and practitioners better address the sexual health risks of youth.

Table A.11.1. Randomized Controlled Trials Included
in Research Synthesis, by Program Type

One-Time Consultations

1. *ASSESS (Awareness, Skills, Self-Efficacy/Self-Esteem, and Social Support)*
   Boekeloo, B. O., L. A. Schamus, S. J. Simmens, et al. 1999. "A STD/HIV Prevention
   Trial among Adolescents in Managed Care." *Pediatrics* 103(1): 107–15.
2. *Untitled—Reproductive health consultation*
   Danielson, R., S. Marcy, A. Plunkett, et al. 1990. "Reproductive Health Counseling
   for Young Men: What Does It Do?" *Family Planning Perspectives* 22(3): 115–21.
3. *Untitled—Nurse-client interaction intervention*
   Hanna, K. M. 1990. "Effect of Nurse-Client Transaction on Female Adolescents'
   Contraception Perceptions and Adherence." Unpublished doctoral dissertation,
   University of Pittsburgh, Pittsburgh, PA.
4. *Untitled—Physician-delivered AIDS education and counseling program*
   Mansfield, C. J., M. E. Conroy, S. J. Emans, et al. 1993. "A Pilot Study of AIDS
   Education and Counseling of High-Risk Adolescents in an Office Setting." *Journal
   of Adolescent Health* 14(2): 115–19.

Sex Education with an Abstinence Focus

5. *Project Taking Charge*
   Jorgensen, S. R., V. Potts, and B. Camp. 1993. "Project Taking Charge: Six-Month
   Follow-Up of a Pregnancy Prevention Program for Early Adolescents." *Family
   Relations* 42: 401–406.
6. *Education Now, Babies Later (ENABL)*
   Kirby, D., M. Korpi, R. Barth, et al. 1995. *Evaluation of Education Now and Babies Later
   (ENABL): Final Report.* Berkeley: School of Social Welfare, University of California.
7. *McMaster Teen Program*
   Thomas, B. H., A. Mitchell, M. C. Devlin, et al. 1992. "Small Group Sex Education at
   School: The McMaster Teen Program." In *Preventing Adolescent Pregnancy: Model
   Programs and Evaluations,* edited by B. C. Miller, J. C. Card, R. L. Paikoff, and J. L.
   Peterson (28–52). Newbury Park, CA: SAGE Publications.

Sex Education with a Contraception Component

8. *Untitled—Clinic-based self-efficacy training program*
   Baker, C. 1990. "Self-Efficacy Training: Its Impact upon Contraception and Depression among a Sample of Urban Adolescent Females." Unpublished doctoral dissertation, Seton Hall University, South Orange, NJ.
9. *Untitled—HIV/STD prevention curriculum*
   Blake, S. M., R. Ledsky, D. Lohrman, et al. 2000. *Overall and Differential Impact of
   an HIV/STD Prevention Curriculum for Adolescents.* Washington, DC: Academy for
   Educational Development.
10. *Draw the Line/Respect the Line*
    Coyle, K., D. Kirby, B. Marin, et al. 2000. *Effect of Draw the Line/Respect the Line
    on Sexual Behavior in Middle Schools.* Santa Cruz, CA: ETR Associates. Coyle,
    K. K., D. B. Kirby, B. V. Marin, et al. 2004. "Draw the Line/Respect the Line: A Ran-

Table A.11.1. *(Continued)*

domized Trial of a Middle School Intervention to Reduce Sexual Risk Behaviors."
American Journal of Public Health 94(5): 843–51.

11. *Untitled—HIV prevention intervention*
DiClemente, R. J., G. M. Wingood, and K. F. Harrington. 2004. "Efficacy of an HIV
Prevention Intervention for African American Adolescent Girls." *Journal of the
American Medical Association* 292(2): 171–79.

12. *Keepin' It R.E.A.L.!*
Dilorio, C., K. Resnicow, F. McCarty, et al. 2006. "Keepin' It R.E.A.L.!: Results of a
Mother-Adolescent HIV Prevention Program." *Nursing Research* 55(1): 43–51.

13. *Teen Talk*
Eisen, M., G. L. Zellman, and A. L. McAlister. 1990. "Evaluating the Impact of a
Theory-Based Sexuality and Contraceptive Education Program." *Family Planning
Perspectives* 22(6): 261–71.

14. *Family Support*
Herceg-Baron, R., F. F. Furstenberg, J. Shea, and K. M. Harris. 1986. "Supporting
Teenagers' Use of Contraceptives: A Comparison of Clinic Services." *Family
Planning Perspectives* 18(2): 61–66.

15. *Be Proud, Be Responsible (two interventions: abstinence and safer sex)*
Jemmott, J. B. III, L. S. Jemmott, and G. T. Fong. 1998. "Abstinence and Safer Sex
HIV Risk-Reduction Interventions for African American Adolescents: A Randomized
Controlled Trial." *Journal of the American Medical Association* 279(19): 1529–36.

16. *Project SNAPP*
Kirby, D., M. Korpi, C. Adivi, and J. Weissman. 1997. "An Impact Evaluation of
Project SNAPP: An AIDS and Pregnancy Prevention Middle School Program."
AIDS Education and Prevention 9(A): 44–61.

17. *Youth AIDS Prevention Project (YAPP)*
Levy, S. R., C. Perhats, K. Weeks, et al. 1995. "Impact of a School-Based AIDS
Prevention Program on the Risk and Protective Behavior for Newly Sexually Active
Students." *Journal of School Health* 65(4): 145–51.

18. *Focus on Kids—AIDS prevention program*
Li, X., B. Stanton, S. Feigelman, and J. Galbraith. 2002. "Unprotected Sex among
African-American Adolescents: A Three-Year Study." *Journal of the National Medical
Association* 94(9): 789–96. Stanton, B. F., X. Li, I. Ricardo, et al. 1996. "A Randomized,
Controlled Effectiveness Trial of an AIDS Prevention Program for Low-Income African-
American Youths." *Archives of Pediatric Adolescent Medicine* 150(4): 363–72.

19. *Healthy for Life (HFL)*
Moberg, D. P., and D. L. Piper. 1998. "The Healthy for Life Project: Sexual Risk
Behavior Outcomes." *AIDS Education and Prevention* 10(2): 128–48.

20. *Untitled—Cognitive behavioral group training program*
Schinke, S. P., B. J. Blythe, L. D. Gilchrist, et al. 1981. "Primary Prevention of
Adolescent Pregnancy." *Social Work with Groups* 4(1&2): 121–35.

21. *Untitled—Workshop and community-level HIV prevention interventions*
Sikkema, K. J., E. S. Anderson, J. A. Kelly, et al. 2005. "Outcomes of a Randomized,
Controlled Community-Level HIV Prevention Intervention for Adolescents in Low-
Income Housing Developments." *AIDS* 19(14): 1509–16.

(continued)

Table A.11.1. *(Continued)*

22. *Focus on Kids—West Virginia replication*
    Stanton, B., C. Harris, L. Cottrell, et al. 2006. "Trial of an Urban Adolescent Sexual Risk-Reduction Intervention for Rural Youth: A Promising but Imperfect Fit." *Journal of Adolescent Health* 38(1): e25–e36.
23. *RIPPLE Study*
    Stephenson, J. M., V. Strange, A. Oakley, et al. 2004. "Pupil-Led Sex Education in England (RIPPLE study): Cluster-Randomised Intervention Trial." *The Lancet* 364: 338–46.
24. *Project BART (Becoming a Responsible Teen)*
    St. Lawrence, J. S., T. L. Brasfield, K. W. Jefferson, et al. 1995. "Cognitive-Behavioral Intervention to Reduce African American Adolescents' Risk for HIV Infection." *Journal of Consulting and Clinical Psychology* 63(2): 221–37.
25. *SHARE (Sexual Health and Relationships: Safe, Happy, and Responsible)*
    Wight, D., G. M. Raab, M. Henderson, et al. 2002. "Limits of Teacher-Delivered Sex Education: Interim Behavioural Outcomes from Randomised Trial." *BMJ* 324(7351): 1430–35.

Multicomponent/Youth Development Programs

26. *Teen Outreach Program (TOP)*
    Allen, J. P., S. Philliber, S. Herrling, et al. 1997. "Preventing Teen Pregnancy and Academic Failure: Experimental Evaluation of a Developmentally Based Approach." *Child Development* 64(4): 729–42.
27. *Summer Training and Education Program (STEP)*
    Grossman, J. B., and C. L. Sipe. 1992. *Summer Training and Education Program (STEP): Report on Long-Term Impacts.* Philadelphia, PA: Public/Private Ventures.
28. *Peer Power Project*
    Handler, A. S. 1987. "An Evaluation of a School-Based Adolescent Pregnancy Prevention Program." Unpublished doctoral dissertation, University of Illinois, Chicago, IL.
29. *Untitled—"Client-centered" approaches*
    McBride, D., and A. Gienapp. 2000. "Using Randomized Designs to Evaluate Client-Centered Programs to Prevent Adolescent Pregnancy." *Family Planning Perspectives* 32(5): 227–35.
30. *Reach for Health Community Service Intervention (RFH CYS)*
    O'Donnell, L., A. Stueve, C. O'Donnell, et al. 2002. "Long-Term Reductions in Sexual Initiation and Sexual Activity among Urban Middle Schoolers in the Reach for Health Service Learning Program." *Journal of Adolescent Health* 31: 93–100.
31. *Children's Aid Society—Carrera Program*
    Philliber, S., J. Kaye, and S. Herrling. 2001. *The National Evaluation of the Children's Aid Society–Carrera Model Program to Prevent Teen Pregnancy.* Accord, NY: Philliber Research Associates. Philliber, S., J. W. Kaye, S. Herrling, and E. West. 2002. "Preventing Pregnancy and Improving Health Care Access among Teenagers: An Evaluation of the Children's Aid Society–Carrera Program." *Perspectives on Sexual and Reproductive Health* 34(5): 244–51.

Table B.11.1. Sample and Intervention Characteristics of Studies Included in the Review

Intervention type, study, author(s), and location	Program name	Sample and Intervention Characteristics				
		Predominant gender(s) served[a]	Sexually experienced at intake (%)	Focal level in school targeted[b]	School-based setting	Approximate hours duration
One-time consultation						
Boekeloo et al. (1999)	ASSESS	Both	>21	Middle	No	1
Danielson et al. (1990)	None	Males	37	High	No	1
Hanna (1990)	None	Females	92	High	No	0.25
Mansfield et al. (1993)	None	Females	100	High	No	0.5
Sex education with abstinence focus						
Jorgensen et al. (1993)	Project Taking Charge	Both	45	Middle	Yes	22
Kirby et al. (1995): site 1 (teen-led)	ENABL	Both	10	Middle	Yes	5
Kirby et al. (1995): site 2 (adult-led)	ENABL	Both	10	Middle	Yes	5
Kirby et al. (1995): site 3 (adult-led)	ENABL	Both	10	Middle	Yes	5
Thomas et al. (1992)	McMaster Teen Program	Both	19	Middle	Yes	10
Sex education with contraception component						
Baker (1990)	None	Females	100	High	No	5.5
Blake et al. (2000)	None	Both	51	High	Yes	11
Coyle et al. (2000, 2004)	Draw the Line/ Respect the Line	Both	4	Middle	Yes	15
DiClemente et al. (2004)	Untitled HIV prevention	Females	100	Mixed	No	16
Dilorio et al. (2006)	Keepin' It R.E.A.L.!	Both	9	Middle	No	14

(continued)

Table B.11.1. (Continued)

Intervention type, study, author(s), and location	Program name	Sample and Intervention Characteristics				
		Predominant gender(s) served[a]	Sexually experienced at intake (%)	Focal level in school targeted[b]	School-based setting	Approximate hours duration
Eisen et al. (1990)	Teen Talk	Both	37	Mixed	Partial	12–15
Herceg-Baron et al. (1986)	Family Support	Females	87	High	No	5
Jemmott et al. (1998)	Be Proud, Be Responsible	Both	25	Middle	Yes	8
Kirby et al. (1997)	Project SNAPP	Both	8	Middle	Yes	8
Levy et al. (1995)	Youth AIDS Prevention Project	Both	35	Middle	Yes	11
Li et al. (2002)	Focus on Kids	Both	36	Middle	No	18
Moberg and Piper (1998)	Healthy for Life	Both	< 22	Middle	Yes	40
Schinke et al. (1981)	None	Both	Not reported	High	Yes	14
Sikkema et al. (2005): workshop	None	Both	73	Mixed	No	6
Stanton et al. (2006)	Focus on Kids: West Virginia	Both	21	Mixed	Partial	12

Study	Program	Gender		Grade		
Stephenson et al. (2004)	RIPPLE Study	Both	7	Middle	Yes	8
St. Lawrence et al. (1995)	BART	Both	50	Mixed	No	14
Wight et al. (2002)	SHARE	Both	17	Middle	Yes	15
Multicomponent/youth development						
Allen et al. (1997)	Teen Outreach Program (TOP)	Females	Not reported	High	Yes	71
Grossman and Sipe (1992): cohort 2	STEP	Both	45	Mixed	No	295
Grossman and Sipe (1992): cohort 3	STEP	Both	45	Mixed	No	295
Handler (1987)	Peer Power	Females	12	Middle	Yes	150
McBride and Gienapp (2000): site E	None	Females	63	High	No	27
McBride and Gienapp (2000): site F	None	Females	63	High	Yes	31
McBride and Gienapp (2000): site G	None	Females	63	High	Yes	22
O'Donnell et al. (2002)	Reach for Health	Both	25	Middle	Yes	146
Philliber et al. (2001): New York	Carrera Program: NYC sample	Both	26	Mixed	No	242
Philliber et al. (2001): replications	Carrera Program: Replications	Both	24	Mixed	No	205
Sikkema et al. (2005): multicomponent	None	Both	73	Mixed	No	>10

a. A program is labeled as predominantly serving a particular gender if more than 90 percent of the sample is of one gender.

b. A program is labeled as serving middle school– or high school–age adolescents if it specifically targeted younger or older adolescents. If all school-age adolescents were targeted, then the program is labeled "mixed."

Table B.11.2. Methodological and Outcome Characteristics of Studies Included in the Review

Intervention type, study, author(s), and location	Methodological Characteristics		
	Units randomized	Total youth (baseline)	% response at follow-up[a]
One-time consultation			
Boekeloo et al. (1999)	Students	215	92.0
Danielson et al. (1990)	Students	1,195	81.3
Hanna (1990)	Students	51	74.0
Mansfield et al. (1993)	Students	90	92.0
Sex education with abstinence focus			
Jorgensen et al. (1993)	Classes	91	100.0
Kirby et al. (1995): site 1 (teen-led)	Classes	4,652[d]	66.3
Kirby et al. (1995): site 2 (adult-led)	Classes	4,652[d]	66.3
Kirby et al. (1995): site 3 (adult-led)	31 schools	5,244	73.7
Thomas et al. (1992)	21 schools	3,289	78.1
Sex education with contraception component			
Baker (1990)	Students	62	76.0
Blake et al. (2000)	30 teachers	1,349	68.9
Coyle et al. (2004)	19 schools	2,829	87 and 71
DiClemente et al. (2004)	Students	522	88.1
Dilorio et al. (2006)	11 B and G clubs	582	90.2
Eisen et al. (1990)	Mixed	1,444	61.5
Herceg-Baron et al. (1986)	Students	469	78.0
Jemmott et al. (1998)	Students	659	78.3
Kirby et al. (1997)	102 classes	~2,100	72.7
Levy et al. (1995)	15 districts	2,392	69.8
Li et al. (2002)	76 peer grps	383	73.0
Moberg and Piper (1998)	21 schools	2,483	74.1
Schinke et al. (1981)	Students	53	100.0
Sikkema et al. (2005): workshop	10 housing dvp	820	67.4
Stanton et al. (2006)	110 groups	1,131	79.9
Stephenson et al. (2004)	29 schools	8,766	75.9
St. Lawrence et al. (1995)	Students	246	91.5
Wight et al. (2002)	25 schools	7,616	76.9

Months of follow-up since baseline[b]	Control group services	Outcomes Included in This Review[c]		
		Initiated sex	Pregnancy risk	Pregnancy
9	Health exam		X	X
12	None	X	X	
3	Video/pamphlets		X	
2	10 minute session		X	
6	None	X		
17	Regular sex ed	X	X	X
17	Regular sex ed	X	X	X
17	Regular sex ed	X	X	X
48	Regular sex ed	X	X	X
6	Clinic services		X	X
6	Regular sex ed	X		
24 and 36[e]	Regular sex ed	X		
6 and 12	General health ed		X	X
4, 12, and 24	1 hour session	X	X	
13	Regular sex ed	X	X	
15	Clinic services		X	X
3 and 12	General health ed	X	X	
17	Regular sex ed	X	X	X
21	Regular sex ed	X	X	
12	Regular sex ed		X	
29	Regular sex ed	X	X	
12	None		X	
3 and 18	Video and discussion	X	X	
3, 6, and 9	General health ed		X	
12 and 24	Regular sex ed	X	X	X
14	Regular sex ed	X	X	
24	Regular sex ed	X	X	

(continued)

Table B.11.2. *(Continued)*

Intervention type, study, author(s), and location	Methodological Characteristics		
	Units randomized	Total youth (baseline)	% response at follow-up[a]
Multicomponent/youth development			
Allen et al. (1997)	Mixed	695	81.0
Grossman and Sipe (1992): cohort 2	Students	1,635	77.2
Grossman and Sipe (1992): cohort 3	Students	1,591	84.7
Handler (1987)	Students	63	79.4
McBride and Gienapp (2000): site E	Students	292	77.4
McBride and Gienapp (2000): site F	Students	166	77.1
McBride and Gienapp (2000): site G	Students	232	65.9
O'Donnell et al. (2002)	18 classes	255	76.5
Philliber et al. (2001): New York	Students	598	80.9
Philliber et al. (2001): replications	Students	565	80.9
Sikkema et al. (2005): multicomponent	10 housing dvp	744	65.7

a. Response rates reported in this table are based on the data available for use in the meta-analysis. Response rates therefore may be slightly different from primary authors' reported response rates.

b. Follow-up length noted in this table is based on the latest follow-up with less than 40 percent sample attrition.

c. Outcomes included in this table are only those that met the criteria for inclusion in the meta-analysis.

d. Separate baseline sample sizes and response rates were not reported for the two sets of programs randomized at the classroom level.

e. Latest follow-up for this study was 36 months. However, due to sample retention of less than 60 percent, outcome for males in the study are based on the 24-month follow-up measure (87% retention). 36-month effects were included for the female sample where attrition was within acceptable range (71%).

Months of follow-up since baseline[b]	Control group services	Outcomes Included in This Review[c]		
		Initiated sex	Pregnancy risk	Pregnancy
9	Unknown			X
42	Summer job	X		X
42	Summer job	X		X
12	Regular sex ed	X		X
8	Little to no svcs	X	X	
8	None	X	X	
6	None	X	X	
45	Regular sex ed	X		X
36	Recreation svcs	X	X	X
36	Recreation svcs	X	X	X
3 and 18	Video and discussion	X	X	

NOTES

1. Narrative reviews include Bennett and Assefi (2005), DiClemente and Crosby (2006), Frost and Forrest (1995), Grunseit et al. (1997), Kirby (2001), Manlove et al. (2002), NHS Centre for Reviews and Dissemination (1997), Oakley et al. (1995), Pedlow and Carey (2004), Solomon and Card (2004), Thomas (2000), and Visser and Van Bilsen (1994). Meta-analytic reviews include DiCenso et al. (2002), Dolan Mullen et al. (2002), Franklin et al. (1997), Johnson et al. (2003), Kim et al. (1997), and Silva (2002). Scher, Maynard, and Stagner (2006) summarize the findings and policy recommendations for each of these reviews.

2. Kirby (2007), a recently published update to the 2001 review, uses similar narrative synthesis methods to strengthen and support the findings from the earlier review.

3. For a more detailed description of the program methods, go to http://www.campbellcollaboration.org/doc-pdf/scherteenpregnancyprot.pdf. See Scher et al. (2006) for a fuller discussion of methods, data sources, and findings.

4. One study (Sikkema et al. 2005) evaluated two different types of programs: one sex education program with a contraception component, and one multicomponent program. The effects of these programs are analyzed separately in the meta-analysis.

5. If available, an anchor measure of "always" using contraception was used to compute pregnancy risk. If this measure was not available, then use of contraception at most recent intercourse was used. In the rare cases where neither of the above measures was available, any use/nonuse of contraception was used. Sensitivity analyses showed that the estimated impacts did not depend on how this variable was measured.

6. Scher and colleagues (2006) present study-specific findings from the current evidence base of rigorously evaluated programs that explore impacts on sexual experience rates, pregnancy risk, or pregnancy rates. In comparing the results from this review with the results from the original studies, there are cases where the original authors found differences statistically significant and the Scher and colleagues analysis fails to find significant effects. This discrepancy results largely from two issues: (1) Some studies randomized at cluster levels (for example, classrooms or schools) but analyzed the data at individual student levels. Intraclass correlations within these clusters can lead to an underestimate of the variance across outcomes. After adjusting for clustering, impacts that originally appear statistically significant are no longer significant. (2) Some studies report outcomes for conditional subsamples such as pregnancy rates only among the sexually active. This review assesses outcomes based on the full original study samples (sexually active and inactive).

7. Statistically significant heterogeneity tests from these analyses suggest that the effect sizes differ beyond what would be expected from sampling error. This heterogeneity exists because certain studies have significantly larger or smaller effect sizes than the overall "average" effect size. This variation may result from differences in methodological characteristics, program models, target populations, or subgroups served. For the most part (unless otherwise noted), heterogeneity tests were not statistically significant when pooling studies by program type. For this reason, the bulk of results presented from this analysis focuses on outcomes by program type.

8. Before adjusting for clustering within groups, there was a statistically significant effect favoring the intervention group for sex education programs with a contraception component.

9. Numerator is having unprotected sex, denominator includes the sample of both sexually active and sexually inactive adolescents.

10. There is considerable heterogeneity for impact estimates related to the one type of program for which a sizeable number of studies was represented—sex education programs with a contraception component (Q=51.3, df=18, $p < 0.001$).

11. Since this review was conducted in 2006, it did not include the most recent experimental findings of abstinence-only programs published in 2007. Most notably, Mathematica Policy Research, Inc., published rigorous experimental evaluation findings for four programs that met federal abstinence-until-marriage guidelines, and failed to find positive or negative impacts on sexual initiation, sexual activity rates, or pregnancy rates (Trenholm et al. 2007).

12. Comparisons across intervention types have not been derived experimentally, and thus it is not possible to use the information from this analysis to suggest that one particular intervention type is more or less effective than another. For example, intervention types could be confounded with other study features such as study design and methods or subgroups served.

13. For example, since sex education is nearly universal, often adolescents who are part of the "control group" are actually receiving some type of sex education and/or pregnancy prevention services in their schools and communities. Thus, instead of exploring the *overall* impacts, often intervention studies measure the *relative* impacts of newer or more focused programs as compared to "usual" services.

REFERENCES

Bennett, Sylvana E., and Nassim P. Assefi. 2005. "School-Based Teenage Pregnancy Prevention Programs: A Systematic Review of Randomized Controlled Trials." *Journal of Adolescent Health* 36:72–81.

Blake, Susan M., Rebecca Ledsky, David Lohrman, Laurie Bechhofer, Pat Nichols, Richard Windsor, Stephen Banspach, and Sandra Jones. 2000. *Overall and Differential Impact of an HIV/STD Prevention Curriculum for Adolescents.* Washington, DC: Academy for Educational Development.

Darroch, Jacqueline E., and Susheela Singh. 1999. *Why Is Teenage Pregnancy Declining? The Roles of Abstinence, Sexual Activity, and Contraceptive Use.* New York: The Alan Guttmacher Institute.

Darroch, Jacqueline E., David J. Landry, and Susheela Singh. 2000. "Changing Emphases in Sexuality Education in U.S. Public Secondary Schools, 1988–1999." *Family Planning Perspectives* 32(5): 204–12.

DiCenso, Alba, Gordon Guyatt, A. Willan, and L. Griffith. 2002. "Interventions to Reduce Unintended Pregnancies among Adolescents: Systematic Review of Randomised Controlled Trials." *BMJ* (*British Medical Journal*) 324(7351): 1426–30.

DiClemente, Ralph J., and Richard A. Crosby. 2006. "Preventing Sexually Transmitted Infections among Adolescents: 'The Glass Is Half Full'." *Current Opinion in Infectious Diseases* 19:39–43.

Dolan Mullen, Patricia, Gilbert Ramirez, Darcy Strouse, Larry V. Hedges, and Ellen Sogolow. 2002. "Meta-Analysis of the Effects of Behavioral HIV Prevention Interventions on the Sexual Risk Behavior of Sexually Experienced Adolescents in Controlled Studies in the United States." *Journal of Acquired Immune Deficiency Syndromes* 30 (Supplement 1): 94–104.

Doniger, Andrew S., Edgar Adams, Cheryl A. Utter, and John S. Riley. 2001. "Impact Evaluation of the 'Not Me, Not Now' Abstinence-Oriented, Adolescent Pregnancy Prevention Communications Program, Monroe County, New York." *Journal of Health Communication* 6(1): 45–60.

Flanigan, Christine. 2001. *What's Behind the Good News: The Decline in Teen Pregnancy Rates during the 1990s*. Washington, DC: National Campaign to Prevent Teen Pregnancy.

Franklin, Cynthia, Darlene Grant, Jacqueline Corcoran, Pamela O'Dell Miller, and Linda Bultman. 1997. "Effectiveness of Prevention Programs for Adolescent Pregnancy: A Meta-Analysis." *Journal of Marriage and the Family* 59(3): 551–67.

Frost, Jennifer J., and Jacqueline Darroch Forrest. 1995. "Understanding the Impact of Effective Teenage Pregnancy Prevention Programs." *Family Planning Perspectives* 27(5): 188–95.

Grunseit, Anne, Susan Kippax, Peter Aggleton, Mariella Baldo, and Gary Slutkin. 1997. "Sexuality Education and Young People's Behavior: A Review of Studies." *Journal of Adolescent Research* 12(4): 421–53.

Guyatt, Gordon H., Alba DiCenso, Vern Farewell, Andrew Willan, and Lauren Griffith. 2000. "Randomized Trials versus Observational Studies in Adolescent Pregnancy Prevention." *Journal of Clinical Epidemiology* 53:167–74.

Johnson, Blair T., Michael P. Carey, Kerry L. Marsh, Kenneth D. Levin, and Lori A. J. Scott-Sheldon. 2003. "Interventions to Reduce Sexual Risk for the Human Immunodeficiency Virus in Adolescents, 1985–2000." *Archives of Pediatric Adolescent Medicine* 157:381–88.

Kaiser Family Foundation. 2000. *Sex Education in America: A Series of National Surveys of Students, Parents, Teachers, and Principals*. Menlo Park, CA: Kaiser Family Foundation.

Kim, Nina, Bonita Stanton, X. Li, Kay Dickersin, and Jennifer Galbraith. 1997. "Effectiveness of the 40 Adolescent AIDS-Risk Reduction Interventions: A Quantitative Review." *Journal of Adolescent Health* 20(3): 204–14.

Kirby, Douglas. 2001. *Emerging Answers: Research Findings on Programs to Reduce Teen Pregnancy*. Washington, DC: National Campaign to Prevent Teen Pregnancy.

———. 2007. *Emerging Answers 2007: New Research Findings on Programs to Reduce Teen Pregnancy—Full Report*. Washington, DC: National Campaign to Prevent Teen Pregnancy.

Manlove, Jennifer, Elizabeth Terry-Humen, Angela Romano Papillo, Kerry Franzetta, Stephanie Williams, and Suzanne Ryan. 2002. "Preventing Teenage Pregnancy, Childbearing, and Sexually Transmitted Diseases: What the Research Shows." Research brief. Washington, DC: Child Trends.

NHS Centre for Reviews and Dissemination. 1997. "Preventing and Reducing the Adverse Effects of Unintended Teenage Pregnancies." *Effective Health Care* 3(1): 1–12.

Oakley, Ann, Deirdre Fullerton, Janet Holland, Sean Arnold, Merry France-Dawson, Peter Kelley, and Sheena McGrellis. 1995. "Sexual Health Education Interventions for Young People: A Methodological Review." *British Medical Journal* 310(6973): 58–162.

Pedlow, C. Teal, and Michael P. Carey. 2004. "Developmentally Appropriate Sexual Risk Reduction Interventions for Adolescents: Rationale, Review of Interventions, and Recommendations for Research and Practice." *Annals of Behavioral Medicine* 27(3): 172–84.

Santelli, John S., Joyce Abma, Stephanie Ventura, Laura Lindberg, Brian Morrow, John E. Anderson, Sheryl Lyss, and Brady E. Hamilton. 2004. "Can Changes in Sexual Behaviors among High School Students Explain the Decline in Teen Pregnancy Rates in the 1990s?" *Journal of Adolescent Health* 35(2): 80–90.

Scher, Lauren Sue, Rebecca A. Maynard, and Matthew Stagner. 2006. *Interventions Intended to Reduce Pregnancy-Related Outcomes among Teenagers.* Copenhagen, NO: Campbell Collaboration Social Welfare Group.

Sikkema, K. J., E. S. Anderson, J. A. Kelly, et al. 2005. "Outcomes of a Randomized, Controlled Community-Level HIV Prevention Intervention for Adolescents in Low-Income Housing Developments." *AIDS* 19(14): 1509–16.

Silva, Monica. 2002. "The Effectiveness of School-Based Sex Education Programs in the Promotion of Abstinent Behavior: A Meta-Analysis." *Health Education Research* 17(4): 471–81.

Solomon, Julie, and Josefina J. Card. 2004. *Making the List: Understanding, Selecting, and Replicating Effective Teen Pregnancy Prevention Programs.* Washington, DC: National Campaign to Prevent Teen Pregnancy.

Sonfield, Adam, and Rachel Benson Gold. 2001. "States' Implementation of the Section 510 Abstinence Education Program, FY 1999." *Family Planning Perspectives* 33(4): 166–71.

St. Lawrence, Janet S., Ted L. Brasfield, Kennis W. Jefferson, Edna Alleyne, Robert E. O'Bannon III, and Aaron Shirley. 1995. "Cognitive-Behavioral Intervention to Reduce African American Adolescents' Risk for HIV Infection." *Journal of Consulting and Clinical Psychology* 63(2): 221–37.

Thomas, Mark H. 2000. "Abstinence-Based Programs for Prevention of Adolescent Pregnancies." *Journal of Adolescent Health* 26(1): 5–17.

Trenholm, Christopher, Barbara Devaney, Ken Forston, Lisa Quay, Justin Wheeler, and Melissa Clark. 2007. *Impacts of Four Title V, Section 510 Abstinence Education Programs.* Princeton, NJ: Mathematica Policy Research, Inc.

U.S. Department of Health and Human Services. 2000. *National Strategy to Prevent Teen Pregnancy: Annual Report 1999–2000.* Washington, DC: U.S. Department of Health and Human Services.

Ventura, Stephanie J., William D. Mosher, Sally C. Curtin, Joyce C. Abma, and Stanley Hershaw. 2001. "Trends in Pregnancy Rates for the United States: 1976–97: An Update." *National Vital Statistics Reports* 49(4). Hyattsville, MD: National Center for Health Statistics.

Visser, A., and P. Van Bilsen. 1994. "Effectiveness of Sex Education Provided to Adolescents." *Patient Education and Counseling* 23:147–60.

Walker, Karen E., and Lauren J. Kotloff. 1999. *Plain Talk: Addressing Adolescent Sexuality through a Community Initiative.* Philadelphia, PA: Public/Private Ventures.

About the Editors

Saul D. Hoffman is Professor of Economics and Department Chair at the University of Delaware, where he has taught since 1977. He is also a core faculty associate for the Program in Women's Studies, University of Delaware, and a research associate at the Population Studies Center, University of Pennsylvania. Hoffman has published widely on welfare policy, teen pregnancy, and issues in employment and earnings. He is the author of two books on the earned income tax credit published by the W. E. Upjohn Institute; an economics textbook on women's issues, *Women and the Economy: Family, Work, and Pay,* published by Addison Wesley in 2005; and *By the Numbers: The Public Costs of Teen Childbearing,* published in 2006 by the National Campaign to Prevent Teen Pregnancy. He serves on the research advisory board of the National Campaign to Prevent Teen Pregnancy.

Rebecca A. Maynard is University Trustee Chair Professor of Education and Social Policy at the University of Pennsylvania, Senior Program Associate at the W. T. Grant Foundation, and Affiliate Scholar at Abt Associates. She teaches courses in research methods, economics, and education policy and maintains an active research agenda focused on youth risk reduction and skills attainment. Maynard has published widely on welfare policy, educational innovation, employment and training, teenage pregnancy and parenthood, and evaluation design. Her research has appeared

435

in a wide range of journals and has been published by a wide range of presses including the Brookings Institution Press, Urban Institute Press, the National Academy of Sciences, Russell Sage Foundation, University of Michigan Press, and University of Wisconsin Press. She has testified before Congress on welfare policy, teenage pregnancy prevention, and child care policy and has advised states and foreign governments on various aspects of social welfare policy.

About the Contributors

Michael Brien is a senior manager in the Economic and Statistical Consulting group in Deloitte Financial Advisory Services LLP's Forensic & Dispute Services practice. He has conducted research in labor economics, policy analysis, and economic demography and has been published in peer-reviewed economics journals. His litigation work includes cases related to pharmaceutical rebates, employment and credit discrimination, and insurance liability disputes stemming from asbestos claims. He earned a doctorate in economics from the University of Chicago.

Robert M. Goerge is a research fellow at the Chapin Hall Center for Children at the University of Chicago. Central to his research is the goal of improving the available information on all children and families, but particularly those who are abused or neglected, disabled, poor, require mental health services, or come to the attention of service providers. He is the principal investigator of the Integrated Database on Children's Services in Illinois project. In addition to his work on children's services, he has recently begun to focus on how the provision of services to children and their well-being is affected by neighborhood conditions. He also has conducted research on understanding the effects of out-of-school programs on youth.

Jeffrey Grogger is the Irving Harris Professor in Urban Policy in the Harris School. He specializes in labor economics, applied microeconomics,

437

applied econometrics, and economics of crime. His recent work has examined the effects of welfare time limits and racial profiling. He is a coeditor of the *Journal of Human Resources* and an associate editor for the *Journal of Population Economics.*

Allen W. Harden is a senior researcher with the Chapin Hall Center for Children at the University of Chicago. His areas of research interest include child welfare, poverty, urban ecology, and social change.

Robert H. Haveman is John Bascom Emeritus Professor of Economics and Public Affairs at the University of Wisconsin–Madison, where he is also a research associate in the Institute for Research on Poverty. He is also an adjunct professor at Australia National University, Canberra. His research is in the economics of poverty and social poverty, where he has published widely. His most recent book is *Human Capital in the United States from 1975 to 2000: Patterns of Growth and Utilization* (with Andrew Bershadker and Jonathan A. Schwabish), published by the W. E. Upjohn Institute for Employment Research.

V. Joseph Hotz is the Arts and Sciences Professor of Economics at Duke University. His areas of specialization are labor economics, economic demography, evaluation of the impact of social programs, and applied econometrics, and he has published extensively in these areas. Hotz is a fellow of the Econometric Society and a research associate of the National Poverty Center, the Institute for Research on Poverty, and the National Bureau of Economic Research.

Bong Joo Lee is associated with Chapin Hall Center for Children at the University of Chicago and the Department of Social Welfare at Seoul National University. His research interests are the statistical modeling of the patterns of human service use, issues of childhood poverty, and demography of children and families.

Jennifer Manlove is a senior research scientist and area director for Fertility and Family Structure at Child Trends. She is a sociologist and has worked on multiple projects examining relationship context, sexual activity, contraceptive use, pregnancy, and childbearing among adolescents and young adults. She has also been involved in research identifying effective pregnancy prevention and STI-prevention programs.

Susan Williams McElroy is associate professor of economics and education policy at the University of Texas at Dallas, School of Economic, Political and Policy Sciences. She has conducted research on and written about the economic and social consequences of teenage pregnancy and childbearing, economics of education, and poverty and economic inequality. She received her Ph.D. in economics of education from Stanford University.

Lisa Mincieli is a project analyst at Harvard University. Before her position at Harvard, she was a research analyst at Child Trends. She has conducted research on teen and nonmarital childbearing, unintended childbearing, and adolescent sexual behavior.

Kristin Anderson Moore, a social psychologist, is a senior scholar and Senior Program Area Director of the Research-to-Results program area at Child Trends. She has been with Child Trends since 1982, studying trends in child and family well-being, the effects of family structure and social change on children, the determinants and consequences of adolescent parenthood, fatherhood, the effects of welfare and welfare reform on children, and positive development. From 1992 to 2006, she served as president, before choosing to return to full-time research. In recent years, Dr. Moore has established the Research-to-Results program at Child Trends, which focuses on the conceptualization, design, implementation, improvement, evaluation, and dissemination of information about effective programs to policymakers, funders, practitioners, and other researchers. For 10 years, she was a principal investigator on the Family and Child Well-being Research Network established by the National Institute of Child Health and Human Development to examine factors that enhance the development and well-being of children.

Elaine Peterson is associate professor in economics at California State University, Stanislaus. She has been a research assistant in the Financial Structure Section of the Federal Reserve Board and the Institute for Research on Poverty. Her research includes work on neighborhood quality and children's success, and on policy-related determinants of teen nonmarital childbearing. She completed her Ph.D. at the University of Wisconsin–Madison.

Emilie McHugh Rivers received her master's degree in economics from the University of Wisconsin–Madison. She is currently a staff economist at Laurits R. Christensen Associates.

Seth G. Sanders is professor of economics and public policy studies in the department of economics and the Terry Sanford Institute of Public Policy at Duke University. He has four broad research programs: the economic consequences of teenage childbearing on women and children, economic shocks and the effects on workers and families, gay and lesbian families and their performance in the U.S. economy, and gender and racial wage differences among the highly educated. His work combines insights from many fields and has appeared in economics, sociology, and statistics journals.

Elizabeth Terry-Humen is a research scientist at Child Trends. She has conducted research on adolescent sexual activity, contraceptive use, pregnancy, and childbearing. She received a master's in public policy from Georgetown University.

Robert J. Willis is professor of economics at the University of Michigan, where he also is a research scientist at the Institute for Social Research and research associate of the Population Studies Center. Willis is currently the principal investigator on two large longitudinal surveys, the Health and Retirement Survey and the Assets and Health of the Oldest Old Survey, which are collecting data on Americans over age 50. He is an authority on the economics of the family, marriage, fertility, labor economics, human capital and population, and economic development.

Barbara Wolfe is professor of economics and preventive medicine and director of the Institute for Research on Poverty at the University of Wisconsin–Madison. She is also a research associate of the National Bureau of Economic Research. Her research interests are poverty, health economics, and disabilities. She is coauthor, with Robert Haveman, of *Succeeding Generations: On the Effects of Investments in Children* (Russell Sage Foundation, 1994) and has published widely in professional journals and edited monographs.

Index

Abecedarian early childhood program, 164
Abortion
    fertility rate trends and, 7, 42–44, 79
    teen mothers study and, 61–62,
        113*nn*4–5
    underreporting of, 64
Abstinence-focused sex education, 405,
    410–11, 415–16, 420
"Abstinence plus" programs, 405–6
Academic achievement. *See* Cognitive
    development; Educational attain-
    ment
Acute health conditions, 225, 231, 239,
    246. *See also* Health and health care
    for children
Adolescent Health Survey, 261
Adolescent outcomes
    academic achievement, 183–84
    behavior outcomes, 184–85
    cognitive development, 183–84
    home and family environment, 186–87
    overview, 11–12
    physical health and well-being, 189
    relationship quality, 187–88
Adoption and Foster Care Reporting Sys-
    tem (AFCARS), 263

Adoption and Safe Families Act of 1997
    (ASFA), 258, 259, 261
AFDC (Aid to Families with Dependent
    Children). *See* Public assistance
AFQT. *See* Armed Forces Qualifying Test
African Americans
    abortion and, 43, 44
    academic achievement of children of
        teen mothers, 183
    behavior outcomes and, 184
    birth rate trends for, 265
    child abuse and, 260, 276
    child support obligations and, 142
    contraceptive use, 37
    fertility rate in, 26, 39
    foster care placements of, 260, 270, 273
    health issues and, 189
    incarceration rate, 295, 312
    nonmarital births and, 30–31, 45,
        128–30, 334
    relationship quality outcomes, 188
    sexual activity of, 33
Aid to Families with Dependent Children
    (AFDC). *See* Public assistance
American Public Human Services Associ-
    ation (APHSA), 286*n*5